PLAGUES, PANDEMICS AND VIRUSES

FROM THE PLAGUE OF ATHENS TO COVID-19

ABOUT THE AUTHOR

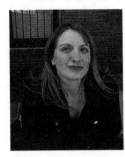

(photo: Richard Haynes)

Heather Quinlan studied English literature at Ithaca College. She broke into the professional world as a children's book editor for Sterling Publishing, launching its successful biography series for middle schoolers. She is now a freelance writer and filmmaker. Her writing has been features in PBS's *MetroFocus, The Wall Street Journal, Medium*, and *The New York Daily News*. She's been featured in *The New York Times, The New Yorker, CBS This Morning*, and NPR's *All Things Considered*, and she was nominated for an Emmy Award for her work on NatGeo Kids' *Weird but True!* series. She lives in New Jersey with her husband, writer Adam McGovern.

PLAGUES, PANDEMICS AND VIRUSES

FROM THE PLAGUE OF ATHENS TO COVID-19

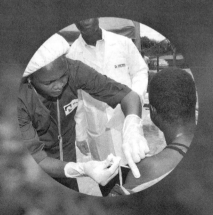
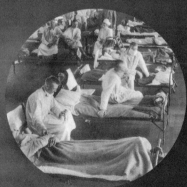
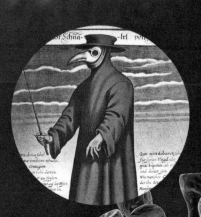

HEATHER E. QUINLAN

ALSO FROM VISIBLE INK PRESS

The Handy Psychology Answer Book, 2nd edition
by Lisa J. Cohen, Ph.D.
ISBN: 978-1-57859-508-2

The Handy Religion Answer Book, 2nd edition
by John Renard, Ph.D.
ISBN: 978-1-57859-379-8

The Handy Science Answer Book, 5th edition
by The Carnegie Library of Pittsburgh
ISBN: 978-1-57859-691-1

The Handy State-by-State Answer Book: Faces, Places, and Famous Dates for All Fifty States
by Samuel Willard Crompton
ISBN: 978-1-57859-565-5

The Handy Supreme Court Answer Book
by David L Hudson, Jr.
ISBN: 978-1-57859-196-1

The Handy Technology Answer Book
by Naomi E. Balaban and James Bobick
ISBN: 978-1-57859-563-1

The Handy Western Philosophy Answer Book: The Ancient Greek Influence on Modern Understanding
by Ed D'Angelo, Ph.D.
ISBN: 978-1-57859-556-3

PLEASE VISIT THE "HANDY ANSWERS" SERIES
WEBSITE AT WWW.HANDYANSWERS.COM.

PLAGUES, PANDEMICS AND VIRUSES: FROM THE PLAGUE OF ATHENS TO COVID-19

Visible Ink Press®
43311 Joy Rd., #414
Canton, MI 48187-2075

Visible Ink Press is a registered trademark of Visible Ink Press LLC.

Most Visible Ink Press books are available at special quantity discounts when pur-chased in bulk by corporations, organizations, or groups. Customized printings, special imprints, messages, and excerpts can be produced to meet your needs. For more information, con-tact Special Markets Director, Visible Ink Press, www.visibleink.com, or 734-667-3211.

Managing Editor: Kevin S. Hile
Art Director: Graphikitchen, LLC
Typesetting: Marco Divita
Proofreader: Shoshana Hurwitz
Indexer: Larry Baker

Cover images: Ebola vaccination (UC Rusal Photo Gallery), 1918 flu pandemic (Armed Forces Institute of Pathology/National Museum of Health and Medicine), plague doctor (Johannes Ebert and others, *Europas Sprung in die Neuzeit, Die große Chronik-Weltges-chichte*), smallpox victim (Illinois Department of Public Health), background images (stock.adobe.com and Graphikitchen, LLC).

Cataloging-in-Publication Data is on file at the U.S. Library of Congress.

Printed in the United States of America.

10 9 8 7 6 5 4 3 2 1

CONTENTS

PHOTO SOURCES

ACKNOWLEDGMENTS

Writing a book, even on a topic that you're drawn to, can be complicated, and this is not a project I could've completed on my own. As such, I want to thank my husband, Adam McGovern, for listening to the entire book read aloud and offering his insight, support, and good cheer. Also cheering me on and sending me the latest pandemic news was my mother, Catherine Christman, and my stepfather, Ken Christman, who sadly passed away before this book was finished and to whom it's dedicated.

Also, a huge thank you to Lori Wark for her work on the *Decameron* section; Kevin Hile, my editor, for his patience and direction; and Roger Jänecke, my publisher, for *his* patience, good will, and for talking to me at BEA in the first place.

Finally, I heartily appreciate the thoughtfulness and honesty of those who agreed to be interviewed for this book: Pastor Stephen C. Butler, Prof. Sharon DeWitte, Dr. Greg Galvin, Kristen Ficarra Huetz, Barbara Fisher Coughlin, Anita Ghatak, Imam Wesley Lebron, Jeanette Mallett, Prof. Richelle Munkhoff, Rabbi Ariann Weitzman, those who are co-parenting during a pandemic, and last but not least, Dr. Anthony Fauci, who took time out of a horrendously busy day in the middle of a pandemic to talk to me about viruses and why he majored in Classics.

DEDICATION

To anyone who ever failed science class.
And to Ken, who taught me the answer always has to make sense.

THE BEGINNING OF THE END

Ivy is not a parasite or a virus, yet it behaves like one. In fact, ivy arguably performs better than many microscopic killers—instead of infecting its host and then dying along with it, ivy kills the host and survives. Tales of people leaving their windows open on summer nights only to find that ivy had crept in by morning is enough to make one invest in herbicides, and yet, even the deadliest of chemicals don't always do the trick.

Look around, and you'll see the survival of the fittest. Humans, trees, dogs, fish, even guinea pigs that are currently alive are descended from ancestors that survived hundreds, thousands, or sometimes even millions of years of disease, environmental change, warfare—anything that nature could throw at it to thin the herd. We're all survivors—and yet, we all still die, sometimes quietly and peacefully and sometimes violently. This book is about those who died in droves, powerless to diseases of the mind, body, and even spirit—diseases that are so powerful, they can fell the strongest of any species, just as a gentle-looking ivy can bring down a mighty oak.

The sheer quantity of these deaths affects not only individuals but communities, economies—even the arts. Without the Great Plague, *Canterbury Tales*, *The Decameron*—not even *The Seventh Seal*, a film that was released centuries later—would exist.

When the Old World first met the New World en masse in the sixteenth century, they proceeded to destroy it with the help of horses, cows, and chickens while also believing they were saving the indigenous people from a godless life. AIDS brought the outing of the gay community: because they were dying, suddenly, the manliest of Hollywood actors were forced to confess that they loved their fellow manliest of Hollywood actors. In all these scenarios, death reached into places no one had ever imagined it could.

This book will cover plagues, pandemics, and all manner of viruses, bacteria, buboes, vaccines, and diseases that felled entire civilizations—but within are also stories of heroism, of art, of warfare, and of healing because plagues are more than sickness. They reshape borders, create literature, push us to learn what we can about medicine … hopefully in time to stop diseases whose potential to destroy is only just being realized.

A PREFACE TO THE BLACK DEATH

Let's start with the reason you might have picked up this book: the Black Death.

"God is deaf nowadays and will not hear us. And for our guilt he grinds good men to dust," wrote William Langland in his poem "Piers Plowman." Langland was one of the lucky few who survived the Black Death, though "lucky" may not be the correct word because once the Black Death disappeared, what remained was a land in ruins and its people insane with grief and confusion. Where did this plague come from? Why did God allow this to happen? Will it come back again? These are all questions we're still asking today in one form or another.

Traditionally, the study of history hasn't focused on disease partly because it's been too mysterious to write about decisively and partly because it doesn't fit in with our idea of history being written by humans. Sometimes, bacteria or viruses do, in fact, do the writing.

A fourteenth-century person's lack of understanding about medicine also meant that they didn't record in detail what happened, and when they did, it wasn't reported particularly well. Frequently, diseases were seen as the result of God's wrath over … something. Lack of prayer, overall heresy—even Jews were named as potential causes. Widespread death was also blamed on miasma, which we know today as an oppressive feeling, but back then, it was a synonym for "bad air." Therefore, a lot of speculating as to just what went on had to be done centuries later.

Despite these roadblocks, the medical community was able to piece together several clues; today, we largely believe that plague was caused by bacteria and turned into a pandemic through international trade. Nothing spreads disease like trade. Trade is great for the economy and terrible at keeping people alive. In this case, the bacterium *Yersinia pestis* (aka *Y. pestis*) hitched a ride on fleas, which hitched a ride on rats, which hitched a ride on ships that started in the Far East and made their way to the Mediterranean, bearing cloth, spices, and plague. Death was coming, and people could not do anything to stop it. The rest is history.

BACTERIA AND VIRUSES

Let's take a minute and look into what *Y. pestis* is about. *Y. pestis* is a bacterium. The flu is a virus. Are bacteria and viruses the same thing? No. Bacteria are to viruses what you are to a potato. Both bacteria and viruses can ruin your day by giving you a cold or explosive diarrhea, but that's where the comparison ends. You and a potato actually have more in common because you're both living organisms with complex cells and are capable of reproduction and metabolism; you even both have "eyes," so to speak. A virus is not capable of reproduction and metabolism. In some circles, a virus isn't even considered alive. Nor is it dead. It exists, so to speak, in a gray area.

Bacteria are cellular creatures that you can easily see under a microscope. They were among the first life forms to appear on Earth. They're mostly made of cytoplasm, that is a clear, jelly-like fluid that houses all the biochemical reactions that keep bacteria alive. To prevent the cytoplasm from floating away, bacteria are surrounded by cell membranes, also known as cell walls. Though a bacterium is just a tiny, single cell, the weight of all the bacteria in the world is more than that of every living plant and animal.

Bacteria live everywhere: in the water, on you—trillions are around you right now—on your furniture, in your bed, on your skin, and even inside you. You have 10 times more bacterial cells inside you than your own cells.

Bacteria live everywhere: in the water, on you—trillions are around you right now—on your furniture, in your bed, on your skin, and even inside you.

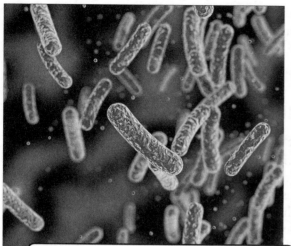

Bacteria such as these salmonella bacteria, are cellular organisms that possess all the qualities of other types of cells, such as a membrane, a nucleus, and cytoplasm. Most bacteria are benign, but some can cause illness.

Bacteria have a bad reputation, but most are actually good—roughly 80 percent, as a matter of fact. For example, the bacteria that live in your gut create conditions that keep "bad" bacteria away and aid in digestion.

When bacteria grow big enough, they reproduce asexually through a process called binary fission. This means that bacteria copy their DNA and then split into "daughter cells," which are exact duplicates of their parent. Note that it's "parent," not "parents," as only one parent cell is involved (hence the word "asexual"—*a* being the Greek prefix for "non").

Viruses are even simpler. They have the dubious distinction of being the simplest life form on Earth. Scientists don't even know where they came from. For starters, they're smaller than bacteria. Much smaller. Like you next to the Statue of Liberty. Their average size is 100 nanometers; to put that into context, an inch is 254,000 nanometers, meaning a quarter of a billion viruses can fit into one inch. Louis Pasteur called the virus "a microbe of infinite smallness." This is why millions of types of viruses exist, but we only know of a few thousand.

Bacteria may reproduce on their own, but viruses cannot. They need you: the host.

Viruses have no cytoplasm and no chemical processes. A virus is just genetic code, either DNA or RNA, and some proteins packaged inside a shell called a capsid. This genetic code is like HTML for a web page. It is what drives a virus to invade. Viruses are the great invaders, better than Genghis Khan, Attila the Hun, or "Space Invaders": they invaded long before them, have continued to do so long after, and have killed far more people.

The outer shell of every virus is designed to attach to a particular host cell's receptors. It could be a cell that's part of your nervous system, which is what the rabies virus attaches to, or a cell that's part of your respiratory system, which is what the COVID-19 virus attaches to. Not all host cell receptors look alike, so therefore, not all viruses look alike. (A coronavirus is round, while a rabies virus looks like a dumbbell.) When a virus does find a host cell with the right receptors, the virus will bind to it, enter a cell, link its genetic material to the host cell's genetic material, then use the host cell's own parts to turn it into a virus factory.

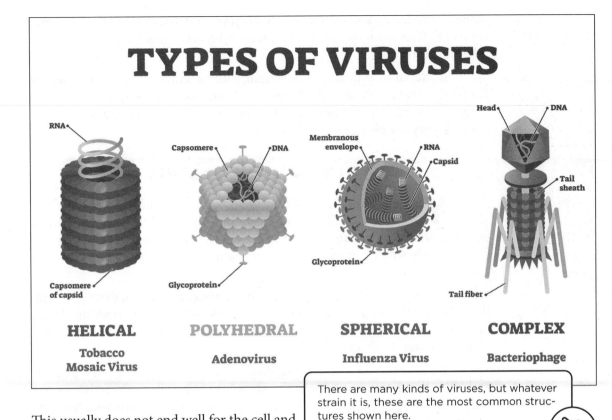

TYPES OF VIRUSES

HELICAL	POLYHEDRAL	SPHERICAL	COMPLEX
Tobacco Mosaic Virus	Adenovirus	Influenza Virus	Bacteriophage

There are many kinds of viruses, but whatever strain it is, these are the most common structures shown here.

This usually does not end well for the cell and leaves the host facing a viral infection. Even bacteria aren't safe from viruses.

So, say one person is sick with a bacterial infection, and another is sick with a viral infection. Both people have been "infected," or contaminated, but by different pathogens (as viruses and bad bacteria are collectively known). When you determine the type of pathogen, then you will know how to treat it if treatment is available.

Bacterial infections can be fought with antibiotics—medicines that destroy bacteria by wrecking their biochemical processes. The biochemical processes of the patient's cells are different enough from those of bacteria, so they largely won't be hurt by antibiotics.

We can't do the same with a viral infection because, as you'll recall, viruses have no biochemical processes, so antibiotics have nothing to attack. It would be like an army going to battle in an empty field. Antiviral drugs can block a virus from entering your cells, but even antiviral drugs don't work the same way on every type of virus. However, we have another weapon—that weapon is called a vaccine. Vaccines won't *cure* viral diseases, but they will *prevent* them. This is why people get flu vaccines before winter comes to lessen the odds of getting the flu.

Bacterial infections can be fought with vaccines as well, but generally speaking, vaccines are used more frequently against viruses because, as a rule of thumb, the simpler the pathogen, the more effective the vaccine, and viruses are very, very simple.

YOUR IMMUNE SYSTEM

You've been under attack every second of your life since the day you were born. Bacteria, viruses, fungi—billions of them—are trying to build a home in your body. However, we've evolved a complex army that includes guards, soldiers, intelligence—everything but the cavalry—to protect you from dying.

This military of immunity not only identifies enemies, it destroys them, then keeps tabs on them if they ever come back. While most organisms living in your body—even bacteria—are actually helpful, bacteria and viruses called pathogens want to destroy you.

We have two ways of stopping this: innate immunity, which just goes out and kills all unknown pathogens the same way, regardless of whether or not your body has seen them before; and acquired immunity, which is your immune system, which has learned certain pathogens' strategies to avoid danger. Every animal has an innate immune system—even sponges—but only vertebrates have the acquired kind.

The first barriers of your immune system are your skin—which we think of as keeping our organs inside, though its other responsibility is to keep invaders out—and the mucous membranes. Mucous membranes line all the internal surfaces that come into contact with the outside, like your nostrils, mouth, and lungs. Mucous membranes produce mucus, which is a thick fluid that traps microbes and helps get rid of them when you cough or blow your nose.

Most of the immune system within your body consists of white blood cells called leukocytes, a word from the Greek *leuk*, meaning "white," and *cyt*, meaning "cell." They can go almost anywhere in the body they want except places like the brain and the spinal column—which, for obvious reasons, are highly guarded areas.

Different types of leukocytes exist—those that are part of the innate immune system are called *phagocytes* (*phago* is the Greek word for "eating").

PLAGUES, PANDEMICS AND VIRUSES

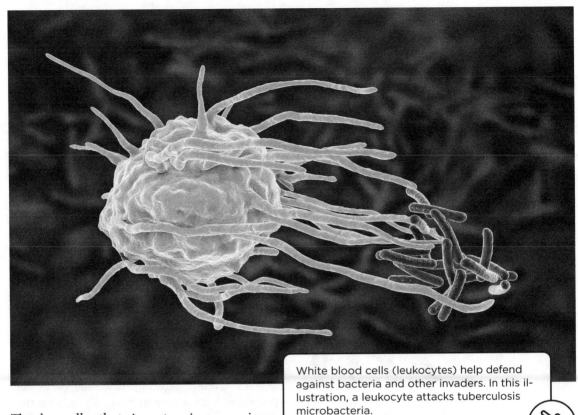

White blood cells (leukocytes) help defend against bacteria and other invaders. In this illustration, a leukocyte attacks tuberculosis microbacteria.

They're cells that ingest microorganisms through what's called phagocytosis. They will chase down invading cells, grab them, and swallow them.

The grandest phagocytes are the *macrophages*, which means "big eaters." They don't travel around the body looking to help out but stand guard by your various organs. They will kill invading microbes and also destroy cells that have gone rogue, like cancer cells. They swallow them whole, then trap them inside a membrane, where they get torn apart by enzymes.

If that isn't enough destruction, neutrocytes are the most abundant of the white blood cells; about 100 billion are made every day in the bone marrow. Neutrocytes also move through the bloodstream and can quickly get to where the action is after receiving an SOS signal from cells that line the bloodstream. This is called "neurocyte recruitment"; neurocytes are akin to the first responders of the immune system. They will also signal other cells for backup by emitting proteins called cytokines. The neutrophils fight so furiously that they can kill healthy cells in the process.

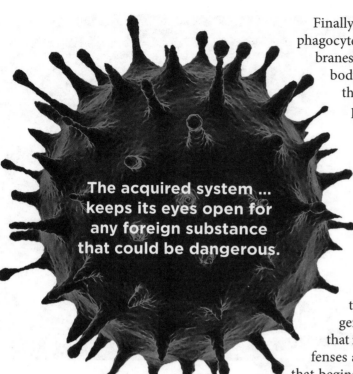

The acquired system ... keeps its eyes open for any foreign substance that could be dangerous.

Finally, dendritic cells are a type of phagocyte that, as with mucous membranes, hang out on the parts of your body that come into contact with the environment. They devour pathogens, but their work doesn't end there. Dendritic cells then pass along intelligence about these pathogens to the lymph nodes, thus bridging the gap between innate immunity and acquired immunity.

In order to be effective, the acquired immune system has to learn everything it can about every pathogen it comes across, then store that information so it can build defenses against it. This isn't a process that begins over time—at birth, you already started to assemble one tough acquired immune system, taking in both the good bacteria that can help you and also harmful ones that can hurt you. This is especially crucial because as a newborn, you were bombarded with bacteria and pathogens that you hadn't had to worry about in the sterile environment of the womb. The acquired system therefore keeps its eyes open for any foreign substance that could be dangerous.

Dangerous foreign substances are also known as antigens, a word that means "antibody generator." Antigens are proteins produced by intruders that incite an immune response from your body, such as creating antibodies that bind to the antigens, tagging the pathogen as an enemy for the immune system to attack.

Your acquired immune system includes a type of blood cell that is different from phagocytes—these are called lymphocytes. Lymphocytes go after specific pathogens they already know about, like tackling a "Most Wanted" list. The two major types of lymphocytes are T cells and B cells.

T cells lead most of the entire acquired immune system. Like a dendritic cell, when a macrophage finds a pathogen and destroys it, the macro-

PLAGUES, PANDEMICS AND VIRUSES

phage will then keep some of the pathogen's antigens, shred them into pieces, carry them on their surface, and bring them to the T cell. This activates the T cell, causing it to release cytokines, which induce it to make tons of copies of itself. Some of these new T cells will track down infected cells and go on the attack, while others will become helper T cells that sound the alarm to attract more white blood cells and release a chemical that allows other white blood cells to multiply.

Now, let's go back and say that something specific has penetrated that first barrier, like a rusty nail in your foot. Bacteria from the nail capitalize on this sudden opportunity and enter the wound. At first, their small numbers help them go unnoticed, but after continuously multiplying, they will reach a population threshold, whereby they change their behavior and start damaging the body. The immune system then has to switch into high gear and go on the attack as soon as possible.

Two types of cells that defend your body are macrophages, which literally consume intruders, and T cells, which work by injecting granules into diseased cells, killing them.

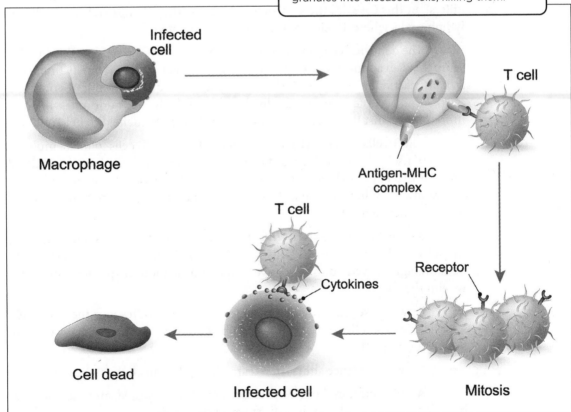

Infected cell

Macrophage

T cell

Antigen-MHC complex

T cell

Cytokines

Receptor

Cell dead

Infected cell

Mitosis

First, the phagocytes begin to swallow up the intruders. Then, the big eaters, the macrophages, intervene—they guard every border region of the body. Most of the time, they alone can stop an attack because they can eat 100 pathogens in one gulp, as it were.

When the macrophages start to wear out, they release proteins that tell other phagocytes where they are and call for backup to come ASAP. Neutrophils leave their patrol in the blood route and move to the battlefield.

Neutrophils generate barriers that trap and kill bacteria. They are so deadly that they've evolved to self-destruct in order to stop them from causing too much damage. (Dead neutrophils gather together in what we call "pus.") If this is not enough to stop the invasion, the head of the immune system kicks in.

Both the dendritic cells and more macrophages get active. They destroy the enemies and start collecting enemy samples. They rip them to pieces and keep them on their outer layers. It's here that a crucial decision is made: should they signal for antiviral forces that call for antibody cells or an army of bacteria killers? In this case, it's the antibacterial forces. They then travel to the closest lymph node, where T cells are waiting to be activated.

The dendritic cell or macrophage is on its way, looking for a T cell with a setup that can connect to the specific enemy's antigen. When it finally finds one, a chain reaction takes place. The T cell is activated; it quickly duplicates over and over. Some become memory T cells that stay in the lymph node and will bring immunity against this enemy, and some travel to the battlefield to help out.

The T cells release cytokines, which activate the B cells to make multiple copies of itself, and these B cells start making antibodies, which are specialized proteins that either to bind to the surface of a pathogen or activate macrophages to swallow it. Billions of them flood the blood and saturate the body, heading to where they're needed.

Meanwhile, at the site of infection, guard and attack cells fight hard, but they also die in the process. T cells work like drill instructors, ordering them to be more aggressive and to stay alive longer, but without help, they can't overwhelm the bacteria.

Now, the second line of defense arrives. Antibodies join the battlefield and disable or kill the intruders. Macrophages are especially good at eating up the bacteria that the antibodies have attached to.

Now, the balance shifts. In a team effort, the infection is wiped out.

At this point, millions of your cells have already died, and the ones that haven't commit suicide, so they don't waste resources.

However, some stay behind, such as memory T cells. If this enemy is encountered again in the future, they will be ready for it and probably kill it before you even notice.

Not every battle is victorious, unfortunately. It takes time for the body to learn where the invaders are, attack, and build up defenses. If a body is too weak (e.g., from age) to fight back, a severe infection could be fatal. This is where vaccines come in.

VACCINES AND ANTIBIOTICS

As great as memory cells are, acquiring them through an infection is always unpleasant and sometimes dangerous. (That's why young children are often sick—they don't yet have enough memory cells.)

Vaccines work by teaching the immune system to learn the different pathogens *before* they cause an infection. One way of doing this is injecting dead invaders—pathogens that have already been killed or even just proteins that belonged to the pathogen. This is called a "killed" vaccine. Our immune system has no problem handling an enemy that's already dead; the vaccine triggers an immune reaction without actually causing the illness. Sometimes, the potency of the memory cells that comes from this type of vaccination diminishes over time, which means that booster shots may be necessary.

Every year as summer comes to an end, pharmacies begin to advertise flu shots for the upcoming flu season. One vaccination for the flu will not give you a lifetime immunity. In fact, the vaccination you get might not even give you immunity for one flu season, but it puts the odds in your favor.

The flu virus mutates quickly and unpredictably, so every year, researchers try to find a pattern of flu mutations and develop the vaccine accordingly.

PLAGUES, PANDEMICS AND VIRUSES

The flu virus mutates quickly and unpredictably, so every year, researchers try to find a pattern of flu mutations and develop the vaccine accordingly. What you get is a "killed" version of what researchers and immunologists believe to be the strain that will come out this year. ("Killed" is in quotes because viruses are neither alive nor dead, but this is the best adjective we have. The same is true for "live" viruses.) The next year, a different flu shot will be given.

Live vaccines include invaders that are quite alive, though they are very weak. They're just enough to wake up the immune system and create even more memory cells than a killed vaccine. Booster shots are usually not needed. These include vaccines for measles, mumps, and rubella. Unlike killed vaccines, live vaccines need to be refrigerated and maintained in a lab, so they have a finite life span. Killed vaccines are easier to store and use.

The first published account of a vaccination—which was against smallpox—took place in 1796 by British scientist Edward Jenner. At the time, physicians had been on the right track—through a process called variolation, they inoculated patients with an injection of bits of smallpox scabs or pus. The idea was that a milder form of the disease would emerge and then subside, leading to immunity; similar practices had previously been done in China, the Middle East, and Africa, though those were done through inhalation instead of injection.

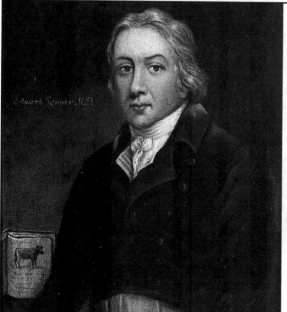

Dr. Edward Jenner not only developed the vaccine for smallpox, he was also greatly responsible for popularizing the use of vaccines in England and the world.

Lady Mary Wortley Montagu, the wife of the British ambassador to Constantinople, had herself been stricken by the disease in 1715, leaving her skin pitted with scars. Later, in the Turkish countryside, she witnessed the practice of variolation and wrote to her friends: "The old woman comes with a nut-shell full of the matter of the best sort of small-pox, and asks what vein you please to have opened," whereupon she "puts into the vein as much matter as can lie upon the head of her needle." Patients retired to bed for a couple of days with a fever and, Lady Montagu noted, emerged remarkably fine. "They have very rarely above twenty or thirty in their faces, which never mark." She reported that thousands of people safely underwent the operation every year and that the disease had largely been contained in the region. "You may believe I am well satisfied of the safety of this experiment," she added, "since I intend to try it on my dear little son." Her son never got smallpox.

Unfortunately, not all patients reacted to the inoculations the same way; some actually did develop full-blown smallpox and died.

However, Jenner noticed that during smallpox outbreaks, milkmaids were not infected. He believed this had to do with their exposure to cowpox, a type of pox that erupted on cow udders. The milkmaids' hands would get cowpox blisters, which were irritating but far less dangerous than smallpox. The blisters eventually went away without leading to agonizing suffering and death. Jenner then hypothesized that an injection of cowpox—a less potent version of smallpox but still in the same viral family—would render a patient immune to smallpox without risking the patient's life.

So, in 1796, Jenner inoculated a young boy named James Phipps, the son of Jenner's gardener. Phipps was Jenner's ideal specimen because he wanted "a healthy boy, about eight years old for the purpose of inoculation for the Cow Pox." Jenner scraped pus from a cowpox pustule located on the hand of milkmaid Sarah Nelmes and used it to inoculate Phipps with two small cuts on each of his arms.

After observing Phipps, Jenner wrote:

> On the seventh day he complained of uneasiness in the [armpit] and on the ninth he became a little chilly, lost his appetite, and had a slight headache. During the whole of this day he was perceptibly indisposed, and spent the night with some degree of restlessness, but on the day following he was perfectly well.

Later, Jenner injected Phipps with pieces of smallpox material, and no outbreak followed. Phipps was immunized from smallpox (and cowpox).

After Phipps grew up, got married, and had children, Jenner gave him and his family a free lease on a cottage in southwest England, which became the Edward Jenner Museum between 1968 and 1982. Phipps went to Jenner's funeral in 1823 and died at the age of 65 in 1835. Both Jenner and Phipps are buried at the Church of St Mary in Berkeley, Gloucestershire, England.

An illustration of Sarah Nelmes's hand—complete with cowpox pustules—from Jenner's *An Inquiry into the Causes and Effects of Variolæ Vaccinæ* can now be seen at Harvard University's Center for the History of Medicine.

In 1979, the World Health Organization (WHO) declared smallpox eradicated, and vaccinations essentially ended. This victory was the result of public-health efforts, with vaccination at the forefront.

PLAGUES, PANDEMICS AND VIRUSES

(For a detailed discussion of smallpox during the European invasion of the Americas, see the chapter "Smallpox in the New World.")

Vaccinations are administered as a preventative way to keep diseases (i.e., measles, mumps, diphtheria, tuberculosis) from attacking or reduce the effects of ones that have already attacked. They largely fight off viral infections, though some work against bacterial ones. Antibiotics are medicines that either work preventively or attack bacteria after they've already invaded.

Unlike vaccines, the practice of administering antibiotics via moldy bread has been around since the times of ancient Egypt, China, Serbia, Greece and Rome, where its healing properties, particularly when pressed against infected wounds, may have been due to raw forms of antibiotics produced by the mold, but it wouldn't be until the twentieth century that mold would completely revolutionize medicine.

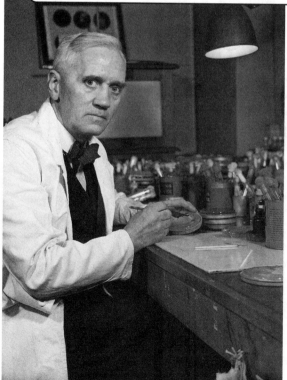

The Scottish scientist and Nobel Prize winner Alexander Fleming discovered the first effective antibiotic, benzylpenicillin, in 1923.

Antibiotics target one pathogen: bacteria—the bad kind, like the ones that can cause strep throat, staph infections, and pneumonia. While your immune system will go after them, sometimes, they can use a little help, just as with a viral infection. That's where antibiotics come in. They can help tear apart bacterial cell walls or block the protein production that is critical to bacterial survival.

In 1928, Scottish scientist Alexander Fleming discovered modern-day penicillin quite by accident. After working with bacteria called staphylococci, he left the lab to go on vacation and didn't quite clean up as well as he should have. This is lucky for us because when Fleming returned, he noticed bits of mold growing on a staphylococci sample. The mold had killed the bacteria. This is penicillin.

Penicillin works by stopping bacteria from renewing while it grows. This weakens the cell wall and causes it to burst, killing the bacteria while leaving the host cells intact.

The results were shocking. In less than three decades, life expectancy in the United States shot up by eight years. It was hailed as a

14

miracle drug during World War II, allowing the Allies to patch up a soldier and have him ready to fight again within weeks. Before penicillin, people died from minor cuts that led to infection. Now, they could survive a war.

Its discovery sent researchers on the hunt for more antibiotics that are used today in everything from vaccines to cancer drugs.

RESISTANCE IS NOT FUTILE

Unfortunately, a resistance has begun, and more and more of our antibiotics have become less effective. Penicillin and erythromycin, for example, which used to destroy many bacterial strains, have become less lethal against pathogens because of their overuse, leading some bacteria to develop their own resistance. Diseases that were once under control have now made a comeback thanks to these resistant strains, known as "superbugs."

Just like any organism, bacteria can undergo random mutations. Most are harmless, but occasionally, one comes along that gives its organism an edge in the survival game. This is part of biologist Charles Darwin's theory of natural selection, which states in part that the "principle by which each slight variation [of a trait], if useful, is preserved." For bacteria, this means mutations that make them resistant to certain antibiotics give them a huge advantage and are therefore passed along to subsequent generation after generation, making them resistant as well, and so on, and so on.

The worry is that other bacteria will join this resistance faster than we can come up with solutions or, worse, that bacteria will become immune....

Reproduction isn't the only way these resistances are passed on. Some bacteria can release their resistant DNA when they die to be picked up by other bacteria. Others use a method called "horizontal gene transfer" to share their resistant genes with nearby bacteria.

Every year, it's estimated that nearly 500,000 new cases of drug-resistant tuberculosis occur worldwide. In the United States, Atlanta, Georgia's Centers for Disease Control and Prevention (CDC) estimate that every year, 200,000 people get sick from these superbugs, leading to more than 23,000 deaths.

The worry is that other bacteria will join this resistance faster than we can come up with solutions or, worse, that bacteria will become immune, leading to all kinds of untreatable diseases. The WHO has characterized antibiotic resistance as a "serious threat [that] is no longer a prediction for the future, it is happening right now in every region of the world and has the potential to affect anyone, of any age, in any country."

Tuberculosis (TB), which infects the lungs, is the number-one infectious disease in the world, killing more than one million people each year. TB is difficult to treat, and some strains need years of daily treatment with multiple drugs. Gonorrhea, a sexually transmitted infection, has, through horizontal gene transfer, developed strains resistant to all but a few antibiotics. *E. coli* can boot out any antibiotics that have entered its cells. Salmonella causes more illnesses, hospitalizations, and deaths than any other foodborne illness. Through horizontal gene transfer, they, too, are able to use certain enzymes to break down antibiotics before they even attack. Meanwhile, overuse of antibiotics can also leave patients susceptible to other illnesses, like *Clostridium difficile*, which can cause colitis, a disease of the colon.

Staphylococci, or "staph," is a group of bacteria that lives everywhere: on our beds, on our skin, up our noses. They're usually harmless, except for certain strains. These won't go down without an enormous fight that might take you with it. Methicillin-resistant *Staphylococcus aureus* (or MRSA; pronounced MER-sa) is another strain that's benefited from horizontal gene transfer. They've become monstrous, resistant to any number of antibiotics. Its victims are often hospitalized patients, whose immune systems are already compromised, because MRSA can get into the skin through spaces created by invasive medical equipment, like catheters or feeding tubes. Prisoners catch MRSA from being in confined spaces with poor hygiene. Treatment is extremely challenging. It's so deadly that researchers have spent years trying to develop a vaccine, though none have yet been approved.

Antivirals are not heard about as much as vaccines or antibiotics, but they're just as vital. They're administered to make viral infections less severe, although many have to be given within a specific time frame after the initial infection in order to be effective.

Many antivirals stop viral replication by preventing the release of viral components into a host cell or preventing the viruses from being released from the cell. This is a delicate operation, as the antiviral needs to be able to stop the virus without harming your cells, which now contain them.

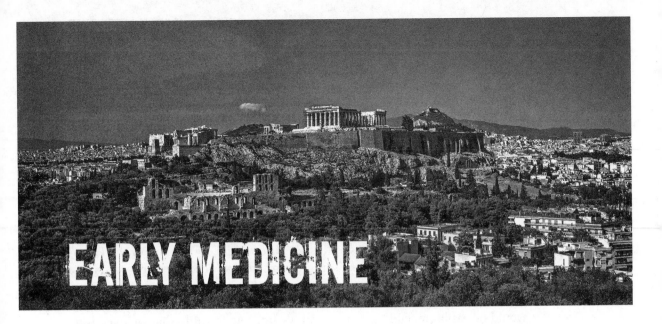

EARLY MEDICINE

The question "Why me?" has been asked about everything from a rogue shopping cart denting a car to a grim health prognosis. It was also asked in the earliest days of humankind, when so much of the world was misunderstood and one's fortune seemed to be in the hands of the fates. Medicine men acted as doctors, seers—even lawyers, pleading the afflicted's case to the gods, and when they weren't arguing for the defense, they were using spells, herbs, and charms to try to heal the sick.

Today, for all of our philosophical studies and medical discoveries, we're still asking "Why me?" Emotions frequently act as the driving force in our decision making, a through line of the human condition, perhaps a holdover from when we were fleeing saber-toothed tigers. In 1943, archaeologist Grahame Clark wrote, "To the peoples of the world generally … I venture to think that Paleolithic Man has more meaning than the Greeks." This means that instinct kept us alive, while philosophy just made us ask a lot of hypothetical questions. (Incidentally, Clark's father, Charles Clark, survived fighting overseas in World War I, only to die in the 1918 flu epidemic.)

PAGING DR. PALEO

Though in modern times, women tend to live longer than men, it was the other way around in Paleolithic times (between 3.3 million–10,000 years ago) due primarily to all the ways a woman could die from childbirth—hemorrhaging, infection, blood clots, or even a baby too large to be born vaginally, with a torturous labor lasting for days until both mother and child died. If the mother lived, chances are that she'd have to endure the same torture multiple times and not always give birth to a baby that was alive. Even with a longer life expectancy than women, though, men lived for only 25 to 40 years; a midlife crisis back then, if such a thing had existed, would've occurred at the same time as adolescence, so perhaps, it's better that such existential terrors did not happen until much later.

The ailments faced by those living during Paleolithic times varied from place to place—note that by now, some populations stayed in Africa, while others moved on to today's Asia, Russia, Europe, and, by the end of the Paleo-lithic era, the Americas. With this migration came new climates, new predators, and new viruses and bacteria that one needed to adapt to or die. Add to that potentially fatal broken bones, rickets due to vitamin deficiency, infections that would be easily treatable today … and it's amazing to think that we lived long enough to have sex and reproduce.

The earliest *Homo sapiens* had certain tools to practice medicine—their hands, knives, and needles made of bone, complete with an eye for thread made of animal sinew. Though we don't know when it began, archaeologists have found evidence of suturing from skeletons that date back to Paleolithic times. These people were also the world's first pharmacists; herbs were discovered in Shanidar Cave in today's Kurdistan; meanwhile, all the way in northern Europe, a mushroom known as *birch polypore*, which induced diarrhea to treat consti-pation, was found among the remains of a man who'd been mummified.

These are all tremendous pharmaceutical and therapeutic leaps and con-nections made when almost nothing in terms of instrumentation was available. Bacteria and viruses were all around but unknown, yet that didn't matter. It was treating the everyday, like arthritis in a twentysomething patient, that was a more pressing matter, but the following will demonstrate how medicine evolved, just as those who were its patients evolved.

HIPPOCRATES AND THE FIRST PHYSICIANS

Imhotep (c. 2667–2600 B.C.E.) was, among other professions, a physi-cian in ancient Egypt who was eventually deified as the god of medi-cine … about 2,200 years after he died (c. 380–343 B.C.E.). He's generally considered the author of what's now known as the *Edwin Smith Papyrus*. (Edwin Smith bought the papyrus from an antiques dealer in 1862. It dates to c. 1600 B.C.E., long after Imhotep's time, but is believed to be a copy of Imhotep's work.) The papyrus contains almost 100 anatomical terms and describes 48 types of injuries along with how to treat them, but the majority of the text deals with surgery, trauma, and insights into gynecology. It also contains eight spells, which may have been used as a last resort when all else failed. Spells and all, the papyrus shows a level of medical knowledge that went well beyond famed Greek physician Hippocrates, who lived 1,000 years later.

It begins with the patient examination, after which treatment was divided into three sections: "An ailment which I will treat"; "An ailment with which I will contend"; or "An ailment not to be treated." Ones that were thought treatable, or at least worth a try, included stitching wounds, bandaging, splints for broken bones, poultices, battling an infection with honey, and using raw meat to stop bleeding. Immobilization was the answer for skull and spinal injuries since the connection had already been made between the brain and conditions like paralysis.

Despite this, it's Hippocrates (c. 460– c. 375 B.C.E.) who is widely considered the father of modern medicine. Hippocrates is thought to be the first person who believed that diseases came from nature, not the gods. In his *On Sacred Diseases*, he wrote, "It is thus with regard to the

Often called the "Father of Medicine," the Greek physician Hippocrates established the first school of medicine, making the science a distinct profession.

disease called Sacred: it appears to me to be nowise more divine nor more sacred than other diseases, but has a natural cause from the originates like other affections. Men regard its nature and cause as divine from ignorance and wonder…."

The Hippocratic Oath, a promise from a doctor to his patient, is still recited by medical school graduates today, some 2,500 years after it was written— even though it's a much different edition, which omits sections like swearing an oath to Apollo.

I swear by Apollo the physician, and Asclepius, and Hygieia and Panacea and all the gods and goddesses as my witnesses that, according to my ability and judgment, I will keep this Oath and this covenant … to teach them this art … without fee or covenant.

I will use those dietary regimens which will benefit my patients … and I will do no harm or injustice to them.

PLAGUES, PANDEMICS AND VIRUSES

I will neither give a deadly drug to anybody who asked for it, nor will I make a suggestion to this effect. Similarly, I will not give a woman an abortive remedy.

I will not use the knife.…

Whatever houses I may visit, I will … remain free of sexual relations with both female and male persons.…

What I may see or hear in the course of treatment … I will keep to myself.

If I fulfill this oath and do not violate it, may it be granted to me to enjoy life and art, being honored … if I transgress it and swear falsely, may the opposite of all this be my lot.

A codified set of medical laws sounds very forward thinking, but we can actually reach all the way back in time to the Code of Hammurabi (Hammurabi was the Babylonian ruler at the time), written in Mesopotamia between 1948 and 1905 B.C.E.—almost 1,500 years before Hippocrates. (Hammurabi was more of a contemporary of Imhotep, if you consider a 600-plus-year difference to be a contemporary.) Here is something similar, if slightly more violent, than the Hippocratic Oath. To wit: "If a surgeon performs a major operation on a nobleman … and caused the death of this man, they shall cut off his hands." This eye-for-an-eye approach reveals much about the differences in the philosophies of both the times and the societies.

Indian medicine also predated the Greeks, culminating in the most famous medical guide of its time, *Suśrutasamhitā, or Suśruta's Compendium*, which covered tooth extractions, prostate removal, cauterization, intestinal obstructions, abscess draining, 12 types of fractures, six types of dislocations, and cataract surgery, just to name a few. Although hard to date—estimates range from 1000 to 1 B.C.E.—its teachings range as far as today's Baghdad, Sicily, and Cambodia.

Continuing eastward, the Chinese *Yellow Emperor's Inner Canon* (2698–2598 B.C.E.) invented, so to speak, the concept of *yin* and *yang*, which we still use today, albeit not always in a medical context. The Chinese of the time believed that all states of being could be classified as *yin*, which corresponds to darkness, cold, and femininity, while its counterpart, *yang*, was associated with light, warmth, and masculinity. Determining the root of an illness meant checking for a balance of *yin* and *yang* or, rather, an imbalance. In this way, it bears more than a passing resemblance to what would be made so popular by the Greeks centuries later—the idea that a healthy body had a balance of four humors.

The Chinese also believed in a life force known as *qi*, which, in a healthy person, would spread easily through a system of internal channels. A blockage in one or more of these channels could be treated by acupuncture, where a series of needles is strategically placed just below the skin, opening up these blocked channels and allowing the *qi* to again flow freely.

The Sicilian philosopher Empedocles (c. 500–430 B.C.E.) introduced the idea of the four humors, which was further developed by Greek Hippocrates and Roman Galen. Here, total health was achieved by the balance of four liquids within the body, known as humors: black bile, yellow bile, blood, and phlegm. These were intertwined with the four elements that formed the basis of our world—earth, air, fire, and water—as well as their associated qualities of dryness, coldness, warmth, and wetness. Hippocrates, though not always correct, at the very least could take a leap beyond the human body to look for a diagnosis, like what made up our world, and how it affected us physically and mentally.

Hippocrates may have been the father of Western medicine, but Galen was not far behind. Born in what is today Turkey in around 131 C.E., Galen was a staunch proponent of the humoral theory, sorting it even further into particular days that were more likely to rebalance humors—a process called *crisis*. A patient who has trouble breathing, according to Galen, would be more likely to be healed on uneven days, especially the fifth and the seventh. (This theory was continued into the nineteenth century when esteemed Canadian physician Sir William Osler [1849–1920] believed that a similar *crisis* was rarely likely to occur before the third or after the twelfth day of any given month).

Given that not many technical breakthroughs in medicine had occurred for centuries and that this was a theory that seemed more plausible than others, Hippocrates and Galen ruled medical thought until the twentieth century until the invention of antibiotics proved to be a better treatment than bleeding a patient.

Galen's, however, was not the only word in ancient Roman medicine, at least not during ancient Roman times. Historian Pliny's *Natural History* cries "Humbug!" at the superstitious character of Roman medicine.

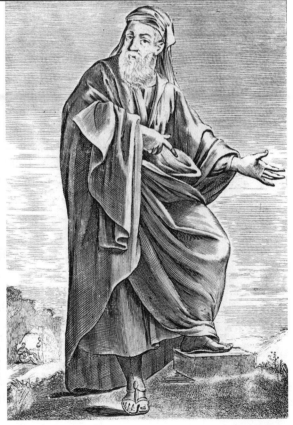

Empedocles introduced the idea of four humors, which need to be in balance in order to maintain a healthy body.

We read, for instance, in the memoirs of Democritus, still extant, that for some diseases, the skull of a malefactor is most efficacious…. Apollonius, again, informs us in his writings, that the most effectual remedy for tooth-ache is to [make incisions in] the gums with the tooth of a man who has died a violent death; and, according to Miletus, human gall is a cure for cataract. For epilepsy, Artemon has prescribed water drawn from a spring in the night and drunk from the skull of a man who has been slain, and whose body remains unburnt. From the skull, too, of a man who had been hanged, Antæus made pills that were to be an antidote to the bite of mad dog. Even more than this, man has resorted to similar remedies for the cure of four-footed beasts even—for [ear infections] in oxen, for instance, the horns have been perforated, and human bones inserted; and when swine have been found to be diseased, fine wheat has been given them which has lain for a night in the spot where a human being has been slain or burnt!

Far from us, far too from our writings, be such prescriptions as these! It will be for us to describe remedies only, and not abominations; cases, for instance, in which the milk of a nursing woman may have a curative effect, cases where the human spittle may be useful, or the contact of the human body, and other instances of a similar nature. We do not look upon life as so essentially desirable that it must be prolonged at any cost, be it what it may—and you, who are of that opinion, be assured, whoever you may be, that you will die none the less, even though you shall have lived in the midst of obscenities or abominations!

MEDICINE FROM THE MIDDLE EAST

Before launching into plagues and pandemics, another group worth mentioning for its medical acumen is the Arabs. Before the Spanish Inquisition, European populations benefited greatly from Arab knowledge of how things worked on the inside and how they were influenced by the outside.

We owe enormous debts of gratitude to the Arab world: they translated much of the Greek writing that would've otherwise been lost to the ages, and they influenced countless numbers of physicians in the Western world in medicine and chemistry. Plus, our adoption of their numerical system meant the end of cumbersome Roman numerals. Imagine having to multiply DCXX and XXIV to get XIVDCCCLXXX as opposed to 620 × 24 = 14,880!

Arab writer Rhazes (c. 841–926 C.E.), known by his contemporaries as "The Experienced," borrowed from Hippocrates and Galen, among others, but added his own unique observation of diseases. His *Liber de Pestilentia* contains the first known description of measles and a brilliant discourse on smallpox, which he was able to distinguish from the former.

Like Rhazes, Avicenna (908–1036 C.E.) was a Muslim physician (and also philosopher) who combined the principles of Greco-Arabic medicine into great writings, the most famous being his *Qanon* or "Canon," which served as the go-to medical textbook for longer than nearly any other work in medical history. He could even be described as the Father of Forceps: "In some cases a difficult delivery—owing to the size of the child—[you must] endeavor to extract it. When this fails forceps are to be applied, and the child is to be extracted by them."

> Avicenna is considered to be one of the greatest scientists of his day. Also known as Ibn Sina, Abu Ali Sina, and Pur Sina, he wrote hundreds of books, 40 of which concern medicine.

Avicenna was so highly prized by Christian writers in the later Middle Ages that he's even mentioned in Geoffrey Chaucer's *The Canterbury Tales*, though not for his work on diseases but on poisons.

However, all this knowledge could not save the mighty city-state of Athens.

THE PLAGUE OF ATHENS

The catastrophe was so overwhelming that men, not knowing what would happen next to them, became indifferent to every rule of religion or law.

—Thucydides

Thucydides (c. 460–c. 400 B.C.E.) was a historian who wrote a firsthand account of the war between the Athenians and the Spartans in the *History of the*

Peloponnesian War. However, his above quote isn't about the effects of war; it's about the effects of plague—specifically, the Plague of Athens.

This was a plague so powerful that, coupled with war, demolished Athens to the point where the home of some of the world's greatest writers, scientists, artists, and armies would never again reach its former glory. It was replaced by another city-state: Sparta. Sparta was all about war. It devoted all its resources toward it. The Spartan mentality was formed by war.

The cities were rivals—or, to put it more realistically, Athenians and Spartans hated each other. War seemed inevitable, and, indeed, in 431 B.C.E., they began fighting each other in what became the Peloponnesian War (431–404 B.C.E.).

At one point, Athens looked like it might actually defeat the mighty Spartan warriors, thanks in a large part to its superior navy. This navy included men whom Athens had recruited from outside the city. This sudden increase in manpower also brought with it a change in population living in close quarters along with poor hygiene and an Athenian port that is believed to have been the entry point of the plague. This port, Piraeus, which was in Athens, was the only way Athenians could get food and supplies.

The plague killed an estimated 75,000 to 100,000 people, including Pericles, ruler of Athens, along with his wife and two sons. His death had terrible consequences, for Athenians soon realized that it was only his leadership that had held them together.

The Plague of Athens came in two waves: Phase one, in 429 B.C.E., killed a reported 33 percent of the population; phase two, between 427 and 426 B.C.E., killed a reported 26 percent of the people who had survived phase one. In total, it reportedly killed close to 100,000 people just in Athens and the nearby areas.

According to Thucydides:

> It began, by report, first in that part of Ethiopia that lieth upon Egypt, and thence fell down into Egypt and Africa and into the greatest part of the territories of the king. It invaded Athens on a sudden and touched first upon those that dwelt in Piraeus, insomuch as they reported that the Peloponnesians had cast poison into their wells (for springs there were not any in that place). But afterwards it came up into the high city, and then they died a great deal faster.

This is where Thucydides's opening quote comes into play. Because the rulers who came after Pericles were incompetent, in addition to the Athenians believing they were under a death sentence, law and order broke down. People

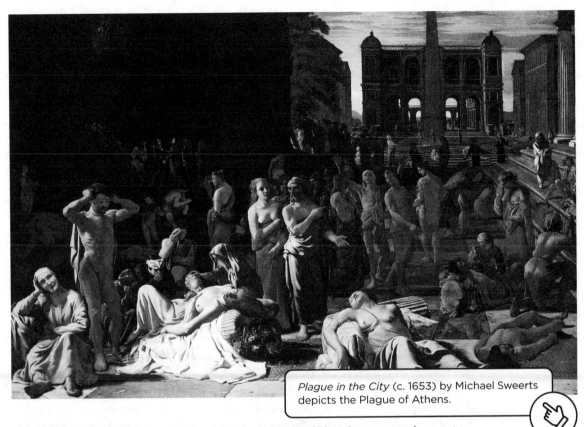

Plague in the City (c. 1653) by Michael Sweerts depicts the Plague of Athens.

spent all their money because they didn't think they'd live long enough to enjoy a savings account, and when they didn't die, they were left broke.

The earliest plague doctors and family members who tended to the ill were among the most vulnerable. The dead were heaped on top of each other, left to rot, or shoved into mass graves. Sometimes, those carrying the dead would come across an already burning funeral pyre, dump a new corpse on it, and walk away. Others stole from preprepared pyres so as to have enough fuel to cremate their own dead. Those lucky enough to survive the plague developed an immunity and became the main caretakers of those who later fell ill.

The site of the many funeral pyres in Athens caused the Spartans to temporarily withdraw from fear of getting the disease.

Homer's Plague

The word "plague" in the header is used loosely because, as we'll later see, scientists, researchers, historians, and all who have studied the Plague of

Athens are not certain if it actually was a plague. They mostly have Thucydides's account to guide them, and while his accounts are descriptive, they can be maddeningly confusing when it comes to describing symptoms. The Greeks were well acquainted with diseases but not how to differentiate them since they were not at all acquainted with germs. Angry gods could cause disease, and any epidemic was called a "plague." In *The Iliad*, the epic poem about the Trojan War recited by Homer in around the eighth century B.C.E., years before the Plague of Athens, "Apollo, the son of Leto and Zeus, angered by the king, brought an evil plague on the army, so that the men were dying, for the son of Atreus had dishonoured Chryses the priest." Apollo was the god of medicine, though he was also a god who caused plague with his arrows.

However, naming epic diseases "plagues" was not due to a lack of medical knowledge solely on the part of the Greeks. This plague is similar to the Bible's Book of Exodus, where God inflicted ten "plagues" or disasters on Egypt in order to force Pharaoh to free the Israelites from slavery; Apollo did so to force Agamemnon to return Chryses's daughter back to him.

Thucydides: Plague Reporter

Unlike other diseases of antiquity or even from a few hundred years ago, the Plague of Athens had Thucydides's firsthand account, which he wrote to teach others how to identify the pestilence should it reoccur. The problem was that the symptoms he described could fit a wide variety of diseases; scholars and physicians alike still debate what exactly caused the Plague of Athens. Measles? Typhus? Smallpox? Actual plague? What they had to go on was that the disease came on quickly, initially causing red eyes, a runny nose, and bad breath. "They were taken first with an extreme ache in their heads, redness and inflammation of the eyes," wrote Thucydides. "And then inwardly, their throats and tongues grew presently bloody and their breath noisome and unsavoury."

After that came convulsions, rashes, gangrene, blisters, and the feeling of one's insides being on fire. The final stages were blindness and exhaustion before death. Thucydides reported that "most of them had also … a strong convulsion, and in some ceased quickly but in others was long before it gave over. Their bodies outwardly to the touch were neither very hot nor pale but reddish, livid, and beflowered with little pimples and whelks, but so burned inwardly as not to endure any the lightest clothes or linen garment to be upon them nor anything but mere nakedness, but rather most willingly to have cast themselves into the cold water."

Smallpox was a strong possibility. It's contagious, and its symptoms include fever, rash, and blindness, yet Thucydides's description of gangrene on the arms and legs ("and he that overcame the worst of it was yet marked with the loss of his extreme parts") is extremely rare for smallpox and may even be a symptom of a secondary illness.

Bubonic plague was also a good candidate, but the lack of any description of buboes—painful swellings of the lymph nodes—lessens the odds that the Athenian plague was actually bubonic plague. Scarlet fever? No—it only affects humans (Thucydides wrote that this pestilence sickened dogs) and generally has a very low mortality rate (at least by modern times, although it could have been higher in ancient Greece). Measles was eliminated for the very same reasons and usually only strikes cities with dense populations above 300,000, few of which existed in the ancient world.

The possibility that the Athenian plague was a combination of diseases also existed. Multiple diseases exist simultaneously in any society. It's also possible that the disease that afflicted Athens either went extinct or has mutated in the past several thousand years, along with its various symptoms, so it's simply not recognizable today, especially if one is trying to match the ancient diseases to modern ones in a ratio of 1:1.

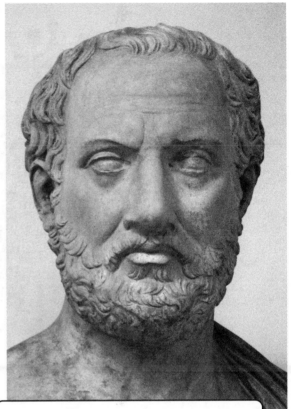

An Athenian general and historian, Thucydides is famous for his writings on the Peloponessian War between Sparta and his native Athens. He is also known as the "Father of Scientific History" and assiduously recorded the events of the Plague of Athens.

"Ancient Athenian Plague Proves to Be Typhoid" declared a 2006 article in *Scientific American*. "Did Ebola Cause the Ancient Plague of Athens?" asked a 2015 article of *The Atlantic* even though the Ebola virus didn't appear in humans until 1976—in Africa. Also, according to a 2019 article by *Target Health*: "It is suggested that the outbreak of the 'plague' in Athens in the 5th century B.C.E. was caused by moldy food containing immunosuppressive mycotoxins, including the irritant T-2 toxin produced by certain Fusarium micro-fungi."

So, when all is said and done, the Plague of Athens is still a mystery. Neither doctors nor researchers have uniformly accepted Ebola, typhoid, smallpox, measles, bubonic plague, cholera, influenza, or countless others as its cause. In addition, Thucydides's descriptions of the symptoms have probably lost something in the translation—for example, the ancient Greek word *phlyktainai* could be "blisters" or "callouses"—or could be completely wrong since Thucydides had no medical training. In 1994, the excavation of mass graves dating back to the time of the Plague of Athens gave some hope that after 2,500 years, a diagnosis would finally happen. DNA samples from the teeth of the dead pointed to typhoid fever as the primary culprit, but the methods researchers used were soon considered flawed, and because, unlike bacteria, viruses degrade quickly, the possibility of ever discovering what happened in Athens 2,500 years ago is unlikely.

> DNA samples from the teeth of the dead pointed to typhoid fever as the primary culprit, but the methods researchers used were soon considered flawed....

As for the Athenians, five years of the plague—or whatever affliction it was—dealt a massive blow to Athens, from which it reportedly never recovered. Their wartime strength and morale were in tatters, and they'd also lost a significant amount of their population. Athens would still put up a fight—the Peloponnesian War lasted 17 years—but they were eventually defeated by Sparta, and Athens's glory as the major superpower of ancient Greece was at an end. Once the strongest city-state in Greece before the Peloponnesian War, Athens never regained its hold, and Sparta became Greece's newly crowned superpower. The economic costs of the war cast a shadow all across Greece; poverty erupted in the Peloponnese region, and war became a common occurrence.

Some final words from Thucydides:

Besides the present affliction, the reception of the country people and of their substance into the city oppressed both them and much more the people themselves that so came in. For having no houses but dwelling at that time of the year in stifling booths, the mortality was now without all form; and dying men lay tumbling one upon another in the streets, and men half-dead about every conduit through desire of water. The temples also where they dwelt in tents were all full of the dead that died within them. For oppressed with the violence of the calamity and not knowing what to do, men grew careless both of holy and profane things alike. And the laws which they formerly used touching funerals were all now broken, everyone burying where he could find room. And many for want of things necessary, after so many deaths before, were forced to become impudent in the funerals of their friends. For when one had made a funeral pile, another getting before him would throw on his dead and give it fire. And when one was in burning, another would come and, having cast thereon him whom he carried, go his way again.

Thucydides's *History of the Peloponnesian War* was still unfinished when he died in 399 B.C.E. It's believed that Xenophon also had a hand in finishing. Xenophon was a Greek soldier and writer who had led 10,000 Greeks safely through the vastness of the Persian Empire after the end of the Peloponnesian War.

THE PLAGUE OF JUSTINIAN

It sates itself on the life-blood of fated men,
paints red the powers' homes with crimson gore.
Black become the sun's beams in the summers that follow,
weathers all treacherous. Do you still seek to know? And what?

—Anonymous (translation by Ursula Dronke, 1997)

The *Poetic Edda* is a series of poems about Norse mythology whose writers are unknown, but their works have had a significant impact on literature, influencing writers like J. R. R. Tolkien and George R. R. Martin.

The above selection comes from *Völuspá*, the *Poetic Edda*'s first section. In it, a fortune-teller reveals to Norse god Odin that Odin and many gods will be killed by fire, and Earth will be destroyed by flood during a final battle of good versus evil. This ending is called *Ragnarök—ragna* meaning "reign" and *rök* meaning "twilight." After *Ragnarök*, the fortune-teller sees the world eventually reappearing from the water, with an eagle soaring over a mountain. The surviving gods reminisce about the past, and the fields begin to grow again.

The *Poetic Edda* was written in the thirteenth century, but it eerily describes an apocalyptic time in the sixth century that took place not only in Scandinavia but around the world.

A global cooling period between 536 and c. 600 C.E. is believed to have occurred at the same time as a massive volcanic eruption that came from Ilopango in today's El Salvador. (Ilopango is now dormant.) Researchers, led by geologist Robert Dull, performed radiocarbon measurements on tree trunks that had been exposed to Ilopango's volcanic deposits.

Their results showed that Ilopango spewed the equivalent of 10.5 cubic miles of dense rock. This means that it was one of the biggest volcanic events in the last 7,000 years. The blast was more than 100 times bigger than Washington State's Mount St. Helens's eruption in 1980 and several times larger than the Philippines's Mount Pinatubo eruption in 1991. It shot sulfuric gases and particles miles into the sky, reflecting sunlight away from Earth's surface ("Black become the sun's beams in the summers that follow"), kicking off a century-long temperature decline, with global temps down by possibly as much as 3.6 degrees Fahrenheit and bringing about the end of the Classic Maya era.

The *Poetic Edda* was written in the thirteenth century, but it eerily describes an apocalyptic time in the sixth century that took place....

Far away in Europe, Irish records described crop failures, bread shortages, and famine. Summer snow was reported in southern Italy and China. In Scandinavia, tree growth was severely stunted because of the climatic seesaw, with tree rings bearing telltale signs of damage from frost in the summer of 536. Similar to the language in the Scandinavian *Poetic Edda*, Byzantine historian Procopius wrote in 536 C.E. that "during this year a most dread portent took place. For the sun gave forth its light without brightness ... and it seemed exceedingly like the sun in eclipse, for the beams it shed were not clear."

The world was beginning to adjust to its new normal when something snapped it back into chaos. It was the Plague of Justinian in 541 C.E. The plague was named for Emperor Justinian I, who ruled the eastern, or Byzantine, portion of the Roman Empire at the time and was best known for directing the construction of the Hagia Sophia, which was originally a Greek Orthodox cathedral and is now a Muslim mosque.

Even though an 800-year gap exists between the Plague of Justinian and the Black Plague, the commonalities are startling. Both came at a time of failing crops and climatic changes (though in the case of the Black Plague, it was torrentially wet weather, not summer snow). Both plagues are thought to come from the same bacteria, and both are thought to have been ignited by trade that started in the Far East and traveled west largely via the Silk Road.

The Silk Road was a channel of trade routes that began in China and branched out through India and the Middle East and ended in southern Europe; another route began in Southeast Asia, branched into East Africa, and ended in southern Europe. These routes lasted in various formations from the second century B.C.E. until roughly 300 years ago.

Its name came from the Chinese silk trade, which was so lucrative that the Great Wall of China was extended to protect it. Paper, spices, philosophies, religions—all were traded along this network. (Even a tapestry uncovered in western China showed a Greek warrior and a centaur.)

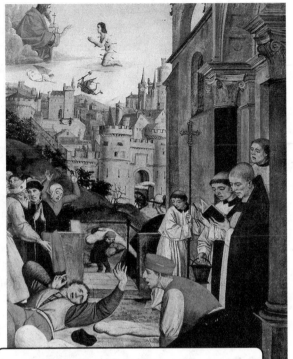

A c. 1498 painting by Dutch artist Josse Liefe-rinxe depicts Saint Sebastian pleading for the life of a man stricken by the Plague of Justinian. The plague reoccurred off and on from the mid-sixth through the mid-eighteenth centuries.

Along with cultural and economic trade, both the Silk Road and commercial boats were great for spreading diseases, especially plagues. Both brought along flea-covered rats; it's believed that the cause of the Plague of Justinian was the bacteria in these rats that was discussed in the introduction: *Yersinia pestis*.

According to Procopius, who was to the Plague of Justinian what Thucydides was to the Plague of Athens:

It reached Byzantium in the midst of spring, where I happened to be staying at the time. And it came thusly … at first those who met these creatures tried to turn them aside by uttering the holiest of names and exorcising them in other ways as best one could, but they accomplished absolutely nothing, for even in sanctuaries, where the most of them fled for refuge, they were dying constantly. But later on they were unwilling to even listen to their friends when they called them, and they shut themselves up in their rooms and pretended not to hear, although the doors were being beaten down, fearing that he who was calling was one of the spirits.

The Plague of Justinian was a pandemic that was one of the deadliest ever, unless reports of its death toll were greatly exaggerated. Researchers still debate the overall mortality rate, which could be anywhere from 25 to 50 million people over the two centuries it supposedly recurred (starting in 541 C.E., with recurrences until 750) and caused the end of the Roman Empire and the birth of the Middle Ages.

However, this theory does not take into account that the Western Roman Empire was already in disarray, and, by contrast, the Byzantine Empire would survive until 1453, when it was invaded—not by disease but by the Ottoman Turks. The very fact that it has garnered little attention over the decades and is virtually unknown today, even though it supposedly killed millions upon millions, may prove that it wasn't as deadly as was once thought.

Let's start with what we do know—here's Justinian.

Justinian I became emperor in 527 C.E. after the Roman Empire had been split in two—a result of the misguided belief that the Roman Empire had grown so large and unwieldy that dividing it into eastern and western halves would make it easier to rule and protect from invaders. Justinian was emperor of what was the Eastern, or Byzantine, Empire—more Greek influenced than Roman. This strategy worked terrifically for the eastern half, as they had a robust economy based on agriculture and long-distance trade, but not so much for the western half, who were spending much of their time and money fending off nearby Germanic tribes and government corruption.

> The Plague of Justinian was a pandemic that was one of the deadliest ever, unless reports of its death toll were greatly exaggerated. Researchers still debate the overall mortality rate....

Justinian wanted to restore the Roman Empire to its glory days, and that meant reuniting the East and West, with himself at the helm. His general, Belisarius, conquered the coastline of North Africa. Then, the Kingdom of the Ostrogoths fell, bringing territories like Dalmatia (today's Croatia), Sicily, and even the crown jewel, Rome, back into the fold. Justinian then reclaimed the southern end of the Iberian Peninsula—today's southern Spain—establishing the province of Spania. These campaigns increased Byzantine control over the Western Mediterranean, and Justinian's dream seemed to be a sure bet.

However, something got in the way of his plans.

The Plague of Justinian began in China and exploded in Constantinople, the capital of the Byzantine Empire. (Previously called Byzantium, Constantinople is now known as Istanbul, the capital of Turkey.) The plague weakened the Byzantine Empire at a critical point, when Justinian's armies were claiming victory after victory.

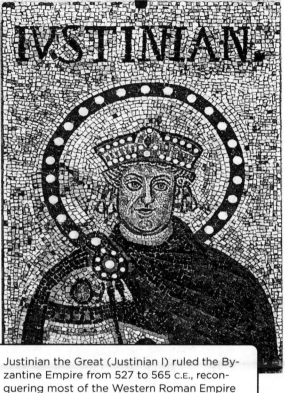

Justinian the Great (Justinian I) ruled the Byzantine Empire from 527 to 565 C.E., reconquering most of the Western Roman Empire in an effort to restore Rome's former glory.

With the onset of the plague came remedies that included cold-water baths and amulets, and physicians were brought in from Alexandria in Egypt. They could not do much, though it probably didn't matter in the long run, as most of the sick who were able to see physicians were only the wealthy sick.

Massive taxation had already occurred in order to retake western Rome as well as for the building of churches, like the Hagia Sophia. Once the plague hit, it cut a wide swath through the farming community and the agricultural trade, which had meant so much to the Byzantines. Fewer people meant fewer farmers which meant less grain, causing prices to soar and tax revenues to decline, but Justinian wasn't going to let the near-collapse of the economic system get in the way of financing his conquests, so in response to his decaying population and territories, Justinian did something unthinkable: he raised taxes and added taxes on the dead, which forced families to pay taxes on behalf of dead loved ones.

According to Procopius:

When pestilence swept through the whole known world and notably the Roman Empire, wiping out most of the farming community and of necessity leaving a trail of desolation in its wake, Justinian showed no mercy towards the ruined freeholders. Even then, he did not refrain from demanding the annual tax, not only the amount at which he assessed each individual, but also the amount for which his deceased neighbors were liable.

Justinian died in 565 C.E. His obsession with rebuilding the empire led to his legacy as the "last Roman." By the end of the century, much of the land in Italy that he had conquered had been lost when the Byzantines changed direction and pushed east into Persia.

The initial plague in 541 C.E. killed close to 40 percent of Byzantium's inhabitants and led to the deaths of up to one-fourth of the Eastern Mediterranean population. Subsequent waves of the plague continued to strike throughout the sixth, seventh, and eighth centuries, though each wave brought fewer fatalities. Competing views claim that the mortality of the Justinian Plague was far lower

THE DIVINE COMEDY

In the *Divine Comedy*, published by Florentine poet Dante Alighieri in 1320, the main character is guided through purgatory and the tortures of hell by ancient Greek poet Virgil, but after the long trek, Dante finally reaches Paradise, where he's guided by his great, unrequited love, Beatrice. Justinian I is in heaven in what's known as Mercury's Sphere, hidden by the rays of the sun. This corresponds to Justinian's desire to unite the Roman Empire but on behalf of his own glory more than that of Rome's. His introduction was "Caesar I was and am Justinian," which means he was Caesar on Earth and Caesar in spirit but just Justinian in heaven, yet he's described as a defender of the Christian faith and the restorer of Rome to the empire; Dante treats him as the consummate emperor.

Justinian brought back the prestige of the Roman Empire, but that prestige was lost in subsequent years because of divisions in Christianity. For making this loss more regrettable, Dante has Justinian summarize the history of the Roman Empire from his own point of view. Justinian then explains why he is in Mercury's Sphere, a place for those who did honorable things in order to gain glory. Now, they enjoy Paradise, but they are eclipsed by the sun.

than previously believed. After the last recurrence in 750, pandemics on the scale of the Plague of Justinian did not appear again in Europe until close to 600 years later with the Black Death.

Speaking of the Black Death, with the help of samples taken from the teeth of Justinian Plague victims in Bavaria, Germany, it was determined that the bacteria called *Yersinia pestis* most probably caused the Plague of Justinian. Since bacteria can sometimes survive in the blood (unlike viruses, hence the inability to diagnose what caused the Plague of Athens), teeth were chosen as samples because they have numerous blood vessels.

The DNA from *Y. pestis* was analyzed and found to be closely related— like a cousin—to the strain of *Y. pestis* that caused the Black Death, a strain that still exists in Central Asia. This suggests that the route of infection was indeed through trade from Asia to Europe.

Scientists believe that the Justinian strain eventually died out, just as some family lines die out. Based upon DNA analysis of bones found in graves, the type of plague that struck the Byzantine Empire during the reign of Justinian was bubonic, although it was very probable that other types of plague, pneumonic and septicemic, were also present. We're about to find out what this means.

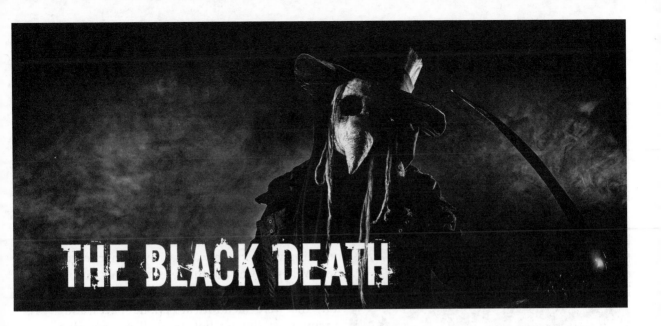

THE BLACK DEATH

If you lived in Europe right before the Black Death, you probably worked on a farm. If you were a man, you were on average 5 feet, 7 inches tall, married, and lived in a two-room house that you built yourself. If you were a woman, you were on average 5 feet, 2 inches tall, had been married since you were about sixteen, and had three to five children, who would live at least until adolescence. You were also part of the feudal system.

Throughout most of medieval Europe as well as parts of Asia were the "Three Estates." These differed somewhat throughout different times and different countries, but essentially, the First Estate was clergy, the Second Estate was nobility, and the Third Estate comprised most of the population: the Peasantry. Taken together, this was called a feudal society. In broad terms, a lord was a landowner and member of the Second Estate who leased his land to a peasant in the Third Estate. The peasant and his family were allowed to live on the land, known as a fief, in exchange for working the land or, in some cases, providing military service. This was never something a vassal could "work off." They were stuck in this strata for life, and they often paid more taxes than the nobility. The obligations and corresponding rights between lord and vassal concerning the fief formed the basis of the feudal relationship.

Aside from being a feudal society, the people of the Middle Ages experienced many of the same problems we do today—overdevelopment, food shortage, and environmental issues. Forests were leveled to make room for the growing populations, and marshes were drained to make room for crops. They didn't have a lot of spare land left, with some parts, like England and the Neth-

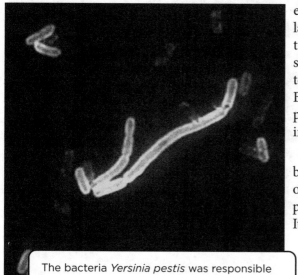

The bacteria *Yersinia pestis* was responsible for both the Plague of Justinian and, eight centuries later, the Black Plague.

erlands, becoming badly overcrowded. Arable land was being broken into smaller and smaller tracts, so peasants were less able to feed themselves and their families. British economic historian Bruce Campbell estimates that before the Black Death, 40 percent of people were at the poverty line and 30 percent were below it. Social inequality is bad for general health.

So, with all this famine, filth, and backbreaking work in the world, why bother to go on? Well, this was not the case for every European. Some enjoyed life in cities like Florence, Italy, that were filled with art, public spaces, and temperate climates, but above all, most Medieval Europeans had a strong belief in God and the Church. Through good works and prayer, a person may not have an easy life on Earth, but after death, they would hopefully enjoy an eternity in Paradise. People attempted to stack the odds in their favor; they carried holy trinkets, like pieces of the Communion wafer, or relics, which were usually phony (i.e., a piece of the true cross; the tooth of a martyred saint). Priests encouraged parishioners to donate as much as they could to the Church and hospitals run by the Church—whether it be money, land, or anything else they had to offer. Since the belief was that God spoke through the clergy, the more people gave, the better their chances were of an eternity in Paradise, even if these were people who had almost nothing to give.

Europe of the 1300s didn't start well. Repeated hot and wet summers destroyed the fields that yielded the crops that populations relied on. Famine ensued, and winters were even worse—colder than usual, farm animals didn't get enough food and starved or froze to death.

Also, few towns had clean drinking water. Most of what families drank came from nearby streams, and much of that was boiled over a flame to wash themselves, dishes, and clothes. Families would sit in front of the fire to stay warm in the winter or dry their wet clothes. Buckets were used as toilets, or people just found a place outdoors to use the bathroom, with a handful of leaves or straw for toilet paper.

It's no shock that illness was common in fourteenth-century Europe. Because their medical knowledge had not changed much since the days of Hippocrates and Galen, fourteenth-century people could catch diseases that would

PLAGUES, PANDEMICS AND VIRUSES

seem shocking today, like leprosy. Only half of medieval babies would reach the age of five, and many of their mothers would die giving birth to them. If you were lucky enough to reach old age, you might be rewarded with arthritis, deafness, blindness, and/or agonizing dental problems along with any number of aches and pains that resulted from a lifetime of illnesses and accidents that were never properly treated.

It's not that medieval people were ignorant or dumb, especially when it came to science. Back then, nobody questioned why objects fell instead of floated. They just fell. The reason wouldn't be addressed for another 300 years with Sir Isaac Newton's law of gravity (which he came up with while in exile during the Great Plague of London). Similarly, people didn't yet know the right questions to ask in medicine, and medical equipment had not evolved to the point where we could see bacteria, or cells, or learn how diseases are transmitted.

The first medical school was founded between 1000 and 1100 in Salerno, near Naples, in southern Italy. Soon, they were springing up in prominent cities like Toulouse, France; Bologna, Italy; and Oxford, England. Becoming a doctor was not unlike becoming a member of the clergy—he (not she) was not allowed to marry and had to obey the word of God. As such, it was a calling. However, they weren't called to minister all the sick—instead, most physicians' patients were of the First Estate and the Second Estate.

So, by the time the plague arrived, it wasn't that patients didn't have enough doctors, it was that their education hadn't really progressed beyond ancient times. Hippocrates and Galen still had enormous influence on the medical community. It would be as though today's doctors were still using medical practices from about the time of the Norman Conquest in 1066.

> **Becoming a doctor was not unlike becoming a member of the clergy—he (not she) was not allowed to marry and had to obey the word of God.**

A SENSE OF HUMOR

On the plus side, both Hippocrates and Galen taught physicians to look for natural causes of illnesses: what the patient ate, what his lifestyle was, how much exercise he got—but they also believed that four elements, known as "humors," controlled the body in much the same way the world was controlled by four seasons. The humors were blood, phlegm, choler (yellow bile) and melancholy (black bile). This theory of humors became so popular that the words even entered our vocabulary: to be "phlegmatic" is to be level-headed; "sanguine" (from blood) is optimistic; "choleric" is ill-tempered; and "melancholy" is sad. Hippocrates and Galen believed that these humors not only had the power to make a person sad but to make them ill.

After the fall of both the Greek and Roman empires, the theory of the four humors fell out of public consciousness until c. 1000 C.E., when it caught on with another branch of physicians—Jews and Muslims, who lived from southern Spain all the way to the Middle East. By 1200 C.E., many of the texts that came from Hippocrates and Galen had been translated by Arabs into Latin, the language of Christian scholars and physicians, so that the theory of the four humors was taught in greater Europe again. There was also the Jewish physician Maimonides, whose work covered everything from hemorrhoids to asthma to aphrodisiacs.

This time, the humors gained a mystical aspect. Now, black bile had Saturn as a corresponding planet, while blood belonged to Jupiter. Both planets were considered evil, while the moon (then considered a planet) was thought to cause mental illness—where we get the word "lunatic" from. Therefore, physicians were also trained in astronomy to calculate the healthy and sickly times in a patient's life as determined by the planets and stars.

When the Black Death began, medieval doctors claimed it was caused by the dangerous planets—Mars, Jupiter, and Saturn—passing through the equally deadly constellation Aquarius.

"Terrible is God toward the sons of men…. He often allows plagues, miserable famines, conflicts, wars and other forms of suffering to arise, and uses them to terrify and torment men and so drive out their sins. And thus, indeed, the kingdom of England, because of the growing pride and corruption of its subjects and their numberless sins … is to be oppressed by the pestilences." This is a letter from a senior monk to the bishop of London dated September 1348.

These were people who were used to tough times, but it was the sheer scale of the plague and its frightening speed that terrified the population. Like the Wheel of Fortune, it was impossible to predict whose fate would take a turn for the worse or who would escape. Only about two out of ten people who caught the plague recovered. Whole families—whole villages—were erased as if they'd never existed.

Father abandoned child, wife husband, one brother another, for this illness seemed to strike through breath and sight. And so they died. And none could be found to bury the dead for money or friendship. Members of a household brought their dead to a ditch as best they could. And in Siena great pits were dug and piled deep with the multitude of dead. And I, Angelo di Tura … buried my five children with my own hands…. And there were also those who were so sparsely covered with earth that the dogs dragged them forth and devoured many bodies throughout the city.

—Angelo di Tura of Siena, Italy

Mal is Latin for "bad" or "evil"; even today, you can put those three letters in front of certain English words and turn them into unhappy words, like *malignant*, *malevolent*, *malodorous*, *malcontent*, even *malware*. Also, the Latin phrase *male habitus* means "ill-kept" or "in a bad way." Over the centuries, *male habitus* evolved into the Old French word *maladie*, meaning "disease" (in fact, it still means disease). This eventually branched off into the English word *malady*.

Malady, though indeed an illness, doesn't come close to describing the horror of the Black Death. Perhaps people didn't yet have the language for it because nothing this destructive had occurred within living memory; the word "pandemic," for instance, wasn't coined until the 1500s (from the Latin word *pandēmus*, meaning "affecting all"). The name itself was not used during the pandemic; people weren't screaming, "It's the Black Death! The Black Death!" Some called it "the Great Mortality," "the Great Pestilence," or even the "the Blue Death" due to the color of many of the corpses, but the term "Black Death"

Only about two out of ten people who caught the plague recovered. Whole families—whole villages—were erased as if they'd never existed.

wasn't used until the eighteenth century, and even then, it was to identify this plague as a kind of death to end all deaths—while several plagues were still to come in subsequent centuries, none would cause as much devastation as this one.

Bubonic plague was part of the worst pandemic in history, killing anywhere from 75 to 200 million people in Europe and Eurasia between 1346 and 1353. That's equal to between 30 to 60 percent of Europe's population. It killed so many that it took more than two centuries for the world's population to recover.

The Black Plague came to Europe on ships bringing trade from the East. Within a few short years, it had ravaged the continent.

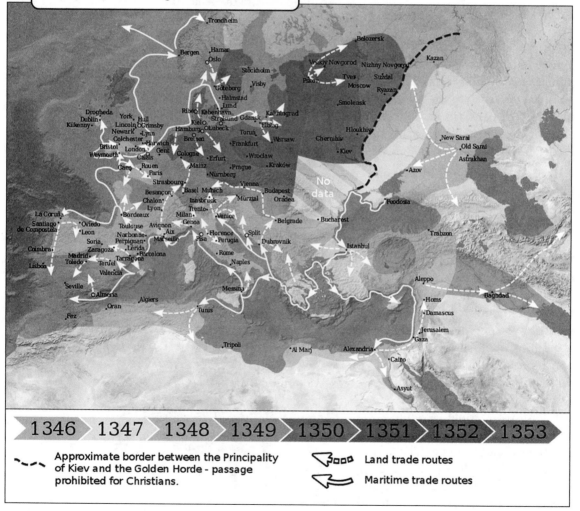

1346 1347 1348 1349 1350 1351 1352 1353

- - - Approximate border between the Principality of Kiev and the Golden Horde - passage prohibited for Christians.

Land trade routes

Maritime trade routes

PLAGUES, PANDEMICS AND VIRUSES

WHERE IT BEGAN

The Black Death boarded ships sailing from ports in Asia, along the trade routes through the Middle East and Turkey, and finally making landfall in Messina, Sicily. Though it was common to personify disease as the Devil or some creature in order to make sense of it, the Black Death had more to do with fleas.

Fleas were a common nuisance in medieval Europe. Whether cottages or castles, homes were often plagued with rat, mice, and flea infestations. Add to that the filthy conditions of towns and villages, where human and animal waste were flung in equal parts onto garbage-strewn streets, and you have the potential for any number of illnesses.

Today, is it generally believed that rats infected with *Y. pestis* boarded trading ships like the ones that sailed from the Far East to the Mediterranean. These rats were then bitten by fleas, and then the fleas caught *Y. pestis*, spreading it by biting a human.

In 1346, ships arrived at the port of Messina with silk and spices; rats and fleas carrying the *Y. pestis* bacteria; and crews covered in boils that oozed blood and pus. Sicilian authorities soon ordered all of these "death ships" out of the harbor, but it was too late—soon, healthy people all over Europe were about to die. The plague was airborne, so it was incredibly, terrifyingly transmissible, spreading easily from person to person, which meant that coughing or sneezing on someone was potentially enough to kill them.

The "death ships" of Messina were not the first instance of plague. It originated in the Far East and had already killed many in countries like China, India,

---

EXCERPT FROM A LATE-MEDIEVAL FRENCH HOUSEKEEPING MANUAL

To Catch Fleas. France c. 1400

Spread two thick slices with paste made of quicklime (crushed and baked limestone mixed with water).

Stand a lighted candle in the center, and place in your chamber at night. Fleas will be attracted by the light, hop onto the lime, be trapped there, and die.

—*The Bourgeois of Paris*, E. Power, ed., Rutledge, 1928

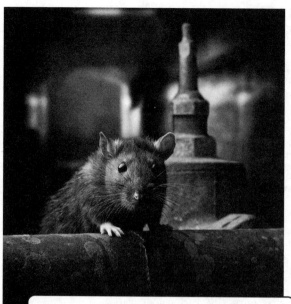

Brown rats served as transportation for fleas that carried the *Y. pestis* bacteria from person to person. Bad sanitation in medieval Europe meant lots of rats were available to do this.

and Egypt, and the Plague of Justinian had prevented the reunification of the Roman Empire 800 years earlier. However, that was 800 years ago, and commerce must go on, so the ships came, seeking a port in the storm.

After Messina, the Black Death reached Marseilles in France and Tunis in North Africa. Then, it spread to Rome and Florence, two Italian cities that were the hub of circuitous medieval trade routes.

How and why did the Black Death spread so quickly and become so destructive? The answer is—we still don't know.

We'll start with *Y. pestis*, though. It's a rod-shaped bacterium covered with a layer called "biofilm," which is really just a clinical term for slime; this slime prevents *Y. pestis* from being eaten by other cells.

A rat may get *Y. pestis* from a flea bite; most often, it's a black rat that will become infected with the bacteria, and the rat becomes a "reservoir" for *Y. pestis*, while the flea is a "vector." ("Vector" is another word for a biting insect that spreads disease from one living thing to another.)

If you're the type to get the heebie-jeebies from seeing a rat, it probably doesn't matter if it's a black or brown rat. One doesn't take the time to investigate; one just sees it and screams, "Rat!" However, from an epidemiological standpoint, particularly when it comes to the Black Death, the color of the rat matters.

Rats belong to the genus *Rattus*. (Despite the name, *Rattus* includes not only rats but hamsters, mice, and gerbils, though we'll concentrate on the rat for right now.) The brown rat, or Norwegian rat (*Rattus norvegicus*), is brown but not Norwegian. It probably originated in China. How it got to be called "Norwegian" is unclear, though it may be English naturalist John Berkenhout who gave it the misnomer, believing it came from Norwegian ships. The name stuck. (See another great misnomer on the chapter on the 1918 flu.)

Brown rats are larger than their cousin, the black rat, and have larger ears and a longer tail. Wherever people are, brown rats are right there with them, scavenging and making more rats.

PLAGUES, PANDEMICS AND VIRUSES

Brown rats are sometimes mistakenly thought to have spread the Black Death, and, indeed, they can suffer from the plague, though researchers believe the major reservoir of bubonic plague is the black rat (*Rattus rattus*). This rat originated in southern and Southeast Asia, then traveled west through the Middle East all the way through Continental Europe and eventually to Great Britain and Ireland. Rats are terrific reservoirs for many diseases because of their ability to hold many infectious bacteria in their blood without dying themselves. What can kill it are cats, owls, weasels, foxes, and coyotes. This certainly doesn't place the black rat at the top of the food chain, but don't worry—black rats run quickly and are fast climbers.

When an uninfected flea bites an infected rat, it ingests the rat's blood and bacteria, including *Y. pestis*. The slime that covers the bacteria causes a backup between the now-infected flea's esophagus and gut, meaning that the flea can get food into its mouth but not into its stomach. The only way the flea avoids starving to death is by vomiting the blood and bacteria into whatever mammal it bites. If that mammal is human, he or she is in danger of contracting the plague. This is what classifies the disease as *zoonotic*, in that it's able to pass from animals to humans. (As we'll see later, barnyard animals are notorious for making people sick as well.)

Rats—who eat everything from pizza to wires—*love* grain, and many of these trading ships were stuffed to the gills with grain. Usually, rats only travel about a mile from where they're born, which is why the plague may have stayed in one place for so long, but these grain ships were possibly the ones that brought the disease west in the first place since Egypt's rat population exploded by feeding on the large granaries there, and now, they were sailing halfway around the world and unknowingly starting a pandemic.

> Rats—who eat everything from pizza to wires—*love* grain, and many of these trading ships were stuffed to the gills with grain.

PLAGUES, PANDEMICS AND VIRUSES

No one knew exactly how the Black Death was transmitted, and no one knew how to prevent or treat it. For example, one doctor claimed that "instantaneous death occurs when the aerial spirit escaping from the eyes of the sick man strikes the healthy person standing near and looking at the sick." Doctors prescribed holding sweet-smelling herbs to one's face to avoid miasma—best defined as "foul air," which came from the aforementioned lack of hygiene at this time. It was believed that plague spread through this miasma, and although certain diseases very well could spread through mounds of filth, plague was not one of them. Baths and sex were frowned upon, as were "heating" or spicy foods, like garlic or pepper, which they believed might cause fever. "Cooling" foods, like vegetables, helped balance the humors.

GERBILS, TOO

Something a bit cuter than *Rattus rattus*: the gerbil. While it's easy to point a finger at and something, well, ratty, gerbils are welcomed as pets, given their own homes, and allowed to crawl all over children. If someone were to do this with a rat, they might be written about in horror stories or police blotters. It's the gerbil's cuddly look and docile nature that lure people into believing they're harmless, and while gerbils wouldn't spread plague with intent—neither would the rat—the result would be the same.

Gerbils, which are relatives of rats, inhabit—among other places—the same parts of Asia that rats do; they also carry fleas and hop on ships bound for parts unknown. Rats have shouldered the blame for the Black Death for several centuries (even more than fleas), but it's only just now that researchers from the University of Oslo are comparing the dates of plague outbreaks with climatic data that were revealed in tree rings. The results showed that major temperature fluctuations in Asia—extreme highs followed quickly by extreme lows—preceded plague outbreaks in Europe by about 15 years. That kind of weather, they believed, would have been too wet for rats to flourish and carry infected fleas across continents, but it was just right for rat cousins, like gerbils and marmots.

Under these conditions, fleas also become more active and gerbils more numerous. Indeed, researchers found that an increase of one degree Celsius doubles the prevalence of plague in Central Asian rodents. Could it be that these furry little friends are rats in gerbil's clothing? The answer is—it's a definite possibility.

PLAGUES, PANDEMICS AND VIRUSES

What we do know for sure is that *Y. pestis* is a type of bacterium that's beyond bad. It's the cause of the plague—and not just one plague but at least three *that we know of*: bubonic, pneumonic, and septicemic.

Bubonic plague is the most common form of the disease. It is marked by the sudden appearance of bulbously swollen, blue, and painful lymph nodes (called buboes) in the groin or armpits, where our lymph nodes are. (In fact, the word *bubon* is Greek for "groin" or "swollen groin.") Bubonic plague is not directly transmitted from one human to another unless direct contact with lymph node tissue or secretions occurs; it's usually caused by the bite of an infected flea. Back then, you had about a 15 percent chance of surviving the bubonic form of plague.

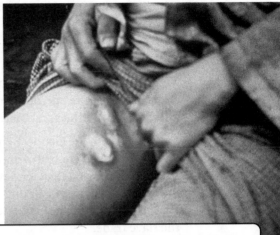

Severe swelling of the lymph nodes (called buboes) in the armpits or, as shown here, around the groin is one symptom of the bubonic plague. Other symptoms include chills, muscle aches, fatigue, fever, and headaches.

Pneumonic plague, the second-most common, can start as bubonic plague but then settle into the lungs, causing a rapid and severe form of pneumonia that leads to respiratory failure, shock, and death. It is the only type that can be spread person to person if someone inhales infected water droplets traveling through the air. No one survived pneumonic plague.

Septicemic plague, the rarest, can also start as bubonic plague but then attacks a person's blood cells, causing skin or other tissue to die and turn black, especially on the extremities, like hands and feet. It's caused by either an infected flea bite or by handling an infected animal. The bad news is that you will most definitely die from septicemic plague, but the good news is that it won't take long, perhaps only a day.

What made the Black Death even more deadly is that the medical community relied on practices that dated as far back as ancient Greece, which would be like the doctors of today practicing the same medicine as they did in medieval times (and by extension in ancient Greek times).

ITALY DURING THE PLAGUE

Italy is a peninsula, meaning it's almost completely surrounded by water. (If it were completely surrounded by water, it would be an island, like Sicily.) The Italy of the Middle Ages is not the Italy we know today, which is an independent country extending from the Alps across the length of the peninsula.

After the fall of the Roman Empire in c. 500 C.E., Italy fractured into what are called city-states, so today's Italian cities, like Florence, Genoa, Pisa, and Venice, were actually independent countries, each with their own government. Because they were surrounded by water, people like the Venetians, Genoese, and Pisans were the great maritime merchants of the Middle Ages.

In 1266, the Genoese entered into an agreement with the Mongols, who had earlier taken control of another peninsula: the Crimea in the Black Sea. The agreement allowed the Genoese to set up a trading center in the Crimean city of Kaffa, making Kaffa an important commercial hub between Europe and the Far East and giving the Genoese a monopoly on the Black Sea trade, particularly the slave trade.

Life wasn't always smooth sailing in Kaffa, though. The Kaffa agreement made a lot of money for both the Genoese and the Mongols, though relations were shaky—they went into business together, but that didn't mean they liked each other, and it was only a matter of time before simmering anger would overtake commerce.

In 1307, the Mongols took back Kaffa because of the slave trade. This had nothing to do with any moral misgivings but rather because the Mongols' new leader, Toqta, realized that the slaves who were being sold by the Genoese from Kaffa could have been used as foot soldiers for Toqta's army. Not only were the Genoese selling them, but they were selling them to the Egyptian Mamluks, who were Mongol enemies. Toqta answered this commercial insult by laying siege to Kaffa—surrounding it as much as possible in order to starve out the Genoese. At first, the Genoese resisted the siege, but they eventually set fire to Kaffa and abandoned it after a year in 1308.

After Toqta died four years later in 1312, a new Mongol ruler, Ozbeg, invited the Genoese back; unbeknownst to either party, the plague was just starting to creep in from China, but at this point, Kaffa was a thriving and quite cosmopolitan city with many ethnic groups and religions, including Greeks, Turks, Mongols, Armenians, and Jews, working and living within its two giant, concentric walls. However, in 1343 this harmony was disrupted by a fight between the Muslim Mongols and the Christian Genoese, which left one Mongol dead. This infuriated the current ruler, Janibeg. (Janibeg was Ozbeg's son—he become ruler after Ozbeg died and Janibeg put his own brothers to death.)

In response, the Mongols again lay siege to Kaffa, and the Genoese stayed until 1344, when Italian reinforcements arrived, killing 13,000 Mongols and de-

PLAGUES, PANDEMICS AND VIRUSES

THE HUMAN PARASITE FACTOR

Today, researchers believe that the numbers behind the rat-to-flea-to-human route of transmission don't work. Nothing is mentioned about large numbers of rats dying off in tandem with humans, as would happen with later plagues. Also, the Black Death spread much farther and faster, and killed many more people, than any other known outbreak. This has led some researchers to speculate that human parasites were just as critical as rats in spreading the Black Death. For example, fleas and lice could have fed on infected humans and then transmitted the disease to other humans.

In a study published in the *Proceedings of the National Academy of Sciences*, researchers used mathematical equations to create different types of plague transmissions during a series of outbreaks in Europe called the second pandemic, which started with the Black Death and recurred through the nineteenth century.

One model has the disease spreading from rats to fleas to people; the second model has the disease spreading from human fleas and body lice to other people; and a third model has the disease spreading from person to person through the air, which occurs only when people develop pneumonic plague.

The result was that the human parasite model best reflected death rates in seven of the nine regions covered.

stroying their weapons. The siege was lifted, yet the Mongols were a people who died hard.

By 1346, Janibeg tried again to drive out the Genoese, but by this point, his army began to die from the plague, which they caught during their travels into Asia and then brought back west. If they were to die, Janibeg thought, they were going to take the city with them. The Mongols proceeded to engage in what is best described as the earliest form of biological warfare: they catapulted their dead over Kaffa's walls and onto the Genoese. Whether the intent was biological or psychological warfare is unknown, but either way, the Genoese eventually caught what the Mongols had, as did the other inhabitants of Kaffa. They fled the city to other ports in Europe, bringing the plague with them.

In October 1347, those who worked at the docks of Messina in Sicily were met with Genoese ships whose sailors were either dead or covered in black boils that oozed blood and pus. The Black Death had arrived.

Many scholars claim the Kaffa ships were the trigger in spreading the pandemic—others believe these ships were just part of several ways the plague entered European ports. Indeed, the major port city of Constantinople had already been leveled in 1346, and in 1347, ports in Crete, Cyprus, Dubrovnik, Pisa, Genoa, Marseilles, Avignon, and Mallorca were the first ones hit in Western Europe. By 1347, it was clear that this pestilence was not going to burn itself out or be limited to port cities, and it began its march inland, beginning in Marseilles, the French gateway to Europe.

> **In October 1347, those who worked at the docks of Messina in Sicily were met with Genoese ships whose sailors were either dead or covered in black boils that oozed blood and pus.**

Gabriele de' Mussi, a clerk from Piacenza in northern Italy, wrote of the plague as though it were some kind of divine punishment; he even mentions buboes.

Tell, O Sicily, and ye, the many islands of the sea, the judgments of God. Confess, O Genoa, what thou hast done, since we of Genoa and Venice are compelled to make God's chastisement manifest. Alas! our ships enter the port, but of a thousand sailors hardly ten are spared. We reach our homes; our kindred and our neighbors come from all parts to visit us. Woe to us for we cast at them the darts of death! Whilst we spoke to them, whilst they embraced us and kissed us, we scattered the poison from our lips. Going back to their homes, they in turn soon infected their whole families, who in three days succumbed, and were buried in one common grave. Priests and doctors visiting the sick returned from their duties ill, and soon were numbered with the dead. O death! cruel, bitter, impious death! which thus breaks the bonds of affection and divides father and mother, brother and sister, son

PLAGUES, PANDEMICS AND VIRUSES

and wife. Lamenting our misery, we feared to fly, yet we dared not remain....

Oh God! See how the heathen Tartar races, pouring together from all sides, suddenly invested the city of Kaffa and besieged the trapped Christians there for almost three years. There, hemmed in by an immense army, they could hardly draw breath, although food could be shipped in, which offered them some hope. But behold, the whole army was affected by a disease which overran the Tartars and killed thousands upon thousands every day. It was as though arrows were raining down from heaven to strike and crush the Tartars' arrogance. All medical advice and attention was useless; the Tartars died as soon as the signs of disease appeared on their bodies: swellings in the armpit or groin caused by coagulating humors, followed by a putrid fever.

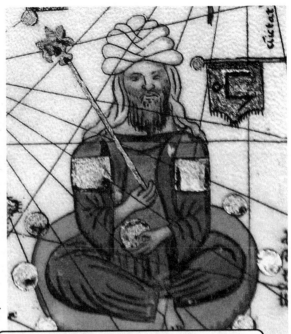

Janibeg (also Jani Beg or Djanibek Khan) was the leader of the Golden Horde, a people who had separated from the Mongols. One story of how the plague came to Europe through Kaffa was that Janiberg's attacking troops catapulted infected corpses into the city.

The dying Tartars, stunned and stupefied by the immensity of the disaster brought about by the disease, and realizing that they had no hope of escape, lost interest in the siege. But they ordered corpses to be placed in catapults and lobbed into the city in the hope that the intolerable stench would kill everyone inside. What seemed like mountains of dead were thrown into the city, and the Christians could not hide or flee or escape from them.... And soon the rotting corpses tainted the air and poisoned the water supply, and the stench was so overwhelming that hardly one in several thousand was in a position to flee the remains of the Tartar army....

THE PLAGUE IN FLORENCE

In 1347, a banker named Giovanni Vilanni happened to be chronicling the history of Florence. His *Nuova Cronica* is a treasure for the amount

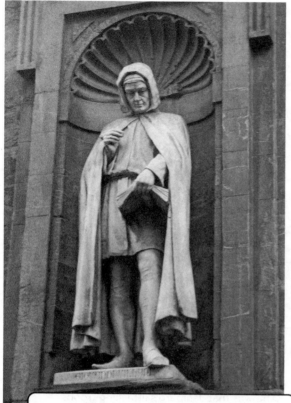

A banker and historical chronicler of Florence, Italy, Giovanni Vilanni recorded the horrors of the Plague of Florence (statue of Vilanni at The Loggia del Mercato Nuovo in Florence).

of detail he gave that other writers would have overlooked: he included the number of banks, bakeries, notaries, and surgeons in Florence and the name of every street, square, bridge, and family.

While the mathematical part of Vilanni's mind hovered over the statistics that made up Florence, the plague is what captured his creative side. In the autumn of 1347, Villani predicted, "This plague was … foretold by the masters in astrology last March…. The sign of Virgo and its master … Mercury … signif[y] death." That winter, earthquakes in Italy and Germany underscored Vilanni's belief that the end was nigh, especially after a "column of fire" glowed over Avignon, France, where the pope held court. Eyewitnesses claimed it was a natural phenomenon produced by "the sun's rays like a rainbow," but Vilanni maintained its appearance "nevertheless [is] a sign of future and great events." By "great," though, Vilanni meant "terrible."

Then, the plague arrived. Vilanni wrote about it as though it were an unwelcome visitor, yet one that couldn't help but admire the beauty of Florence. Stopping to look at "views that resemble paintings" and Florence's "beautiful streets, beautiful hospitals, beautiful palaces and beautiful churches," the plague burst into homes and churches and upon the inhabitants "with the speed of fire racing through a dry or oily substance."

The last line of *Nuova Cronica* says this: "The priest who confessed the sick and those who nursed them so generally caught the infection that the victims were abandoned and deprived confession, sacrament, medicine, and nursing…. And many lands and cities were made desolate. And this plague lasted till _____."

Villani left this part blank so he could fill in the date when it ended, but he died of the plague in 1348. His brother, Mateo, continued the *Cronica* until he, too, died of the plague, but it was finally completed by Mateo's son, Filippo Villani, in 1364.

The fact that the plague brought Florence to its knees was especially poignant because by the fourteenth century, it was arguably the most cosmopolitan, artistic, and influential city on the Italian peninsula. Though one would have thought that title belonged to Rome, the fall of the Roman Empire and, more recently, the pope's move from Rome to Avignon had dimmed Rome's glory. Now, it was Florence that bloomed, a place where works of art were sponsored to beautify the city, and its famed banking industry brought glittering economic prosperity. Florence even got a head start on the Renaissance, thanks to painters like Giotto, writers like Dante, and sponsors like the Medici banking family. Florence also had Orsonmichele, a church featuring a facade adorned with the bronze and stone statues of the saints, carved by sculptors like Donatello.

However, all the beauty, money, and piety in the world couldn't help Italy's wealthiest city. The plague likely entered through Florence's closest port city, Pisa. Once the Florentines realized that the pestilence had begun, city leaders took precautionary measures, like destroying the clothes of the sick and the dead instead of selling them; forcing all prostitutes to leave the city to help cleanse it of sin; and preventing those from Genoa and Pisa from entering.

In June 1348, deaths were occurring at a rate of about 100 per day; by August, it was 400 per day—at least 20 times what was considered normal. By October, the population had been halved from 100,000 to 50,000.

FLORENCE'S BOOK OF THE DEAD

The Grain Office, or *Grascia*, was originally in charge of distributing grain, making sure it got to market, and controlling its price. The *Grascia* later absorbed a judicial office that kept a record of the weekly dead, called the "Book of the Dead" or *Libri di Grascia Morti*. The first book contained the following: the deceased's name, where they lived, cause of death, what parish they were buried in, and the gravedigger who buried them. Depending on who did the recording, a plentiful amount of information could have been recorded or barely a name. The *Grascia Morti* did not take into account those who fled to the countryside to wait out the plague, including city leaders.

However, those who stayed and either avoided or recovered from the plague were often richly rewarded. Members of a guild—which was a type of exclusive union—and those in banking made sure their estates were taken care of. More wills were written than ever before, and this sometimes left the power and money of an entire family consolidated within one family member. The Florentines also had a great spirit of charity, and huge donations were made to help the needy.

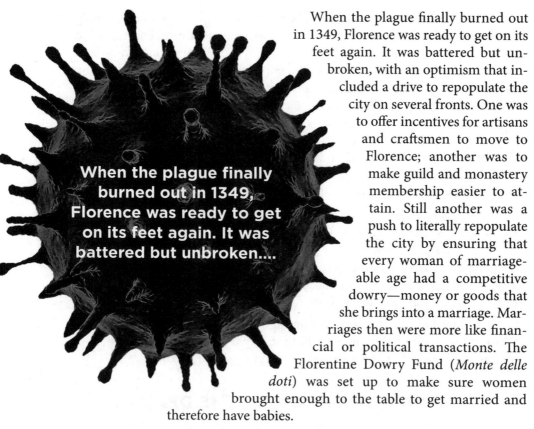

> When the plague finally burned out in 1349, Florence was ready to get on its feet again. It was battered but unbroken....

When the plague finally burned out in 1349, Florence was ready to get on its feet again. It was battered but unbroken, with an optimism that included a drive to repopulate the city on several fronts. One was to offer incentives for artisans and craftsmen to move to Florence; another was to make guild and monastery membership easier to attain. Still another was a push to literally repopulate the city by ensuring that every woman of marriageable age had a competitive dowry—money or goods that she brings into a marriage. Marriages then were more like financial or political transactions. The Florentine Dowry Fund (*Monte delle doti*) was set up to make sure women brought enough to the table to get married and therefore have babies.

From 1363 to the 1420s, Florence endured numerous plague recurrences, and though none of them were anywhere near as destructive as the Black Death (and some may not have actually been the plague), it still hampered Florence's resurgence. It wouldn't be until the late fifteenth century that Florence had returned to its preplague glory days, but the fact that they could do that—sustain that optimism generation after generation, even when the plague itself was a distant memory—is a testament to the inner strength and might of the Florentines.

IS GOD HIDING FROM THE PLAGUE?

After the plague struck Messina in 1347, the Messinese begged the archbishop of Catania—about 60 miles away in Sicily—to let them "borrow" the relics of Catania's martyred St. Agatha in the desperate hope that these relics would protect them from an evil that they had no idea was just beginning. "For we believe," they said, "that with the arrival of the relics, the city of Messina will be completely delivered of this sickness." Not only was the visit fruitless, as the plague raged on through Messina and, indeed, all of Sicily, but even the archbishop died.

This sums up the effect the Church had on the Black Death—which was none—and the effect the Black Death had on the Church—which was enormous. What was essentially the earliest ecclesiastical loss in the war of Church versus Plague would be played out repeatedly over the next several years with devastating results. Even Pope Clement VI was waiting out the plague, sequestered in Avignon, France.

In 1347, the separation of church and state did not yet exist (and "church" was the Catholic Church since Protestantism didn't exist yet, though the plague would be one of several reasons that Protestant thought began). The Church *was* the state. It was the largest landowner in Europe. The pope ruled over all, even kings.

The Church also had a tight grasp on the legal system. Its biblical laws proclaimed who was innocent and who was guilty. In economics, the Church handed over much of banking to the Jewish community not because of any kind of friendly, nondenominational gesture but because the Church believed that loans and their accompanying interest charges went against the Bible. While Jews did not charge interest to other Jews, they considered it permissible to charge interest to non-Jews, so the Church used the Jews as middlemen—loopholes—in order to charge interest on loans.

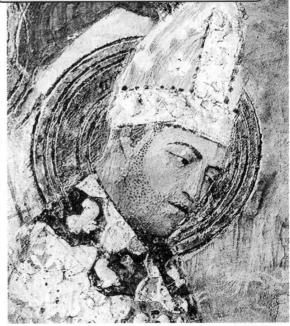

The head of the Catholic Church at the time, Pope Clement VI hid himself in Avignon, France, as he tried to avoid catching the plague.

The Church had its hands in politics, economics, family, the military—the list goes on and on—so when people were dying hideously all over, it was natural that their followers would turn to them for guidance, or even basic comfort, but in the face of such a pandemic, the Church's effectiveness was practically nonexistent.

In fact, to take some of the heat off, Church leaders used this event to remind people that they were sinful and the plague was God's way of punishing them (though they had no explanation for why even the archbishop of Canterbury died of the plague).

Having said all that, the Church wasn't entirely useless. Priests devoted to their calling tended to the sick—so many, in fact, that they presented the Church with a huge problem: they were all dying, too, and many who didn't die abandoned their flock. The Church started to suffer from a shortage of manpower. Whereas before, a life as a monk or priest was only available to the nobility, the Church was now forced to open its doors to anyone. (Any man, that is.) As long as you were alive, you were hired.

This was great for those who were looking for job stability during a plague, but it was not good for the Church or its parishioners. In Winchester, England, nearly 30 men were ordained deacons, promoted to subdeacons, then promoted to priests in just one year instead of the several years it would normally take. They then were sent out to tend to their dying flock with no experience. Add to that the fact that these men joined the clergy because of economic stability, not unshakeable faith, and they were ill-equipped and unschooled as to what it meant to be a priest at a time when people needed spiritual guidance the most.

On an individual level, the response to the plague differed as much as the plague itself. Some did all they could to help the sick. Some did all they could to avoid them. Doctors refused to see patients; priests refused to administer last rites; and shopkeepers closed up shop. Many people fled the cities for the countryside, but even there, they could not escape the disease: it affected cows, sheep, goats, pigs, and chickens as well as people. In fact, the plague killed so many sheep that the Black Death caused a European wool shortage. Scientific studies have suggested that epizootic transmissions—from one animal to another animal—are more likely during cooler summers that follow wet winters, like what happened during the time of the Black Plague.

Y. pestis can still be transmitted to humans from animals in the following ways:

- Flea bites—Plague bacteria are most often transmitted by the bite of an infected flea. Many rodents die, which causes hungry fleas to stop seeking their favorite source of food and look elsewhere. People and animals that visit places where rodents have recently died of the plague are at risk of being infected from flea bites. Dogs and cats may also bring plague-infected fleas into the home. The type of plague most commonly caused by this is bubonic or septicemic.

- Contact with contaminated fluid or tissue—Humans can become infected when handling a plague-infected animal. A hunter skinning a rabbit or other infected animal without using proper precautions could become infected with *Y. pestis*. The type of plague most commonly caused by this is also bubonic or septicemic.

- Infectious droplets—When a person has pneumonic plague, they may cough droplets containing the bacteria into the air. If these droplets are breathed in by another person, they can cause pneumonic plague. Typically, this requires direct and close contact between people. Transmission of these droplets is the only way this plague can spread between people. This type of plague spread has not been documented in the United States since 1924 but still occurs with some frequency in developing countries. Cats are also susceptible to plague and can be infected by eating infected rodents. Sick cats pose a risk of transmitting plague-infected droplets to their owners or to veterinarians. Several cases of human plague have occurred in the United States in recent decades as a result of contact with infected cats.

Not everyone got sick from the plague. The ones who escaped had sequestered themselves as much as possible, with the city of Ragusa (now Dubrovnik in Croatia) even devising the first quarantine. (Today, *quarantine* means "isolation," but the word wasn't coined as such until the 1500s in Venice, where, in the Venetian dialect, *quarantina* means "isolation for 40 days." So, technically, the Ragusans, whose isolation period was 30 days, devised a *trentine*.) Whether you call it quarantine or trentine, these measures, along with strictly patrolled borders, kept the plague at bay, even using spies who sounded the alert when plague had erupted nearby. Ragusa's last plague epidemic was in 1533; in England, it was in 1666; 1733 in the Baltic region; and in the nineteenth century in northern Africa and the Middle East.

Others took a more hedonistic approach, ironically following a biblical phrase from 1 Corinthians: "Eat, drink, and be merry, for tomorrow we shall die." Meaning: we might as well enjoy ourselves now because we won't

Not everyone got sick from the plague. The ones who escaped had sequestered themselves as much as possible, with the city of Ragusa (now Dubrovnik, Croatia) even devising the first quarantine.

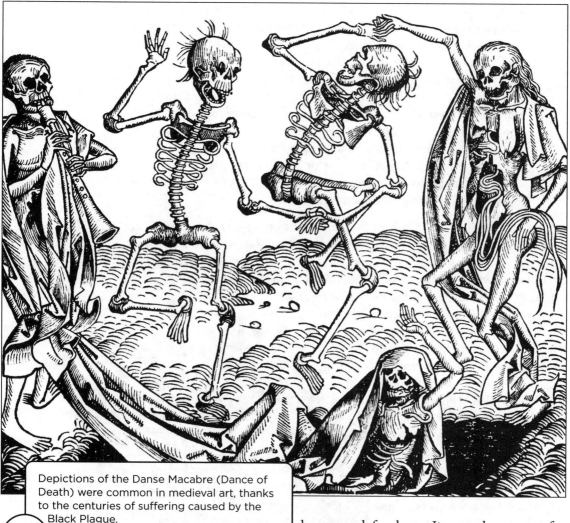

Depictions of the Danse Macabre (Dance of Death) were common in medieval art, thanks to the centuries of suffering caused by the Black Plague.

be around for long. It was also a way for people to avoid facing the sick and dying people all around them, the burial trenches, the smells, the horror, and their own mortality. Perhaps this could be the most enjoyable way to stave off the plague as long as possible. It certainly beat getting bled.

GIOVANNI BOCCACCIO

For the moment, we'll rely on Giovanni Boccaccio to set this scene. Boccaccio was born in 1313 either in Certaldo, a small Tuscan village in Italy, or in Florence. Boccaccio's father was a merchant. Little is known about his mother. Boccaccio was probably born out of wedlock.

Like many families, when it came time for Boccaccio to decide on an occupation, he was expected to follow in his father's footsteps. He was sent to Naples to become a merchant. Boccaccio found this not to his liking. A stint as a banker produced the same result. From an early age, though, Boccaccio had a profound interest in literary pursuits. Away from his father, Boccaccio indulged in his literary passion, which his father most likely found to be foolish since few could make a living solely as a writer.

In 1340, Boccaccio's father brought his son back to Florence. Eight years later, the Black Death arrived. It is not clear whether Boccaccio left his hometown to escape the contagion or witnessed the devastation firsthand. What is known is that, by moving from city to city looking to indeed make a living as a writer, Boccaccio was unintentionally one step ahead of the disease—unlike his father, who died of it.

Of the horror that accompanied the sheer number of dead that was all around him, Boccaccio wrote:

> It was by no means rare for more than one of these [funeral boards] to be seen with two or three bodies upon it at a time. Many were seen to contain a husband and wife, two or three brothers and sisters, a father and son, and times without number it happened that two priests would be on their way to bury someone, only to find bearers carrying three or four additional biers would fall in behind them.

> Such was the multitude of corpses that there was not sufficient consecrated ground for them to be buried in, so when all the graves were full, huge trenches were excavated in the churchyards, into which new arrivals were placed in their hundreds, stowed tier upon tier like ships' cargo, each layer of corpses being covered over with a thin layer of soil till the trench was filled to the top.

Boccaccio began his seminal work, *The Decameron*, in around 1348. The setting? "Many dropped dead in the open streets by day and night, … whilst a great many others, though dying in their own houses, drew their neighbors' attention to the fact more by the smell of their rotting corpses than by any other means. And what with these, and the others who were dying all over the city, bodies were here, there and everywhere." Quite a different view from Villani's Florence.

The Decameron begins with a funeral, after which Pampea, a friend of the narrator, proclaims brightly, "Here we linger for no purpose … [other] than to count the number of corpses being taken to burial…. If this be so (and we plainly perceive that it is), what are we doing here? … We could go and stay together in one of our various country estates…. There we shall hear birds singing … see fresh green hills and plains, fields of corn undulating like the sea."

With that, the narrator invites his band of seven women and three men to the countryside to escape the misery of a hot plague in the city. Surrounded by idyllic seclusion, each participant is tasked with recounting a tale to entertain the group. A story is told each night, except for one day per week for chores and the holy days, during which they do no work at all, resulting in ten nights of storytelling over the course of two weeks. Thus, by the end, they've told 100 stories (even though the word *decameron* is Greek for "ten stories.")

The Decameron is structured as a "frame story," meaning the plague frames the story and is the reason for these ten people to tell their stories. Each daily collection of stories takes a different tone or theme:

Day 1: Witty discussion of human vices

Day 2: Fortune triumphs over its human playthings, but it is trounced by human will

Day 3: People who have attained difficult goals or who have recovered something previously suffered

Day 4: Tragic love stories

Day 5: Happy endings to love that do not at first run smoothly

Day 6: Wit and gaiety

Days 7, 8, and 9: Trickery, deceit, and often bawdy license run free

Day 10: Earlier themes are brought to a high pitch; the widely borrowed story "The Patient Griselda" closes the cycle of tales

All of these stories are rooted in previously told tales, reaching as far away as Persia and India and from *1001 Arabian Nights*. The fact that Boccaccio could write *The Decameron* at a time when people were dying all around him shows a kind of optimism, as though if he continues to write, he will not die, and this plague will one day end.

In his conclusion, Boccaccio says that he wrote the book for "idle ladies," whom he believed needed to have something to pass the time while the men were out working and perhaps also something to take their mind off of what was going on all around them, to escape into their own kind of idyll.

The final chapter, called "The Author's Conclusion," is where Boccaccio admits that he might not have a popular view of the Church. "Since the sermons preached by the friars nowadays in order to rebuke men for their sins are, for the most part, filled with clever quips and jests and gibes, I concluded that such things would not be out of place in my stories." He continues: "And who can doubt that there are still others who will say I have an evil and venomous tongue because in certain places I have told the truth about friars? ... There is no question but that they are moved by the best of motives, seeing how friars are good men who flee hardship for the love of God, do their grinding when the millpond is full, and never blab about it afterward." As if to excuse what he'd just written, Boccaccio ends by informing the reader, "I was told by one of the women next door that I had the best and sweetest tongue in the world."

If Boccaccio leaves us with one lesson, it's that not everyone believes that Church teachings make sense. A new god had arrived in town, and he didn't play by the rules—rules that had been in place as long as anyone could remember. The good deserved to be saved. The evil deserved their death. Now, being good or evil no longer mattered. No one "deserved" to live or die: the plague killed indiscriminately. A woman praying for hours could succumb to the plague while God saved her neighbor who stole from the dead. These random acts occurred before the plague, but it shined a light on the inequities as never before.

A page from Boccaccio's *The Decameron,* a tale about ten people taking shelter from the Black Plague and telling each other stories to pass the time. It is one example of great literature inspired by a time of great tragedy and suffering.

Before the plague, "it was the custom ... for the women, relatives, and neighbors to gather together in the house of a dying person, the last rites were given and prayers were said to help the dying into heaven." Once the plague infected a person, "certain swellings, either on the groin or under the armpits, whereof some waxed of the bigness of a common apple, others like unto an egg, some more and some less, and these the vulgar named plague-boils." (Boccaccio's "vulgar named plague-boils" are now known as "buboes"—hence the name "bubonic plague.")

Without these deathbed traditions, it was believed that the dying could end up in purgatory for an extended stay or find themselves in hell for eternity.

PLAGUES, PANDEMICS AND VIRUSES

"THE RATTLE BAG"

Welsh poet Daffyd ap Gwilym summed up the dualities of sex and death in his poem "Y Rhugl Groen" or "The Rattle Bag" (translated by Joseph P. Clancy). An excerpt here shows how a couple who had just made love, and could potentially procreate, are separated after the woman flees in terror from the plague, embodied as an "imp in shepherd's shape."

And so we were, she was shy,
Learning to love each other,
Concealing sin, winning mead,
An hour lying together,
And then, cold comfort, it came,
A blare, a bloody nuisance,
A sack's bottom's foul seething
From an imp in shepherd's shape,
Who had, public enemy,
A harsh-horned sag-cheeked rattle.
He played, cramped yellow belly,
This bag, curse its scabby leg.
So before satisfaction
The sweet girl panicked: poor me!
When she heard, feeble-hearted,
The stones whir, she would not stay.

"Fear of contagion, kept people away from the dying leaving plague victims to die alone with the knowledge that they were doom in the afterlife."

ENGLAND DURING THE PLAGUE

In 1300, the population of England was about five million but may have been as many as six million people. Their economy was largely based on agricultural production, but trade was growing more and more essential. Producers of both food and other commodities were beginning to diversify or specialize, selling for the greater market and not just for personal and local use. English wool (still available, though the aforementioned shortages did occur) and cloth were major exports.

The English first heard of the Black Death in 1346 through rumors of deaths in the East. Two years later, in June 1348, the Black Death arrived in coastal English towns and reached London in early 1349. Within eight months, about two million of England's five million-plus inhabitants were dead. Despite the very high loss of life, few villages were outright abandoned, and medieval authorities did their best to respond in a timely manner—they'd already known the plague was coming, so they had some time to prepare—yet the economic costs were still astronomical. Work such as construction and mining stopped, though authorities attempted to move ahead with pre-epidemic working conditions. However, the previous years of cold and famine only compounded the economic, social, and spiritual unraveling. In contrast to the earlier times of rapid growth, the English population would not begin to recover for more than a century, and the crisis would dramatically upend the English economy for good, though, in many ways, eventually for the public good.

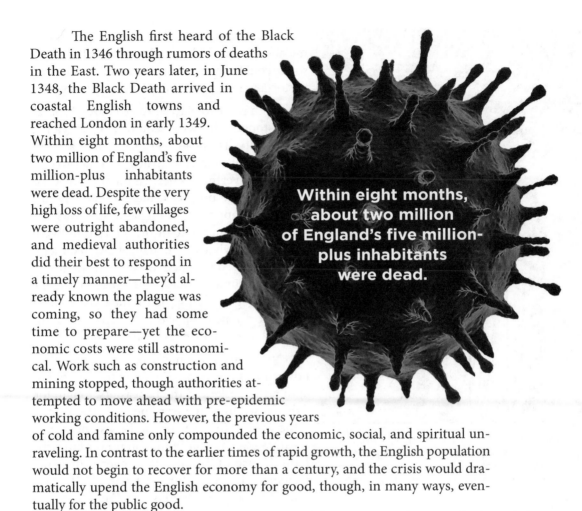

Within eight months, about two million of England's five million-plus inhabitants were dead.

THE DEATH OF A PRINCESS

If the deaths of clergymen revealed that the Black Death could strike anyone, the death of Princess Joan confirmed this. Princess Joan was the daughter of Edward III, the king of England and the leader of the Plantagenet dynasty. The princess was on her way to marry Prince Pedro, heir to the kingdom of Castile. With the marriage, the Plantagenet line would extend from England to Spain. Thanks to a heavily armed retinue, she was, perhaps, the most protected woman of Europe at the time, and it is said that her dowry alone took up an entire ship.

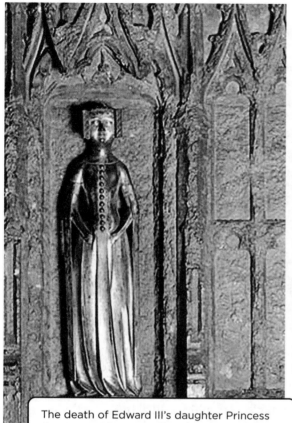

The death of Edward III's daughter Princess Joan was a clear case that the plague did not spare royalty over the commoners. She was only fourteen when the Black Plague ended her life.

Joan was escorted by over a hundred formidable English soldiers and had a portable chapel so she could attend Catholic mass without having to stop and use local churches along the way.

En route to marry Prince Pedro, Princess Joan stopped in what could've been called Plague City: Bordeaux, France. The mayor of Bordeaux, although awestruck at the approaching fleet, nevertheless begged them to leave, so severe was the outbreak, but the Black Death had not yet appeared in England, so it was unlikely that Princess Joan or her retinue were aware of just what kind of danger awaited them, so the party decamped to a castle in town. Within a couple of weeks, members of the entourage began dying. Joan may have been moved to a smaller village, but the plague found her, and in 1348, Princess Joan was dead.

The marriage never occurred, and after Edward III's death in 1377, two branches of the family, the Yorks and the Lancasters, fought for the crown in a civil war known as the War of the Roses. The War of the Roses ended not with a Plantagenet branch in power but with the House of Tudor taking over, which included Henry Tudor, or Henry VIII, who would change England from a Catholic country to a Protestant one in 1532—repercussions no one could have predicted when Princess Joan set sail from Portsmouth.

GEOFFREY CHAUCER

Geoffrey Chaucer was fortunate to escape infection during the Black Death. He was only a child when the plague hit London, and it must have left a definite mark on his childhood, long before he became the "Father of English Literature."

The Chaucer family inherited wealth from relatives who had died in the plague, which struck England five times during Chaucer's lifetime. He first observed the Black Death "in 1348, when he was between five and eight years old.

PLAGUES, PANDEMICS AND VIRUSES

The putrid smell of the thousands of rotting and burning bodies permeated London, and just beyond Chaucer's window, people collapsed on the street," according to Jerry Ellis in his *Walking to Canterbury*. Chaucer used the experience to write about an England where people sought absolution for their sins and the unburdening of their psyches through telling tales.

Geoffrey Chaucer's most famous work is *The Canterbury Tales*. Written between 1387 and 1400, it's similar in form to Boccaccio's *The Decameron*—though instead of the setting being an Italian countryside idyll away from the plague, the characters are English pilgrims who comprise a wide spectrum of occupations and social ranks. This gives their tales a wide variety of voices, dialects, and subjects and reveals their wants and values.

At the Tabard Inn near London, the narrator joins a company of 29 people, who are all traveling to the shrine of martyred Saint Thomas Becket, about 60 miles away in Canterbury. They include a Knight, Squire, Yeoman, Prioress, Monk, Friar, Merchant, Clerk, Man of Law, Franklin, Haberdasher, Carpenter, Weaver, Dyer, Tapestry-Weaver, Cook, Shipman, Physician, Wife, Parson, Plowman, Miller, Manciple, Reeve, Summoner, Pardoner, and Host, who owns the Tabard Inn. The Host suggests that the group ride together and entertain one another with stories. Each pilgrim will tell two stories on the way to Canterbury and two on the way back, and whomever he judges to be the best storyteller will get a free meal at Bailey's tavern.

The Canterbury Tales is the only work of Chaucer's that makes direct reference to the plague, as in "The Pardoner's Tale" and "The Physician's Tale," a portrait of those who would profit during a plague.

Chaucer's Physician in *The Canterbury Tales* is also a plague profiteer: "He kepte that he wan [earned] in pestilence." The Physician cashes in by implying that he has a cure. Also mentioned are the three young drunks in Chaucer's "The Pardoner's Tale," who are so intoxicated that they fail to notice that one of their friends has died of the plague.

The Pardoner's Tale

In medieval times, a pardoner was like a salesman on behalf of the Church. He roamed the countryside offering bishop-endorsed "pardons," or official forgivenesses of sins—for a price. At a time when people had been surrounded by death after death for years, the idea of a pardon in exchange for an eternity in heaven seemed like a pretty great bargain.

Except that it was bogus; no pardons were to be had. As per Catholic dogma, one didn't need pardons if one went to confession. A pardoner wasn't there to save souls; he was there for profit, one of the reasons why the medieval Church as a whole was criticized for caring more about the material world than the spiritual. A pardoner used people's faith and fear to manipulate them and couldn't care less about their spiritual welfare.

Despite that, Chaucer also describes how impressively the Pardoner performs in church, motivated by the fact that such influence will stuff his pockets (perhaps giving rise to the early twentieth-century "medicine shows" of evangelical preachers today).

It's ironic, then, that of all people, "The Pardoner's Tale" should have a *Twilight Zone* comeuppance moral. The Pardoner doesn't care that he's bilking people out of what little they have—in his preaching, he's turning them away from sin. So, who cares if he makes money along the way?

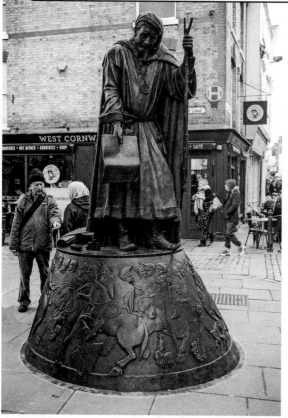

This statue of Geoffrey Chaucer was recently erected in the town of Canterbury, England, which was made famous by the author's book.

In the story, four young men from Flanders are taking on every vice they can at an inn—ones that the Pardoner calls "tavern sins." Not until they hear the death toll of a bell do they realize that one of the members of their party has died of the plague. So, the remaining three, in an alcohol-fueled rage, decide to find Death and kill him.

While on the drunken hunt, they come across an old man, who says they can find Death at the foot of an oak tree. Upon arriving, they find a pile of gold coins and forget about Death. They decide to sleep off the booze at the oak tree and take the coins in the morning. They draw straws to see who should buy some wine and food while the other two sleep. The youngest draws the shortest straw and leaves. While he's away, the other two plan to stab him when he returns. However, the youngest buys wine, which he laces with rat poison in order to kill his cohorts so he can take the gold. When he returns, the two kill him and then drink the poisoned wine, proceeding to die slow and painful deaths.

After he finishes his tale, the Pardoner—who can't help himself—asks for gold and silver from the pilgrims so that they may be pardoned for their sins. The Host tells him that he would sooner cut off the Pardoner's testicles than kiss his relics.

The Old Man in "The Pardoner's Tale" is alternately thought to symbolize Death; Death's messenger; just an old man; or the "Wandering Jew," who is a symbol of Death that will supposedly roam Earth until Jesus returns.

THE JEWISH PERSECUTION

The population also believed that God had the ability to heal and the ability to sicken. Therefore, many reasoned, the plague was God's punishment for people's wickedness. Just as He had sent a flood in the time of Noah, He was now getting rid of the sinful once again.

The Jewish population, the scapegoat for many of the world's ills, did not avoid persecution during the Black Death even though they themselves were dying alongside Christians in some parts, yet concurrently surviving because they were kept apart in ghettoes.

Also, Jewish law stated that people had to wash their hands several times throughout the day, particularly before eating or leaving the bathroom, and at least once a week, a Jew bathed for the Sabbath. These sanitary conditions among the Jewish populations were, for the time, far superior to those in non-Jewish European populations.

Ironic, then, that one of the most popular theories held by Christians during the plague was that Jews were poisoning Christian wells and that Jews were therefore spared from the disease because they lived separate from their Christian neighbors. Many Jews admitted to this under torture.

On July 6, 1348, none other than Pope Clement VI issued the first of two bulls, or edicts, telling Christians not to blame the Jews for the plague. Noting that Jews were also plague victims, Clement announced that people who cast blame on the Jews "had been seduced by that liar, the devil." Clement said that if a plausible reason to hold Jews responsible existed, "we would wish them struck by a penalty of suitable severity." However, no proof existed even though "these same Jews are prepared to submit to judgment before a competent judge." The pope then threatened anyone who harmed a Jew with excommunication.

The pope's edicts had little success and, although the situation varied from town to town and region to region, Clement's efforts were finally undermined by the newly elected Holy Roman Emperor Charles IV, who made the property of those Jews killed in riots up for grabs, giving many "Christians" a

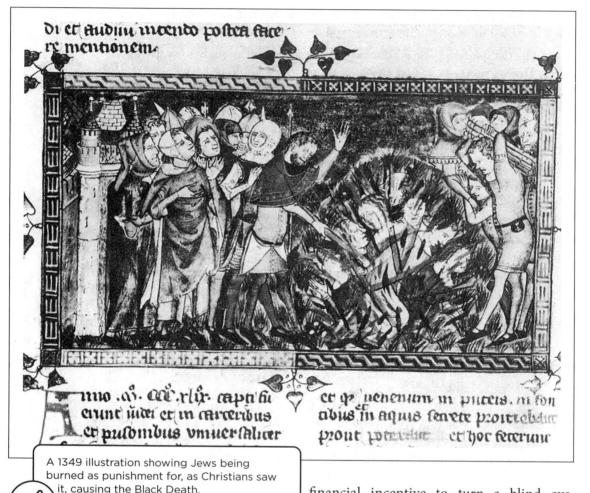

A 1349 illustration showing Jews being burned as punishment for, as Christians saw it, causing the Black Death.

financial incentive to turn a blind eye. Another financial incentive was that many were indebted to Jews for various loans.

So, with fear—economic, religious, and moral—as a powerful motivator, once rumors began that Jews were using the plague to kill Christians, Jews were themselves killed by Christians. In January 1349, the entire Jewish population of Basel, Switzerland—at least 600 people—were forced into a building on an island on the Rhine and burned to death. More than 60 large and 150 small Jewish communities were destroyed in pogroms stirred by these accusations.

From 1349 until about 1390, the Jewish communities of France, Germany, and England almost disappeared completely. In 1350, Frankfurt had over 19,000 Jews. By 1400, fewer than 10 Jews were left. This was typical of several other Jewish communities throughout Western Europe. Many who survived both the plague and persecution fled to today's Poland and Russia, and yet, the plague persisted.

WHO IS DEATH?

As humans, we need a way to create Death as someone we can understand. Not befriend, definitely not enjoy, but at least grasp psychologically. Death is usually personified as a man—although certain cultures do have Death portrayed as a female (i.e., Marzanna in Slavic mythology, Dhumavati in Indian mythology, and La Catrina in Mexico).

In Islam, the archangel Azrael is the *Malak al-Maut*, or "angel of death." He can pull the souls out of bodies and guide them to the afterlife. His appearance depends on how a person lived their life—if it was good, they see a beautiful being, and if it was bad, they see a horrific monster.

In Hebrew scriptures, Death—*Maweth*—is sometimes personified as a devil or angel of death. The *memitim* are angels who decide whether one lives or dies. The name comes from the Hebrew word meaning "executioners."

In Gaelic lore, a female spirit known as a *bean sí* or "banshee" (Irish for "fairy woman") proclaims the death of a person by a kind of beastly shrieking. She can appear in a variety of forms but is typically shown as a white-haired, frightful hag. When several banshees appear at once, it was said to indicate the death of someone great or holy.

The Day of the Dead is a Mexican holiday whose popularity has exploded in both Mexico and the United States, becoming a tradition in both religion and fashion. The holiday involves family and friends gathering to pray for and remember friends and family members who have died and support their spiritual journey. Mexicans see it as a day of celebration because their loved ones arise and celebrate with them. Prior to Spanish colonization, the Day of the Dead occurred at the beginning of the summer. Now, it's associated with October 31,

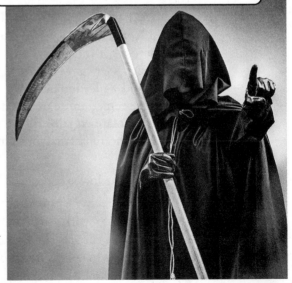

A popular depiction of death is that of the Grim Reaper, a cloaked and hooded figure who carries a scythe representing the harvesting of souls. Anthropomorphizing the concept of death is seen in many world cultures.

November 1, and November 2, or All Saint's Eve/Halloween, All Saint's Day, and All Soul's Day.

In Europe and North America, the idea of the Grim Reaper has become intertwined with Christianity, though no Grim Reaper is mentioned in the Bible. (However, Death is one of the Four Horsemen of the Apocalypse from the Book of Revelation [Revelation 6:7–8].) The Grim Reaper gradually became "Christianized" during the Middle Ages even though its signature features—robe, scythe, and skeleton—came about from folklore. In Norse mythology during the Black Plague, Death was an old woman known as *Pesta*, meaning "plague hag," who wore a black hood. She would go into a town carrying either a rake or a broom. If she brought the rake, some people would survive the plague; if she brought the broom, everyone would die.

The Grim Reaper's look was also largely influenced by the *Danse Macabre* or "Dance of Death." A *danse macabre* painting often showed a group holding hands—alternating the living with the dead—and dancing in a circle. Death is often the leader, or just a chain of alternating dead and live dancers is shown. From the highest ranks of the medieval hierarchy, like the pope, to the lowest, like a beggar, each mortal's hand is held by a skeleton or decayed body.

Scandinavians later adopted the Grim Reaper with the characteristic scythe and black robe. Swedish director Ingmar Bergman's 1957 film *The Seventh Seal* features one of the world's most famous personifications of death chess—here, literally a game of life or death—with a knight who has just returned from the Crusades in time for the plague.

The famous *Totentanz* (literally, "Dance of the Dead") by Estonian artist Bernt Notke was a tapestry that measured 6 feet, 6 inches high and at least 85 feet across. (It was finished in 1466 but destroyed during the Allied bombing of Lübeck, Germany, in World War II.) *Totentanz* showed the dead dancers as lively and agile, looking like they were really dancing, whereas the living dancers seemed more on the dead side, but in most of these paintings, Death is the ultimate equalizer, so a sociocritical element is inherent to the whole genre. In the *Totentanz*, for example, the pope is being led into hell by the dancing Death.

At the lower end of the *Totentanz*, Death calls a peasant to dance, who answers:

I had to work very much and very hard
The sweat was running down my skin
I'd like to escape death nonetheless
But here I won't have any luck

PLAGUES, PANDEMICS AND VIRUSES

The possibility of sudden and painful death increased the religious desire for absolution, but it also evoked a need for gallows humor wherever possible. The *danse macabre* combines both.

THE FLAGELLANTS

The other extremists were the Flagellants. This group believed that the plague was God's punishment for mankind's sinful nature. Far from embracing 1 Corinthians, the Flagellants whipped themselves—repeatedly—with a rope, or "scourge," that had three tails, each embedded with nails. Even the Catholic Church thought they were insane (and no priest was about to start whipping himself with a rope full of nails).

This act was known as the "mortification of the flesh." Today, we think of "mortifi-

A 1349 illustration of Flagellants in Tournai, Belgium. Flagellants whipped themselves until they bled in an effort to gain God's forgiveness for humanity's evils. This, in turn, would hopefully stop God punishing people with the plague.

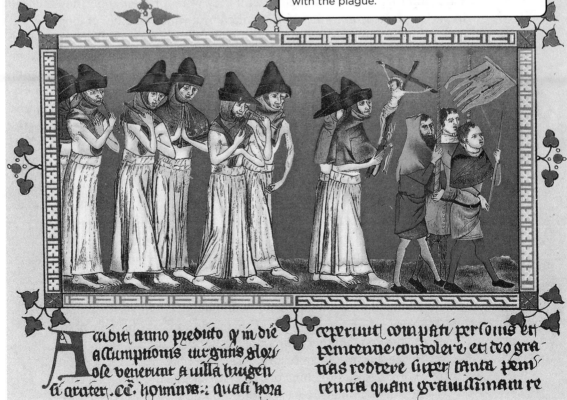

cation" (or, more commonly, the verb "mortified") to describe extreme embarrassment, but here its root stems from *morte* (Latin for "death"), as in metaphorically putting to death the sins of the flesh (rather than metaphorically dying from embarrassment). It stems from Colossians 3:5 in the New Testament (New King James Version): "Therefore put to death your members which are on the earth: fornication, uncleanness, passion, evil desire, and covetousness, which is idolatry." However, the Flagellants followed a more literal interpretation: killing off their flesh.

The Flagellants were first noted in 1259 in Perugia, Italy, after a famine had spread through Europe. Spreading north, sightings occurred in Germany in 1296, and in 1333, a Dominican friar named Venturino of Bergamo tried to revive the movement, gaining momentum and leading roughly 10,000 men into Rome, where they were promptly laughed at and soon dispersed (perhaps because they were mortified). Then came the Black Death, and the Flagellants returned.

Like many zealots, the Flagellants used fear to attract followers. Processions of barefoot, half-naked men marched through the streets, whipping themselves to prove to God how remorseful they were for their sins. They traveled in packs—some wore white robes covered by a white "mantle" or cloak, which gave them the name "doves," and others had a white robe and mantle along with a red cross, symbolizing that they were the Brotherhood of Christ—but when they marched and flagellated, they were bare from the waist up, all whipping themselves into a frenzy. With extraordinary suddenness, the companies of Flagellants appeared again, rapidly spread across the Alps and into Hungary and Switzerland and, by 1349, had crossed into the Netherlands, Bohemia (the Czech Republic), Denmark, and Poland.

The Flagellants gained little traction during the Black Death in one country: England. Robert of Avesbury, a historian who lived in England during this time, described their visit:

> They came to London from Flanders, mostly of Zeeland and Holland origin. Sometimes at St. Paul's [Cathedral] and sometimes at other points in the city they made two daily public appearances wearing cloths from the thighs to the ankles, but otherwise stripped bare.... They marched naked in a file one behind the other and whipped themselves with these scourges on their naked and bleeding bodies. Four of them would chant in their native tongue and, another four would chant in response like a litany. Thrice they would all cast themselves on the ground in this sort of procession, stretching out their hands like the arms of a cross. The singing would go on and, the one who was in the rear of those

PLAGUES, PANDEMICS AND VIRUSES

thus prostrate acting first, each of them in turn would step over the others and give one stroke with his scourge to the man lying under him.

The songs they were singing were known as *Geisslerlieder*, or "Flagellant Songs." The music was simple and unaccompanied because no musical instruments were allowed. They were often sung as call-and-response, where a leader would sing one part followed by the rest singing in unison. (Some of the Flagellant songs survived into the seventeenth century as folk songs in Catholic parts of Central Europe.)

Unlike the Germanic and Slavic people, the English men and women watched the Flagellants as if watching a parade of lunatics; to them, it was more a show than a religious movement one would be compelled to join, but for those who did want to become a Flagellant, they would march for 33.5 days—marking the same number of years that Christ lived. Twice a day, groups numbering anywhere from 100 to close to 1,000 would stop in a field or town—anywhere with an audience—and start with their master reading a letter; this letter was supposedly brought to him by an angel. With medieval fire and brimstone, the master would reveal that Christ was angry at mankind's sinfulness and, in his fury, could possibly destroy the world, but, due to the intervention of the Blessed Virgin, Christ proclaimed that all who joined the Brotherhood for 33.5 days would be saved. Next, the Flagellants would fall to their knees and whip themselves, doing so rhythmically to songs from the *Geisserlieder* while they were bleeding. Sometimes, the blood was soaked up in rags and treated by spectators as a holy relic.

When the Black Death ended, so did the Flagellants for a short time. Like the plague, they would recur and then disappear, both disbursing and facing wrath in the name of God.

Originally, members could only join if they could show that they were able to pay for their own food. However, the movement evolved such that some towns began to notice that sometimes, Flagellants seemed to be bringing the plague with them into towns where it had not yet surfaced. Other troops threatened townspeople if they were not fed. Therefore, later, many were denied entry.

When the Black Death ended, so did the Flagellants for a short time. Like the plague, they would recur and then disappear, both disbursing and facing wrath in the name of God. Some Flagellants were burned at the stake during the Spanish Inquisition of the Late Middle Ages. Processions of hooded Flagellants are still seen today, usually in Catholic countries like Spain, Italy, and the Philippines, where some take it to the extreme of crucifying themselves.

THE END?

All the citizens did little else except to carry dead bodies to be buried.... At every church they dug deep pits down to the watertable; and thus those who were poor who died during the night were bundled up quickly and thrown into the pit. In the morning when a large number of bodies were found in the pit, they took some earth and shoveled it down on top of them; and later others were placed on top of them and then another layer of earth, just as one makes lasagna with layers of pasta and cheese.

—Marchionne di Coppo Stefani

Researchers can only make rough estimates of the total number of deaths from the plague, though it usually ranges anywhere from 75 to 200 million people. A combination of quarantining and the plague burning through everyone it could possibly infect led to its end, after five horrifying years, in 1351. Europe suffered mightily, though deaths were not equally disbursed across the continent. Most of Poland and parts of Hungary, Belgium, and Spain were hardly affected. It was thought that these groups may have had some kind of built-in immunity, though these same groups would endure the pain of the next outbreak between 1360 and 1363 (known as the "little mortality") as well as later ones. Meanwhile, Florence's population went from 120,000 in 1338 to 50,000 in 1351; England may have lost more than 70 per-

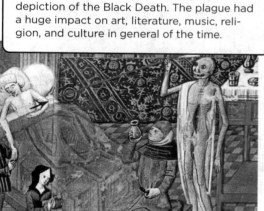

A painting by an unknown Italian artist from the fifteenth century offers yet another depiction of the Black Death. The plague had a huge impact on art, literature, music, religion, and culture in general of the time.

cent of its population, which reportedly declined from seven million before the
plague to two million by 1400.

All social classes were affected, from King Alfonso XI of
Castile to his would-be daughter-in-law, Joan of England,
to the unnamed poorer
classes, but as is the case
here and in subsequent
pandemics and infections,
pathogens may be equal-
opportunity invaders, but
they have more opportunity
among the lower social
classes. During the time of the
Black Death, the latter, living
together in relative squalor, were
the most vulnerable.

After the last of the bodies were buried, those who remained were left with a much different world.

So, what happens when a plague
ends? The answer is that life goes on. What
else is to be done? Mouths still need to be fed,
land to be tilled, markets to be tended. After the last of
the bodies were buried, those who remained were left with a much different world.

However, the number of casualties the Black Death left in its wake resulted in a surprising benefit: an economic boom. Whereas famine, low wages,
and a surplus of workers were the norm before the plague, after the plague, the
few remaining shoemakers, blacksmiths, and the like could demand higher
wages and pay less rent for the land they worked. However, fewer people also
meant less demand for food, so farming itself became less profitable. A mass
migration into towns and villages began with men taking jobs in cloth- or brick-
making. Others became traders or servants. Family farms were abandoned.
Landowners changed their business plans, too—they embraced a new way of
life called capitalism.

WHAT WE GAINED AND WHAT WE LOST

A luck of the draw in genetics helps certain people inherently fight infection better than others. Therefore, people with these genetic gifts

are more likely to live longer and therefore reproduce, giving birth to children who also have strong genes. This is called positive selection, where favored genes survive over time while inferior genes die out. This doesn't mean that we all should be immune to every illness out there, but survivors and their descendants are more likely to survive. In this case, they may have a cluster of three immune-system genes that code proteins that latch on to harmful bacteria, triggering a defensive response. People who lived in places where the Black Death didn't hit—like the Americas—lacked these toll-like receptor genes.

An analysis of bones in London cemeteries from before and after the plague revealed that in the centuries before the Black Death, about 10 percent of the population lived past age 70, said study researcher Dr. Sharon DeWitte, a biological anthropologist at the University of South Carolina. In the centuries after, more than 20 percent of people lived past that age.

The Black Death also transformed the idea of a hospital as a charity home to a place where sick people can go to get better. Simultaneously, important changes occurred in medical practice. The failure of traditional medicine to stop or slow the spread of the plague was analyzed and discussed, and new ideas were put forward. Medicine ceased to be theoretical and became more observational and practical. Studies in anatomy and surgery became part of medical programs in universities. Once being akin to philosophy, medicine evolved into a physical science. With professional doctors becoming more central to a hospital's operations, medical services were specialized, and hospitals or wards specializing in different types of illnesses arose.

Literacy made a tremendous jump after the plague, and among those seeking higher education, the fear of long journeys and being exposed to the plague provided a reason for local universities. The number of universities markedly increased after the plague. Many professors who spoke Latin had died, so those teachers who were fluent in Latin were brought into these new universities. Consequently, the lower-school vacancies were filled up by teachers who had little or no working knowledge of Latin. Instead, they used their local dialects, and the years after the Black Death saw greater use of colloquial speech. Boccaccio, for instance, wrote *The Decameron* in his native Florentine.

The former Third Estate, which had moved up the ranks, also did not know Latin. In 1362, English was declared the official language of the courts, and by 1385, Latin was all but dead after English was made the language of education. When the British Empire took over much of the world, English came with it, and it is now the *lingua franca* of modern society.

Women during and after the Black Death also benefited from the growing importance of writing and fostering the writings of others. In France, Christine de Pisan (1364–1430) became the first European woman to support herself solely by writing.

Of arguably the most importance, feudalism died. The system that burdened peasants with lifetime obligations to their lords was literally turned upside down by the Black Death. So many peasants died during the plague that fields lay abandoned. Lords became desperate for workers. Taking advantage of the scarcity of people, the survivors demanded higher wages—in cash—and fairer treatment. It was like the origins of a labor union since, for the first time, *they* dictated the conditions for their labor. As one nobleman put it, "Servants are now masters, and masters are servants."

In the years after the Black Death, the king and the nobility passed laws that tried to bring back the preplague status quo. (Collective bargaining would be a long way off.) In 1351, the Statute of Laborers was enforced in England, seeking to "prevent laborers from

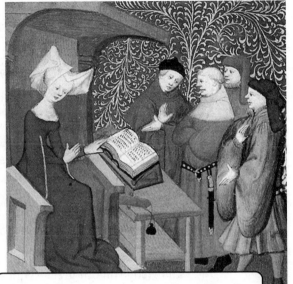

Poet and author Christine de Pisan (aka Christina da Pizzano) worked in the court of King Charles VI of France and was the first woman in Europe to support herself through her writing.

obtaining higher wages," but even the king lacked the power to undo the dramatic changes to the architecture of medieval society. The new freedom of what had been the Third Estate created more job opportunities and more social mobility. The former serfs were now working for themselves, not for their lord. Here was the faint glimmer of the individualism so treasured in our modern Western society.

This individualism gave these former peasants a look at new horizons beyond their tracts of land. Some moved into cities to learn trades. The more successful ones became the new middle class. Cities became popular again as the economy, now firmly on a cash basis, took off. Competition among individual manufacturers slowly replaced the guilds, which had dictated rules of production and the cost of goods. The middle class also used their wealth to become patrons of the arts, science, literature, and philosophy. The result was an explosion of cultural and intellectual creativity that we now call the Renaissance.

The Catholic faith ruled all aspects of medieval life from womb to tomb, but the stranglehold the Catholic Church exercised over people's lives and ways of thinking was broken by the Black Death. With the clergy dying alongside the common folk and with no answers as to why, the Church revealed its lack of

THE PLAGUE CONTINUES

Today, plague still occurs in Central and Far East Asia, Africa, and the Americas. About 2,000 cases have been reported annually in the world for many years. (None of these are epidemics or pandemics, which is why you haven't heard of them.) Most cases occur in rural sub-Saharan Africa and on the island of Madagascar. Usually, about 400 cases of plague occur every year in Madagascar—typically the bubonic type and confined mainly to rural areas. A 2017 plague epidemic that was mostly bubonic started early in the plague season, which normally runs from September through April, which is their hot and rainy season, and led to 2,575 plague cases and 221 deaths.

knowledge on our greatest questions in the face of catastrophe and thereby lost credibility as God's mouthpiece. Many people lost faith or turned to other paths of spirituality. Dogma was increasingly questioned, and people began to think for themselves. This would be the start of the Protestant Reformation.

The fourteenth-century plague was the worst the world had ever seen in terms of loss of life over a given time span, and for centuries, the epidemic, to one degree or another, returned to visit different areas every couple of years or so.

THE PLAGUES OF LONDON

The plague doctor "look" that many are familiar with didn't exist during the Black Death. Prior to the seventeenth century, plague doctors wore protective suits, but it wasn't until 1619 that a uniform was designed, ostensibly to add a barrier between doctor and patient. The man attributed with the invention of this "plague suit" was named Charles de l'Orme, physician to the royal House of Medici and chief physician to three French kings: Henri IV, Louis XIII, and Louis XIV.

> The nose [is] half a foot long, shaped like a beak, filled with perfume with only two holes, one on each side near the nostrils, but that can suffice to breathe and carry along with the air one breathes the impression of the [herbs] enclosed further along in the beak. Under the coat we wear boots made in [goat] leather from the front of the breeches in smooth skin that are attached to said boots, and a short sleeved blouse in smooth skin, the bottom of which is tucked into the breeches. The hat and gloves are also made of the same skin … with spectacles over the eyes.
>
> —Charles de l'Orme

The hat served both form and function. It indicated that the man was a doctor, and it also kept him further covered from the disease. The robe was treated with wax so that no bodily fluids, like pus or blood, could soak into it. The nose (aka "beak") performed dual roles as well: packed with strong-smelling herbs and petals, it kept the foul stench of death, or the miasma, from reaching the doctor—the odor that so many felt was the causing the disease. It should be

PLAGUES, PANDEMICS AND VIRUSES

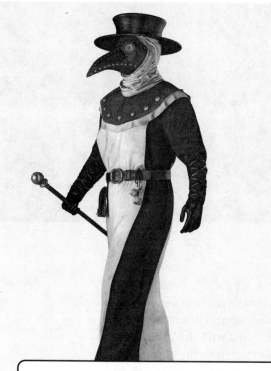

Invented by Charles de l'Orme in 1619, the plague doctor outfit included a mask that looked like a bird with a giant beak. The beak provided room to insert perfumes to protect the doctor from the inevitable bad smells of death.

mentioned that the reason a plague doctor uniform was necessary was because nearly 40 different plagues hit London in the years between 1348 and 1665. The first and last are the best known, but the ones in between did considerable damage, too, as you would imagine a plague would.

It was in the fall of 1635 when another plague struck London in the parish of St. Giles-in-the-Fields. It was greeted with a shrug. Londoners were quite familiar with the carbuncles and sores that had marked the infection from just ten years earlier, when the previous plague struck, so the pestilence lost much of the mystical qualities given to it by those who suffered during the Black Death, though many still carried amulets and tokens that supposedly warded off the disease … just in case.

St. Giles-in-the-Fields was more like a town in the muck. As fall turned to winter, reports of plague among the overcrowded poor started to occur, which were also met with a shrug. Perhaps it was just typhus? (Typhus was a constant presence in London slums.) Then, slowly, creepily, through the dripping walls and streets of filth, the plague began to surface east of the slums of St. Giles—into the slums of the saints: St. Olave's, St. Mary's, and St. Sepulchre-without-Newgate and then into East London, where the miserable conditions of Whitechapel and Stepney were about to become more miserable, surprisingly, as the weather grew warmer.

Cold weather means that people are more likely to stay indoors. This naturally helps to contain the spread of infectious diseases, even extremely infectious ones like the plague, but no matter whether you're a wealthy man about town or a poor family huddling in the tenements, as the days get brighter and cheerier, especially in rainy ol' England, you're stepping outdoors and, therefore, more likely to catch and/or spread diseases.

By April 1636, the plague began to seep through every corner of London. All the precautions from the previous plague were back in effect once more. Law enforcement was called upon to visit every house "wherein lies anyone who has been visited by the plague, to be shut up and watched by day and night." People were forbidden from renting rooms; a tax to aid the sick was levied on each parish; and the infected were quarantined in flimsily constructed sick houses.

The Royal College of Physicians recommended a temporary ban of gatherings, both public and private, quarantining the sick within their own houses and keeping the streets as clean as possible.

However, rules and regulations were difficult to enforce during times of plague. Firstly, they weren't officially laws, as Parliament didn't want to risk the chance of being shut in their own houses. Trash collectors either quit when faced with the mountain of debris or died themselves. Houses whose residents had the plague were marked with a red cross and the words "Lord, have mercy on us." Watchers who stood guard outside these homes, making sure no one went in or out for forty days, were sometimes killed by those gone mad with sickness and cabin fever or sometimes stole from the dead and died themselves. (The sick were often fed by charities with food handed through the window.) Secondly, only nine men comprised what would be called a plague task force; six fled as soon as they could.

God played less of a role in this plague than He did during previous plagues. People still felt that some kind of religious punishment was at work, but it was now part of a set of causes rather than the only one. Plague culprits included deplorable urban hygiene, filth in the streets, rotting food, and stagnant water. The city reeked of filth and death. Now, the thought process went, God may be all-powerful, but our actions decide our fates as well. In his essay "This Time of Pestilentiall Contagion," Francis Herring, a seventeenth-century physician who wrote about both medicine and religion, asserted that plagues were a "stroke of God's wrath for the sinnes of Mankinde" but also advised authorities to provide for the poor, for example, which would then cut back on begging, which would then lead to cleaner streets. Only we could do this, not God. This was a much different way of viewing the world.

London of the 1630s was a Protestant city, so much so that practicing Catholics risked imprisonment or death—not for bringing down the wrath of God on its people but because saying Catholic Mass was an act of treason. Since King Charles I was Protestant, it was assumed that Catholics and those who sought to convert Protestants to Catholicism were putting him in danger. Even worse, if England became Catholic again, then the Protestants would be forced to follow the orders of the pope. In their minds, that was an act beyond treason that was heresy—praying to a false idol. (English Protestants already felt on shaky ground because their queen was French Catholic Henrietta Maria.) So, if you were a practicing Catholic, it was best to practice in the shadows. No Catholic name appeared on parish registers, so no official aid was available to them;

they survived on faith, hope, and definitely the charity of friends, but that was not enough during a time of plague. Therefore, the Catholic community was forced to go public and organize its own charity, and it was decided that this organization should have a leader—one who was chosen in the person of Father Henry Morse.

If one were elected to care for plague victims who were dying hideous deaths in appalling conditions as well as deal with the red tape that accompanies any group who organize them, it wouldn't be surprising if this person would wonder why such a terrible fate had befallen them. But when Morse, normally a reserved sort, heard that he was the chosen one, "he went about in high spirits, unable, it appeared, to restrain himself. No better news, he said, could have been given him. He was chosen for that work—and he hoped that through his means many souls of the dying would be snatched for heaven."

> No Catholic name appeared on parish registers, so no official aid was available to them; they survived on faith, hope, and definitely the charity of friends....

Morse already had plenty of on-the-job training under his belt. He'd spent the previous winter huddled alongside the cold and the sick in the London tenements, nursing plague and typhus victims alike. Now, his elders instructed him to go on a brief retreat before focusing on the enormous task at hand. He spent a week with the Jesuits—a Catholic order devoted to education—in the pleasant village of Surrey, just south of London … though its gardens and country surroundings made it feel worlds away, which was just the type of refuge needed. Jesuit priest William Weston, who died shortly before the Great Plague of London, wrote that it was a place where priests could "refresh their spirit, exhausted after unremitting occupation and anxieties."

Whether Father Morse felt the week went too quickly or was just what he needed, we do not know. However, we do know that he returned, spiritually fit, to a city that had fallen into illness and terror.

A pamphlet had been published at about the same time as Father Morse's return; it listed more than 70 causes of the plague, including everything from drinking beer in a room that was overheated to eating cucumbers. (Cucumbers being one of the many foods that victims reportedly ate before dying and, therefore, were off-limits to those who wanted to stay healthy; actually, if people were to follow the list to the letter, they might have starved to death instead of catching the plague). To us, this list of taboos sounds absurd, but to someone without any knowledge of how plague was spread and who wondered if they were next, any type of guidance was accepted.

As spring turned to summer, conditions changed: they grew worse, at least from the perspective of a human, but grew even better from the perspective of a rat. These are animals that will eat wire—imagine the bounty that flowed through those sewers! What a smorgasbord that had just been served up to them!

The closest that seventeenth-century London came to animal control was an ordinance to kill "cats, dogs, [rabbits,] and tame pigeons" and to prevent swine from "ranging up and down the streets," but they had no way to round up the rats. (In the 400 years since, we've been able to identify bacteria and viruses and cure diseases, but we are still powerless over vermin.) Rats plumped up from the plague-ridden city and its uncollected trash and, with the cats destroyed, the rat population grew as well. The only good thing was that people were literally so sick and tired that no one paid attention to them. This was Dickensian London 176 years before Charles Dickens was born.

In 1636, leaving London was a crime punishable by death. Driven to the brink of madness by the disease and cabin fever, people took their chances anyway. If he or she was discovered outside the borders with sores, they could be made to "suffer the pains of death as in case of felony." No sores outside the borders only meant that one could be "whipped as a vagabond and bound to good behavior." These were fugitives rounded up by the watchers, men who

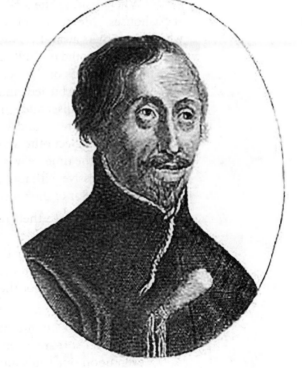

A Jesuit priest, Father Henry Morse was made a saint for devoting himself to helping the sick during the London plague.

PLAGUES, PANDEMICS AND VIRUSES

were like bounty hunters, armed with daggers and axes, who guarded village entrances, returning those who'd escaped. Poet John Taylor wrote of them: "The name of London now both far and near / Strikes all the towns and villages with fear." Of the country folk, Taylor wrote, "Uncharitable hounds, hearts as hard as rock / Who suffer people in the field to sink / Rather than give or sell a draught of drink." An undeclared war broke out between London and its countryside.

THE HEALING HANDS OF FATHER MORSE

"I sent for Mr. Morse when I was visited with the plague," said Margaret Allen, then a resident of St Giles. "And he many times gave alms to me, my husband, and my two little children, who all died of the plague, the parish not giving us anything, we being very poor and seven persons in number shut up." Like a seventeenth-century superhero, Father Henry Morse was a champion of the downtrodden, a man of the cloth who tended to his flock when he was most needed and when others were either running from or murdering this flock, but even greater than a superhero, he did all of this with no fanfare, no headlines, and no priest signal.

When visiting the sick who were boarded up in what were known as "pest-houses," Morse would wear "a distinctive mark on his outer garment," which kept others away. Every week, a list of the newly sick was given to the parish, and Morse would dutifully copy the names into a notebook. He was there to hear the confessions of the sick and dying, give the sacrament of last rites, lay out the corpse to be buried, and go to the burial, which the law dictated had to be done between sunset and sunrise. "Day and night he worked," wrote Belgian priest Father Alegambe, "and although he gave his principal attention to Catholics, he did not neglect others. It is hardly credible what hard work and horrors he endured. All the time he was in close contact with the plague-stricken, entering rooms oppressive with foul and pestilential air, sitting down beside a bed in the midst of squalor of the most repulsive and contagious nature."

In October, with their relief funds dwindling, Father Morse and fellow priest Father John Southworth appealed to the Catholics of London for money that would provide food, medicine, and clothes. This was soon extended to Catholics in all of Great Britain just days after higher taxes had been levied on the healthy parishes to bear the burden of the sick. They could therefore only ask for charity.

Having seen with our eyes the extreme necessity which many of the poorer sort are fallen into.... [W]e do protest to you seriously even upon our souls and consciences, that the greatness of the

FATHER DAMIEN

This brings to mind Belgian priest Father Damien, who lived among lepers in Hawaii who had been quarantined to the island of Molokai; he was their spiritual guide and source of comfort for sixteen years until he finally succumbed to leprosy—now called Hansen's disease—in 1889 at the age of 49.

calamity exceedeth all belief, insomuch as we should never have imagined in the least part of that which really is, had not our own eyes and daily experience attested the same unto us.

It then ends with a quote from 1 John 3:17: "He that hath the substance of this world and shall see his brother in need … how doth the charity of God abide in him?"

Here were two men, waking up every morning knowing that they would be spending that day among the most disgusting of conditions along with the sick and dying and, nonetheless, were able to find a way to say, "Please help us!" that could be felt by their fellow seventeenth-century English Catholics. The response was heartening … and generous. Up until that point, much of the burden had rested on the few relatively wealthy Catholics who lived in London. Catholics from all over the country and even Queen Henrietta Maria, the Catholic queen married to English King Charles I, now helped. "I being a poor laboring woman," said Elizabeth Godwin of St Giles, "never did or was able to keep a servant, and being shut up seven weeks, buried three of my little children, which Mr. Morse relieved with her Majesty's and with diverse Catholics' alms."

Another Catholic gave a similar account. Edward Freshwater, who wasn't even allowed to have Henry Morse as a visitor, received money from Henry Morse through his window. Over the course of two months, his door was only opened twice: each time, it was for a burial cart to retrieve a Freshwater child who had died. This money was used to repay a loan from the local Constable Wilson, who insisted he be paid back.

DOWN WITH THE PAPISTS

Anti-Catholicism was as rampant as disease in plague-addled London, and, looking for a scapegoat, many of its Protestants were happy to find it in the Papists (as Catholics are still known in the United Kingdom and Ireland). The appropriately named Dr. Gouge declared that the main cause of the plague wasn't miasma but Catholics. "Too many seducers are among us," cried Gouge, aimed at men like Father Morse. "And too great countenance is given to them."

Other preachers were happy to have their say as well. "The plague of God is in the land for the new mixtures of religion," said one. As if their lives weren't difficult enough, both Morse and Southworth were also harassed by officials and citizens who saw them as agents of the antichrist.

In February 1636, Morse was arrested and charged with being a priest and "perverting His Majesty's Protestant subjects." He was bailed out by the queen. (Remember, she was Catholic.)

Then, in September 1636, Henry Morse fell ill. This had been after a normal day of hearing deathbed confessions and administering last rites. On his return home, he began shivering. A Catholic doctor named Thomas Turner was sent for. He prescribed a nightly sweat, which involved covering the man in blankets so that he could sweat out the illness. Morse continued his ministrations by day, however, as he believed the need was greater than his immediate health. Whether Morse's illness was the flu, exhaustion, or the plague that was stopped in its tracks is uncertain, but Morse recovered.

> Anti-Catholicism was as rampant as disease in plague-addled London, and, looking for a scapegoat, many of its Protestants were happy to find it in the Papists....

Those who stood as watchers outside the sick houses usually allowed Henry Morse and John Southworth to enter, though one watcher, Robert White—who was also a member of the clergy of London's Church of St Margaret—had his eye on Southworth. (The Church of St Margaret was founded in the 1200s by Catholic monks before it was consecrated a Protestant church in 1614.) "Under pretense of distributing alms," White

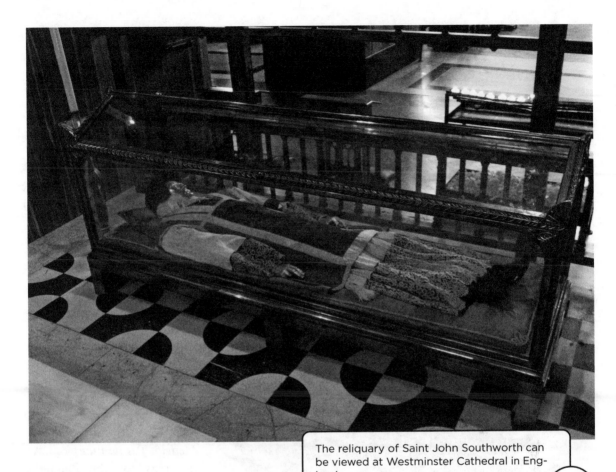

The reliquary of Saint John Southworth can be viewed at Westminster Cathedral in England.

claimed, Southworth "doth take occasion to go into divers visited houses" and then went about the business of trying to convert them. To White, Southworth's work was not extreme selflessness by a man of the cloth but part of the business of spreading Catholic propaganda. White cited one William Baldwin, who was barely clinging to life, as one of Southworth's marks. "[Southworth] set upon him to make him change his religion, whereunto he consented and received the sacraments from the Church of Rome." Furthermore, to stay on target, Southworth would "pay the watchmen to affirm that he comes only to give alms" when, in fact, he was "unsettling poor people in their religion" and, therefore, committing treason.

At the end of October, John Southworth was arrested and charged with treason, which was made possible by Robert White. Sir Dudley Carlton, the clerk of the council, directed a warrant to the keeper of the Gatehouse Prison in Westminster—not far from St Margaret's—to take Southworth into custody, even as the priest maintained that he had "labored only to preserve the poor from perishing which he thought would offend neither his Majesty or the State." For the rest of the year, while the plague continued to rage, Father Morse was left to tend the sick alone, while Father Southworth withered in prison.

One night, a young Protestant girl asked for Morse. Sick with the plague, she wished to be received into the Catholic Church, but she died before Morse could arrive. Her mother, seeing Morse's distress at the timing and understanding that it was because he could not help her daughter, asked to be received into the Catholic Church. "Her neighbors," the account continues, "getting knowledge of this, gathered before her door and begged her not to abandon her old beliefs.... The woman answered them, that even if she should be torn to pieces by wild horses, she would never forsake the Catholic faith, in which alone there was hope of salvation." Later, Morse received her surviving children into the faith before the woman caught the plague herself and died—a Catholic.

While Morse no doubt entered a Protestant home and left it a Catholic one, it was largely because many of the parish officials had left the city, and many who stayed neglected their duties as members of the clergy. Morse looked within scripture to find the evidence for charity, yet some preachers used it to find evidence that the sick should be left alone. In his pamphlet *Medela Pestilentiae*, or "A Remedy for the Plague," Reverend Richard Kephale maintained that elected officials (to whom he dedicated his pamphlet) were bound to the society at large, not the individual. He then argued that the "whole civic body would suffer if their life were taken away by infection." As a direct consequence, in April 1636, the London Council threatened that "if there be any person, ecclesiastical or lay, that shall hold or publish any opinions that it is a vain thing to forbear to re-

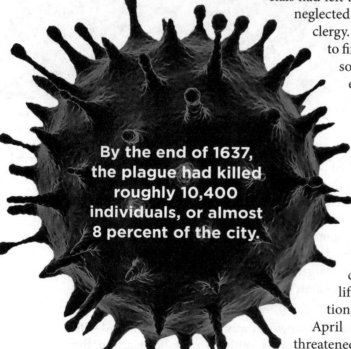

By the end of 1637, the plague had killed roughly 10,400 individuals, or almost 8 percent of the city.

PLAGUES, PANDEMICS AND VIRUSES

sort to the infected … pretending that no person shall die but at the time pre-fixed, he shall be apprehended." It was to these exact people, regardless of religion, that Father Morse attended.

By the end of 1637, the plague had killed roughly 10,400 individuals, or almost 8 percent of the city. In addition to nearly decimating the region, the plague created physical, psychological, and economic suffering for thousands more people.

AFTER THE PLAGUE

In 1641, King Charles I was pressured into forcing the exile of all Catholic priests. Father Morse went to Flanders and resumed his work as chaplain of the Catholic English soldiers there, but two years later, his Jesuit superiors sent him to northern England, and, dutifully, he went. Perhaps he knew he was about to greet certain death, or perhaps he felt that since he survived the plague as a Catholic priest in a Protestant city, he could survive anything, or perhaps he just put his fate in God's hands. So, Father Morse entered northern England and was arrested a year and a half later in Durham. He escaped with the help of the Catholic wife of one of his captors, but after six weeks, he was caught again, imprisoned in Newcastle, and sent by boat to London to meet his fate. Tried once more, people like Margaret Allen and Edward Freshwater—whose quotes in this book come from testimony they gave on behalf of Father Morse—did their best to clear his name by publicly testifying as what we'd call "character witnesses."

Morse was sentenced to death in accord with the law that forbade exiled priests to return to Great Britain. (Indeed, the queen's husband, King Charles I, was executed in 1649 after a series of political conflicts and the belief that he was becoming more tyrant than king. He was made a martyr by the Anglican Church in 1660. Father Southworth was executed in 1654.)

February 1, 1645, was the day of Father Morse's execution. He was able to celebrate Mass. Then, four horses were harnessed to the wicker hurdle on which he was dragged to the gallows that stood on Tyburn Hill—a popular place for hanging. Among the spectators was a crowd of the curious and those who wanted to witness Morse's death, but also in the crowd were the ambassadors of the Catholic countries of Spain, Portugal, and France and the Flemish count of Egmont.

In his last moments, Morse declared that he was being executed solely for his religion. He denied any connection with conspiracies against the king and promised that his chief concern was the welfare of his fellow people. He was then hanged.

THE GREAT PLAGUE OF LONDON

A seventeenth-century Londoner was actually quite well informed about the appearance and progress of the plague. A weekly pamphlet was handed out to the public that recorded the previous week's dead and the causes of their death. It was titled "London Weekly Bill of Mortality"; it had originated roughly a century before the Great Plague of London and was commonplace by the time this plague hit. Like Florence's *Libri della Grascia morti*, it was a weekly collection from the 120 parishes across the city, made possible by the clerk of each parish, who passed the information on to Parish Clerk's Hall every Tuesday.

Unlike Florence's *Libri della Grascia morti*, the London bills were written out, printed, and distributed first to the mayor, aldermen, and privy council on Thursday morning before being made available to the public.

The bill was a double-sided sheet with the date at the top, followed by information on the burials by parish, including parishes inside and outside its walls. (London at the time was a walled city; its wall was built by the Romans in c. 200 C.E. as a defensive measure back when it was a settlement known as "Londinium" and stood until the late 1760s.) By the time of the Great Plague of London, these parishes were subdivided into 97 parishes within the walls, sixteen parishes outside the walls, twelve "outparishes" in the counties of Middlesex and Surrey, and five Westminster parishes.

The other side of the pamphlet, "The Diseases and Casualties this Week," listed the causes of death, how far burials had risen or fallen compared to the previous week, and the value of a loaf of bread. (The value of bread, set by the lord mayor and aldermen of London, was made available to the public in this manner to prevent salesmen from price gouging, particularly during plague times.)

A London Bill of Mortality dated December 19, 1665, showing records of those who have died and the cause. The list shows 68,596 dead from the plague alone that year.

PLAGUES, PANDEMICS AND VIRUSES

A given list of diseases could include "dropsie," or what we used to call "dropsy"—a kind of umbrella term for swelling or edema; "flux," which is today's dysentery; and "childbed," or sudden infant death syndrome. Because these lists recorded London's burials rather than deaths, they're not a complete list, but they still give tremendous insight into the lives and deaths of the city's seventeenth-century population.

Like today, the bills were available for sale at an individual rate or subscription rate (four shillings). They also served as a topic of conversation and correspondence. It was during the plague epidemics, though, that the bills saw a huge uptick in readership. In 1662, London haberdasher John Graunt published a book about the bills called *Natural and Political Observations on the Bills of Mortality*, which became the first book that analyzed London's demographics.

Graunt recognized a need for his book because:

[I] observed that most of them who constantly took in the weekly Bills of Mortality, made little other use of them, then to look at the foot, how the Burials increase, or decrease; And, among the Casualties, what had happened rate, and extraordinary in the week currant; so as they might take the same as a text to talk upon, in the next Company; and withal, in the Plague time, how the Sickness increased, or decreased, so that the Rich might judge of the necessity of their removal, and Trades-men might conjecture what doings they were like to have in their respective dealings.

If this were written today, it would sound something like this: "I noticed that people who read the Bills of Mortality use them as some kind of fodder for water-cooler gossip, especially when it comes to deaths that seem strange or unusual. And when it's plague time, the rich use them to determine if they should get the heck out of town, and businessmen use them to determine if they might go out of business."

Graunt, meanwhile, saw the bills' statistical usefulness: its subtitle was *With reference to the Government, Religion, Trade, Growth, Air, Diseases, and the several Changes of the said City*. Graunt's book reached five editions by 1676—two years after Graunt himself died of liver disease. His burial probably made the weekly bill, though that particular one is lost to history.

Graunt was correct in that people had a morbid fascination with the Bills of Mortality, but it was also a useful tool for officials and physicians to see if a plague was on the horizon. A sustained rise in death tolls during the onset of warmer weather, for example, could be a good indication, and those who were in charge could strategize what to do next. In other words, get a jump on the plague

Perhaps the greatest chronicler of the Great Plague was Samuel Pepys, a wealthy member of Parliament who's most famous today for his detailed diary.

before it ran rampant across the city (and across the country as well since it should be noted that the plague did spread to parts of England over the course of a year or two before it died out, though London, due to its relative size and importance, usually dominates the story).

Meanwhile, ordinary Londoners could track the plague from parish to parish and see if they might be next. Perhaps the greatest chronicler of the Great Plague was Samuel Pepys, a wealthy member of Parliament who's most famous today for his detailed diary. Pepys wrote that he first heard about the Great Plague of London through the weekly Bill of Mortality. In 1665, he recorded the following:

• 27 July. At home met the weekly Bill, where above 1000 encreased in the Bill; and of them, in all, about 700 of the plague.

• 10 August ... to the office, where we say all the morning, in great trouble to see the Bill this week rise so high, to above 4000 in all, and of them, about 3000 of the plague.

• 14 August. Great fears we have that the plague will be a great Bill this week.

• 7 September ... to the Tower; and there sent for the Weekly Bill and find 8252 dead in all, and of them, 6978 of the plague—which is a most dreadfull Number—and shows reason to fear the plague hath got that hold that it will yet continue among us.

• 20 September ... the Duke showed us the number of the plague this week, brought in the last night from the Lord Mayor—that it is increased about 600 more than the last, which is quite contrary to all or hopes and expectations from the coldness of the late season; for the whole general number is 8297; and of them, the plague 7165—which

PLAGUES, PANDEMICS AND VIRUSES

is more in the whole, by above 50, then the biggest Bill yet—which is very grievous to us all.

- 27 September. Here I saw this week's Bill of Mortality, wherein, blessed be God, there is above 1800 decrease, this being the first considerable decrease we have had.

- 30 November. Great joy we have in the weekly Bill, it being come to 544 in all, and but 333 of the plague so that we are encouraged to get to London as soon as we can.

By May 1665, the plague was burning through London's population. Within six months, roughly 7,000 people were dying every week. In August 1665, Pepys took a trip around London, where he was told the story of a man he knew named Will, whose wife and three children had all died "I think, in a day." This made Pepys decide to curtail his trips around London.

Daniel Defoe, the English writer known for his novel *Robinson Crusoe*, was about five years old when the Great Plague of London hit (and his house was one of the few left standing after the Great Fire of London occurred the following year). It was the plague that influenced his 1722 work called *A Journal of the Plague Year*; indeed, the author bases much of the work on the recollections of his uncle, Henry Foe (Daniel Defoe was born "Daniel Foe"), along with the diaries of Samuel Pepys and the Bills of Mortality. However, if published today, it would probably be shelved in the historical fiction section.

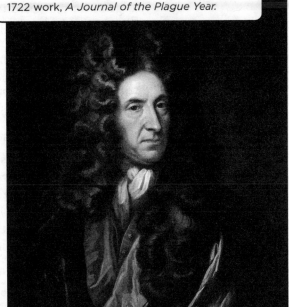

Daniel Defoe, the renowned author of *Robinson Crusoe,* wrote about the plague in his 1722 work, *A Journal of the Plague Year.*

Defoe seamlessly incorporated actual Bills of Mortality that were published during the plague into his own work:

It was about the beginning of September, 1664, that I, among the rest of my neighbours, heard in ordinary discourse that the plague was returned again in Holland; for it had been very violent there, and particularly at Amsterdam and Rotterdam, in the year 1663, whither, they say, it was brought, some said from Italy, others from the Levant, among some goods which were brought home by their Turkey fleet; others said it was brought from Candia; others from Cyprus. It mattered not from whence it came; but all agreed it was come into Holland again.

We had no such thing as printed newspapers in those days to spread rumours and reports of things, and to improve them by the invention of men, as I have lived to see practised since. But such things as these were gathered from the letters of merchants and others who corresponded abroad, and from them was handed about by word of mouth only; so that things did not spread instantly over the whole nation, as they do now. But it seems that the Government had a true account of it, and several councils were held about ways to prevent its coming over; but all was kept very private. Hence it was that this rumour died off again, and people began to forget it as a thing we were very little concerned in, and that we hoped was not true; till the latter end of November or the beginning of December 1664 when two men, said to be Frenchmen, died of the plague in Long Acre, or rather at the upper end of Drury Lane. The family they were in endeavoured to conceal it as much as possible, but as it had gotten some vent in the discourse of the neighbourhood, the Secretaries of State got knowledge of it; and concerning themselves to inquire about it, in order to be certain of the truth, two physicians and a surgeon were ordered to go to the house and make inspection. This they did; and finding evident tokens of the sickness upon both the bodies that were dead, they gave their opinions publicly that they died of the plague. Whereupon it was given in to the parish clerk, and he also returned them to the Hall; and it was printed in the weekly bill of mortality in the usual manner, thus— Plague, 2. Parishes infected, 1.

It almost looked like a scorecard. Defoe continued:

This increase of the bills stood thus: the usual number of burials in a week, in the parishes of St Giles-in-the-Fields and St Andrew's, Holborn, were from twelve to seventeen or nineteen each, few more or less; but from the time that the plague first began in St Giles's parish, it was observed that the ordinary burials increased in number considerably. For example:

From December 27 to January 3	St Giles's 16	St Andrew's 17
January 3 to 10	St Giles's 12	St Andrew's 25
January 10 to 17	St Giles's 18	St Andrew's 28

January 17 to 24	St Giles's 23	St Andrew's 16
January 24 to 31	St Giles's 24	St Andrew's 15
January 30 to February 7	St Giles's 21	St Andrew's 23
February 7 to 14	St Giles's 24	

Besides this, it was observed with great uneasiness by the people that the weekly bills in general increased very much during these weeks, although it was at a time of the year when usually the bills are very moderate.

THE SEARCHERS

Ever heard of the searchers? They killed Romeo and Juliet. Confused? Read on....

The watchers reappeared during the plague, standing guard at the homes of the sick so that the sick didn't leave and kept the population as a whole (except for the wealthy) from leaving London, but before and after the watchers were the searchers. They were first appointed during the plague outbreaks of 1568. According to Dr. Richelle Munkhoff, whose work on searchers has been widely published, "Searchers were always women on poor relief ... they were widows, but you could be widowed at 20. They weren't usually elderly, so if someone got the job they kept it for 30 years or more." Call it job security—and it not just anybody landed this job. "It was somebody who was respected," said Dr. Munkhoff. "It wasn't given to someone who didn't have any standing. In general, a poor but respectable member of the parish. On the dole but with enough skills to do the job. They weren't reviled until a plague."

Searchers worked in pairs regardless of whether or not a plague was occurring, often to find out if plague was on the horizon. "How do you know when a hotspot is going to happen if you're not looking at all times?" asked Dr. Munkhoff. "So when they first start it's 'plague or not plague,' but by Shakespeare's time the government wanted all causes of death. It was all for economics. There was a constant threat of bubonic plague, they had minor ones every other or every fifth year." Women often kept the job within their family across generations, such as mother to daughter or mother-in-law to daughter-in-law, almost like an apprenticeship or family knowledge that was passed down.

With the stroke of a pen, the searchers could condemn a household to a 40-day quarantine. Therefore, according to none other than John Graunt—

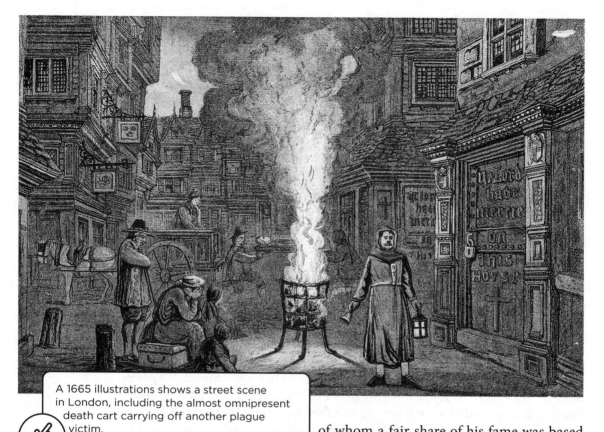

A 1665 illustrations shows a street scene in London, including the almost omnipresent death cart carrying off another plague victim.

of whom a fair share of his fame was based on the data the searchers gathered—dismissed them as unreliable and at the mercy of "a cup of ale, and the bribe of a two-groat [coin] fee." This beer-fueled, two-groat bribe was meant to persuade searchers to call a sick house clean and therefore free of quarantine. Whether they were actually bribed is up for debate, though Dr. Munkhoff asserts, "There was so much riding on that decision that I'm sure there were cases. Not so simple as the searchers are corrupt. These people are your neighbors and you might have a positive relationship with them...."

Physician Nathaniel Hodges asserted that they were "wretches [who] out of greediness to plunder the dead, would strangle their patients and charge it to distemper in their throats." This reputation followed them like miasma. They were also accused of "secretly convey[ing] the pestilent taint from sores of the infected to those who were well."

Though it can't be proven, it certainly seems like William Shakespeare took a dim view of searchers as well. Toward the end of *Romeo and Juliet*, Juliet

PLAGUES, PANDEMICS AND VIRUSES

NATHANIEL HODGES

Nathaniel Hodges, while short on sympathy for the searchers, was quite long on intellect and, it could be said, also maintained a strong constitution, for he got sick twice during the Great Plague but survived even though plague was all around him. Hodges used his observational tools as a way to learn more about the plague and even noted that some pustules were "not easily distinguishable from a Flea-Bite." He was also dismissive of medical treatments of the time, including the famous act of bloodletting. Each morning when he awoke, Hodges ate a kind of medicinal paste that included nutmeg; nutmeg is now known to be an effective flea repellent.

is given a potion by Friar Laurence which will make it appear as though she died so that she would be put in the family crypt. The friar promises to send another friar to tell Romeo of the plan so that he can be with her in the crypt when she wakes up, and then they'll both live happily ever after. Unfortunately for the "star-cross'd lovers," this is one of Shakespeare's tragedies.

ACT V SCENE II	**Friar Laurence's cell.**
[Enter FRIAR JOHN]	
FRIAR JOHN	Holy Franciscan friar! brother, ho!
[Enter FRIAR LAURENCE]	
FRIAR LAURENCE	This same should be the voice of Friar John. Welcome from Mantua: what says Romeo? Or, if his mind be writ, give me his letter.
FRIAR JOHN	Going to find a bare-foot brother out One of our order, to associate me, Here in this city visiting the sick, And finding him, the searchers of the town, Suspecting that we both were in a house Where the infectious pestilence did reign, Seal'd up the doors, and would not let us forth; So that my speed to Mantua there was stay'd.
FRIAR LAURENCE	Who bare my letter, then, to Romeo?

FRIAR JOHN	I could not send it,—here it is again,— Nor get a messenger to bring it thee, So fearful were they of infection.
FRIAR LAURENCE	Unhappy fortune! by my brotherhood, The letter was not nice but full of charge Of dear import, and the neglecting it May do much danger. Friar John, go hence; Get me an iron crow, and bring it straight Unto my cell.

So, what happened? "The searchers of the town / Suspecting that we were both in a house / Where the infection pestilence did reign / Seal'd up the doors, and would not let us forth / So that my speed to Mantua there was stay'd." You'd be forgiven for missing the entire story here given that the searchers, unlike Macbeth's witches, didn't even get any stage time, and

In Shakespeare's famous tragedy *Romeo and Juliet* the fate of the lovers is sealed because of the actions of the searchers who stop Friar John from telling Romeo that Juliet is not really dead.

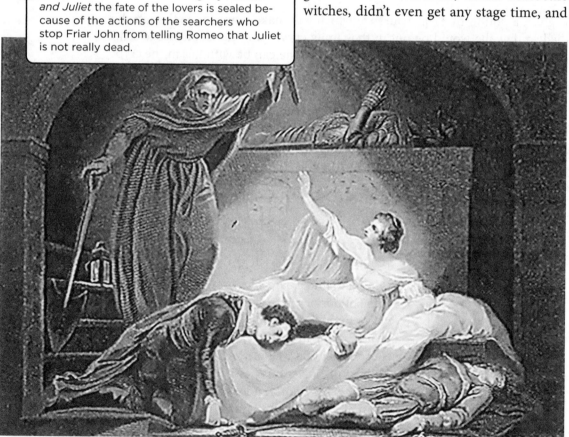

PLAGUES, PANDEMICS AND VIRUSES

even if they had, hardly anyone today would have known the context. (Truth be told, Italy, where *Romeo and Juliet* took place, never had searchers. They were only in England and parts of Scotland.)

Friar John was never able to deliver the message that Juliet was alive because searchers thought he'd been in a house with the plague and they prevented him from leaving, so his letter did not reach Romeo. Had they let him go on his way, the lovers would not have wound up both dying. (In director Baz Luhrmann's 1996 film version, *Romeo + Juliet*, the note gets held up by FedEx.)

Stop Searching

Much of these opinions on the searchers are due to a) misogyny: a woman dictating how a man must behave, and b) socioeconomic status. What right does a widow on the dole have to tell me what to do? So, similar to Father Henry Morse, the searchers faced persecution while being an essential worker during the grimmest and most morbid of times, and it was recorded that children of the searchers died of the plague, so they always risked bringing the pestilence home to their families.

"If they thought someone was sick or had died, the only kind of control they had was to shut up the house," said Dr. Munkhoff. "They got the constable to come, lock the doors with everyone in there, and the family wasn't able to come out for 28–40 days.

"If anyone got sick during that time the house remained closed until you're all dead or you're all better. People had to hand food through the window. It was a huge interference for the household. So here are these two poor women in your neighborhood suddenly deciding your fate. A lot of urban legends started, like searchers declared a woman dead who then began to breathe [in, a way, similar to *Romeo and Juliet*] and they became like witches."

As the earliest medical examiners, searchers examined corpses to find the cause of deaths. They were given a list of symptoms to check for, like swelling around the neck, pustules, and blotches. Their responsibilities were later divided into three essential functions: those who determined whether or not a sickness was associated with the plague; those who cared for the general sick; and those who viewed corpses in an attempt to link deaths to specific diseases. They identified themselves by carrying a red wand.

Their written documents containing statistical data linking sickness to fatality were then recorded in the Bills of Mortality. The searchers' records have enabled historians and researchers to estimate the living conditions and the influence of diseases like the plague on a given population at a time when homes were not required to provide this information to the parish registrars. The searchers' work continued until the Registration Act of 1836, which first required all marriages in England and Wales, then all births and deaths, to be well documented—an act that began the modern era of vital statistics in England and Wales.

ISOLATION IS THE MOTHER OF INVENTION

Medically, Londoners had plenty of schools of thought about the plague. The traditional philosophy of humors was slowly beginning to fall out of favor but still maintained a foothold on English society. It was hard to shake that long-held idea that plague was caused by an imbalance of the humors, so purging and bleeding played a large role in their treatment. (This is why Henry Morse was prescribed a nightly sweat when he became ill during the previous plague.) Meanwhile, those who followed a chemical route looked to nature for the cure. London also had its share of nonprofessional practitioners, like herbalists and wisewomen, and apothecaries, which were like pharmacies, held a wide variety of remedies.

King Charles II was mired in the Second Anglo–Dutch War (1665–1667), which was fought over maritime trade routes. The war, along with the plague, was destroying England's economy, but in addition to wanting his trade routes, Charles II was also a king with a keen interest in medicine. It was most likely for this reason that he called for social distancing (though it wouldn't have that name for another 354 years). In 1666, Charles II ordered all public gatherings, even funerals, to stop. Theaters were shut, and only a few pubs were allowed open. Oxford and Cambridge universities closed.

Isaac Newton had just received his B.A. degree from Trinity College, Cambridge, when the university shut down, but his family was among the wealthy who were allowed to flee the cities for the relative safety of their country homes. Newton spent this plague year 60 miles north of London at his family estate, Woolsthorpe Manor, doing calculus and coming up with the law of gravitation. The latter happened because of an apple tree outside his window.

The story of an apple bonking Newton on the head, causing him to realize that gravity exists, isn't quite true, but, according to an account of Newton's life by his assistant John Conduit, "In the year he retired again from Cambridge on account of the plague ... whilst he was musing in a garden it came into his thought that the same power of gravity (which made an apple fall from the tree to the ground) was not limited to a certain distance from the earth but must ex-

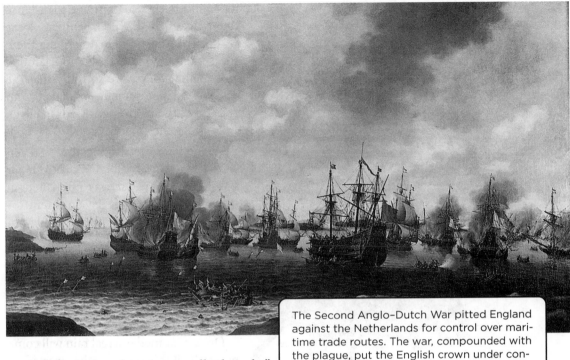

The Second Anglo-Dutch War pitted England against the Netherlands for control over maritime trade routes. The war, compounded with the plague, put the English crown under considerable financial stress (*Attack on the Medway* by Pieter Cornelisz van Soest [1667]).

tend much farther than was usually thought." This means that he was able to conclude that not only did a force exist that kept a falling apple from flying into outer space, that same force pulled the moon toward Earth and, to a lesser extent, Earth toward the moon. As the law states: "The force is proportional to the product of the two masses, and inversely proportional to the square of the distance between them." Sometimes, it's easier just to remember that things fall.

Not content to stick to one breakthrough, Newton also developed the earliest forms of calculus. As Newton himself said, "For in those days I was in the prime of my age for invention & minded Mathematics & Philosophy more than at any time since."

BLAME THE POOR

Regardless of time and place, if disease is afoot, the poor will get hit the worst. Bacteria and viruses are equal-opportunity infectors in that they don't care about your socioeconomic status, but some opportunities are more easily presented than others. During the Great Plague of London, a pathogen had plenty of poor people to choose from, and to distance themselves from the poor, some took the low road of not only describing them in inhumane terms but proclaiming that they were so filthy that the plague actually emanated from them. The poor were, in effect, the plague.

Physician Steven Bradwell's *A Watch-Man for the Pest* was published in 1625, yet its sentiment toward the poor had not changed by the time the Great Plague of London arrived 40 years later. In fact, it was a sentiment echoed about 350 years later by Travis Bickle in Martin Scorsese's 1976 film *Taxi Driver*: "Someday a real rain will come and wash all this scum off the streets."

> Bradwell took the Galenic approach to medicine, so he advised his readers to avoid the miasma of "filthy sincks, stincking sewers, channells, gutters, privies, sluttish corners, dunghills, and uncast ditches."

Bradwell took the Galenic approach to medicine, so he advised his readers to avoid the miasma of "filthy sincks, stincking sewers, channells, gutters, privies, sluttish corners, dunghills, and uncast ditches." Most dangerous of all were the "*Poore People* (by reason of their great want) living sluttishly, feeding nastily on offals, or the worst & unholsomest meates; and many times too long lacking food altogether; have bothe their bodies much corrupted, and their Sprits exceedingly weakened: whereby they become (of all others) most subject to this Sicknesse. And before we see the *Plague* sweeps up such people in greatest heapes."

What's worse is Badwell's assessment that people either contract the plague from without or essentially generate it from within. "From within they are most apt, whose veins and vessels are full of grose humours and corrupt juices, the evil matter (being thicke, and therefore cannot breath out through the pores) increaseth her putrefication (by the heat within) unto the greater malignity, and so become Pestilent."

This was from the point of view of a physician—someone who, in theory, was supposed to tend to the sick, not brand them as the embodiment of disease and leave them to die.

HOT OFF THE PRESSES

It's not surprising that at the time of the Great Plague, the British publishing world was overwhelmed with similar plague books and pamphlets. This is from *Directions for Prevention and Cure of the Plague Fitted for the Poorer Sort*:

> Abstain from the boiled herbs of Colliflowers, Cabbage, Coleworts, Spinage, and Beets; also from all wallowish and lushy fruits, as sweet Plums, sweet Apples, Pears, Peaches, Mallacotoons, Cucumbers, Pompions, Mellons, ripe Gooseberries, ripe Grapes, Apricocks unless eaten with the kernels; also from raw herbs, as Reddish, Spinage, &c. But all fruits baked or thoroughly corrected by the fire, are better than raw.

These publications were as vast in size, quantity, and price as the treatments they proposed. We don't know who wrote *Directions for Prevention and Cure of the Plague Fitted for the Poorer Sort*, but we do know that it's a six-page booklet that draws its content from Galen. It also strikes a tone of authority in terms of telling those of a higher social status how the poor should be treated (and some if its instructions were actually then mandated).

Gideon Harvey was another physician who followed Galen's teachings. His *A Discourse of the Plague* is presumed to have been published in the summer of 1665, when the Great Plague was at what he termed its second stage, or "augment," when the numbers of sick and dying were growing larger. (Its next stage, "the state," would be when casualties from sickness reach their height. That, he predicted, would be in the late summer to early fall, which was proven correct by the Bills of Mortality. September 1665 was the deadliest month of the Great Plague of London, when 7,165 people died in one week.)

The *Loimologia* is a pamphlet about the 1665 London plague that, in part, criticizes the famous local physicians who fled the city rather than help the sick.

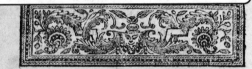

LOIMOLOGIA:

OR, AN

ACCOUNT, *&c.*

SECTION I.

Of the Rise and Progress of the late
PLAGUE.

THE Plague which we are now to give an Account of, discovered the Beginnings of its future Cruelties, about the Close of the Year 1664; for at that Season two or three Persons died suddenly in one Family at *Westminster*, attended

B

Harvey believed that "the Plague is a most Malignant and Contagious Feaver, cause through Pestilential Miasms, insinuating into the humoral and consistent parts of the Body." He also wrote that it was spread through the air by "flaming Arsenical corpuscules floating in the air … attracted into the Body by inspiration through the Lungs and Nostrils; or otherwise they pierce through one's clothes, and so penetrate into the pores of the entire body." His remedies included … purging and bleeding.

In 1665, George Thomson published *Loimologia: a Consolatory Advice, and some brief Observations concerning the present Pest*, in which he reflected on the conduct of those members of the Royal College of Physicians who left the city during the plague, "leaving this great city destitute of their help, when it most needed it." Even the college's president, Sir Edward Alston, left town, but *Loimogia*'s greater purpose was to publicize what Thomson thought was the correct way to treat this new plague (as he believed it to be). Not a man who followed Galen, Thomson challenged those still practicing purging and bleeding.

Thomson's views were not acquired from a distance—he even dissected the body of a plague victim. He believed the disease was airborne and attacked the *archeus*, or a kind of force responsible for the growth of living things. In his eyes, a person must be mentally as well as physically fit in order to battle the plague.

> To conclude, my advice is, that those who desire to preserve themselves from this present Pest, do drinke every morning either Sulphurated Wine, Strong Beer, or what Liquor they please, wherein hath been steeped a large quantity of Horse-Radish-root, with five, six, seven, eight, nine or ten drops of good Spirit of Salt; and no doubt they will find a far better effect, then from a Galenical Electuary of London-Treacle and Wood-Sorrel.

For their part, the Royal College of Physicians printed what we would think of today as some kind of Wiccan cookbook, with directions such as: "[Take] the leaves of Sage, Scordium, Celandine, Rue, Rosemary, Wormwood, Ros solis, Mugwort, Burnet, Dragons, Scabious, Agrimony, Baum, Carduus, Betony, Centery the less, Marygolds leaves and flowers, of each one handful; Let them all be cut, bruised, and infused three days in eight pints of White wine in the month of May, and distilled." (For the record, not all of the "recipes" sounded like something that came out of a witch's spell book; shopkeepers asked customers to drop their coins in dishes of vinegar to sterilize them, the closest thing to hand sanitizer in 1600s England.)

Nevertheless, the plague persisted. Quarantining was back in full force, as it had been in the previous London plague, and a new generation of searchers went to work. Red crosses were painted on the doors of quarantine homes alongside a paper notice that read, "Lord have mercy upon us." Not everyone stayed indoors, however. In April 1665, Charles II ordered a severe punishment for those who took the cross and paper off their door "in a riotious manner" so they could "goe abroad into the street promiscuously, with others." By the time Charles II fled the city in July, the plague was killing about 1,000 people a week.

The plague lasted through most of 1666, with a death toll of about 100,000 people in London and possibly as many as 750,000 in England.

Nighttime burials were still the law, though in the summertime, the darkness didn't last long enough to bury everyone, and the task had to seep into the morning hours. This is when the "dead carts" would hobble through town with the cries of "Bring out your dead!" accompanying them. (This was parodied centuries later in the 1975 film *Monty Python and the Holy Grail*.)

The plague lasted through most of 1666, with a death toll of about 100,000 people in London and possibly as many as 750,000 in England. After peaking in the fall of 1665, the city's plague deaths began to taper off that winter. In February 1666, King Charles II believed that the city was safe enough for him to return.

London would still report plague victims until 1679, but those were mostly in the outlying areas; the major outbreak was mostly over by September 2, 1666, the night a baker named Thomas Farriner unwittingly started the Great Fire of London.

THE GREAT FIRE OF LONDON

London in the seventeenth century was the largest city in Great Britain, with a population of about half a million, and although the

Great Plague of London had brought that population down, Londoners were still cramped within its city walls. A contemporary diarist of Samuel Pepys named John Evelyn wrote that London, compared to Paris, was a "wooden, northern, and inartificial congestion of Houses."

Its street plan was still medieval, with overcrowded, cobbled alleys, and although Londoners had endured several major fires, they still used wood for buildings and thatch for roofs. They weren't legal, but they were cheap, so no one paid much attention. Stone-built homes were only for the wealthy, where mansions were surrounded by a ring of overcrowded parishes. Therefore, fire was common in the teeming, wood-built city, with its countless fireplaces, candles, and ovens.

Back then, firefighters, so to speak, did not yet exist, but the Trained Bands, a British military unit, was available for general emergencies, and watching for fire was one of the jobs of the watchmen, or "bellmen," who patrolled the streets nightly. Community procedures were in place for dealing with fires, and they were usually effective: citizens would be alerted to a house fire by church bells, and many would congregate hastily to fight the fire.

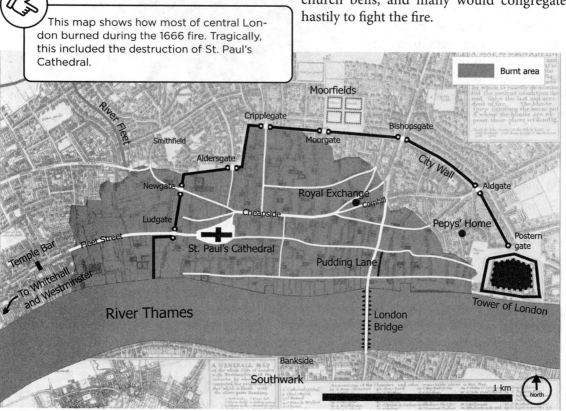

This map shows how most of central London burned during the 1666 fire. Tragically, this included the destruction of St. Paul's Cathedral.

PLAGUES, PANDEMICS AND VIRUSES

The Great Fire started at Thomas Farriner's bakery on Pudding Lane shortly after midnight on September 2, 1666, and spread rapidly west. The major firefighting technique of the day was to create firebreaks—demolishing buildings ahead of the fire's path so that the fire couldn't spread, but the lord mayor of London was indecisive in the face of this catastrophe, so demolitions weren't ordered until the following night, and by that time, the wind had already turned the fire into an inferno that made conventional firebreaks useless.

By Tuesday, the fire had spread over most of the city, destroying St. Paul's Cathedral, which had taken more than 200 years to build in the years between 1087 to 1314. Battalions, such as they were, finally got a handle on the fire that day as the winds died down, and gunpowder that was shot from the Tower of London created gigantic enough firebreaks to stop the spread.

Though the Great Fire of London caused enough damage to earn its name, it did little to end the Great Plague of London, which was already on the decline and whose hot spots, like Whitechapel, Clerkenwell, and Southwark, were largely untouched by the fire, so even if the fire drove out rats in the 436 acres it burned, it didn't spread far enough to drive out all of the plague rats in greater London.

The fact is, historians aren't really sure why the Great Plague of London ended. After the fire, London began to use brick over wood, and brick is also harder for rats to burrow into, but no hygienic or sanitary improvements occurred at the time that might have explained the death of the plague.

THE LEMON THAT SAVED PARIS

The Great Plague of London didn't only strike London. It made its way to France after rumors had begun of its impending arrival. It hit Normandy, Picardia, Sasson, and Amiens, then traveled down the Seine to Rouen. Parisians knew they had to be next, so they imposed quarantines, realizing that they couldn't stop it but were hopeful that they were prepared for it. As far as plagues go, the one in Paris fizzled, while cities like Vienna and Prague would both see casualties of 80,000 people and Amiens 30,000. Paris—a city that had all the same sanitation issues as London—barely felt a scratch. Author and cookbook historian Tom Nealon, in *Food Fights and Culture Wars*, posits that the reason for this was that "when life gave Parisians plague, they went and made *limonade*."

Citrus fruits like lemons are largely grown in warmer climates and had been rare in northern cities, but by the mid-1600s, lemons were being grown and imported to cities that could afford them, like Paris. As a stroke of good timing, lemonade had just become popular in Paris around the time of the Great Plague of London. Men known as *limonadiers* would stroll the city with a tank of lemonade on their backs, offering cups for sale, and where these *limonadiers* went, lemon zest was sure to follow. Lemon peels piled up in the sewers, delighting rats and disgusting fleas. Even though it's difficult to prove that lemonade was the definitive reason why the plague bypassed Paris in the mid-1600s, it certainly didn't hurt.

The legend of the lemon lives on. Lemon peels contain limonene, which is used in food products, soaps, and perfumes for its lemony flavor and scent. It's also an EPA-approved natural bug repellent. Limonene kills insects on contact, suffocating them by damaging their respiratory systems, and is lethal to pests such as fleas, fire ants, and flies. Limonene also is an active ingredient in pesticides used for flea and tick control on pets.

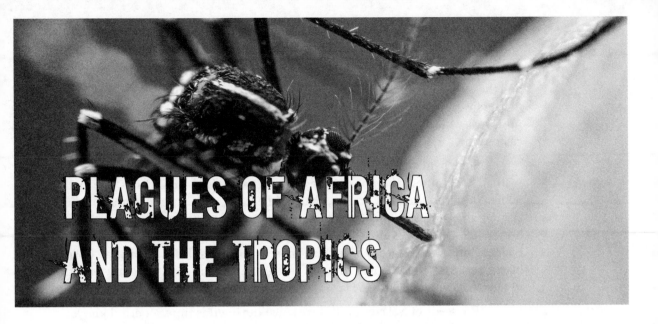

PLAGUES OF AFRICA AND THE TROPICS

As European explorers and colonizers ventured into Africa and the New World, they encountered new diseases in these warmer climates that killed tens of thousands of men and women. Such diseases as yellow fever would have the power to change the course of world history.

YELLOW FEVER

The second-largest Caribbean island is Hispaniola. (Cuba is the largest.) Politically, about one-third of Hispaniola is known as Haiti, where French is spoken, and the other two-thirds is known as the Dominican Republic, where Spanish is spoken. However, centuries ago, the island was called Saint-Domingue. The French controlled the western third (today's Haiti), and Spain influenced the eastern portion (today's Dominican Republic).

What Haitian plantation owners earned financially from sugar production was nothing compared to the toll they took on human dignity. Because slaves suffered from diseases like malaria and yellow fever, the French repeatedly brought in tens of thousands more to make up for the loss. In 1787, the French imported about 20,000 slaves from Africa into Saint-Domingue, while the British "only" imported 38,000 slaves to *all* of their Caribbean colonies. At least 50 percent of slaves died within a year of arriving, so French planters worked them as hard as they could in order to get the most out of them before they'd inevitably die. The death rate was so high that one female slave would often be "married" to several men at the same time, and since slaves had no rights, rape by overseers and the overseers' sons was the rule. Even by plantation standards, French slave masters were insanely cruel. This cruelty masked the white man's fear of slave uprisings, which they appeared to quell with violence, whippings, burnings, and castration.

French historian Paul Fregosi wrote: "Whites, mulattos and blacks loathed each other. The poor whites couldn't stand the rich whites, the rich whites despised the poor whites, the middle-class whites were jealous of the aristocratic whites, the whites born in France looked down upon the locally born whites, mulattoes envied the whites, despised the blacks and were despised by the whites; free Negroes brutalized those who were still slaves, Haitian born blacks regarded those from Africa as savages. Everyone—quite rightly—lived in terror of everyone else … Haiti was hell, but Haiti was rich."

The seeds of a slave revolt were sown during this time, a period known as the Enlightenment. The Enlightenment, which lasted from the seventeenth to the nineteenth century, was a robust time of intellectualism and great thinkers in philosophy, science, literature, and law. Many of those who were part of the Enlightened movement fought against slavery on the basis that it was contrary to the law of nature. In essence, a person's freedom is absolute—no one can take it away—and slaves were, indeed, people.

Toussaint L'Ouverture

Toussaint L'Ouverture (who gave himself that surname—it means "opening") was a free black man and eventual general from Saint-Domingue who was familiar with the ideals of the Enlightenment. Many in the West believed that the world was divided into "enlightened leaders" and "ignorant masses"; L'Ouverture wanted to bridge this gap between the popular masses—who were not necessarily ignorant—and the enlightened view of abolition as a way to liberate his people. L'Ouverture wrote a constitution for Saint-Domingue that abolished slavery, something that had been ignored by the French prior to the French Revolution. L'Ouverture addressed this inconsistency directly in his constitution, which Enlightenment scholars devoured because of his brilliance.

After the establishment of the French First Republic alongside radical changes to French laws, the French National Assembly published the Declaration of the Rights of Man in August 1789, declaring all men free and equal. The declaration, however, did not make it clear whether or not this equality applied to women, slaves, or citizens of the colonies, and it left a loophole that meant that freedom and equality might actually be possible in Saint-Domingue.

Saint-Domingue's colonial overseers were all for independence from the French, as they wanted to set their own rules when it came to slavery and foreign trade. For their part, the African population mostly allied with the British since they knew that if Saint-Domingue became independent from France, it would mean an even more horrible future than the inconceivably horrible one they were living in. The planters would be free to operate slavery as they pleased without being accountable to their own French overlords.

In 1791, the slaves revolted and fought the French, the Spanish, and each other for control of the island. France ignored the plantation owners, and in May 1791, with L'Ouverture on their minds, France granted citizenship to wealthy, free people of color. White planters refused to comply with this decision, and fighting continued to break out between the former slaves and their former white owners.

Meanwhile, the unhappy French plantation owners arranged with Great Britain to declare British sovereignty over the colony, believing that the British would maintain slavery. The British had another agenda. British prime minister William Pitt the Younger feared that the success of a slave revolt would inspire insurrections in the British Caribbean

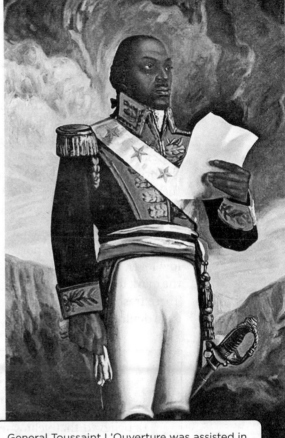

General Toussaint L'Ouverture was assisted in his struggle to free Haiti from the French by the fact that yellow fever killed many of France's troops.

colonies. He also believed that if Great Britain was able to lay claim to Saint-Domingue, which was the richest of the French colonies, its wealth would end up in the British treasury.

American journalist James Perry noted that the great irony of the British campaign in Saint-Domingue was that it ended as a complete debacle, costing the British treasury millions of pounds and the British military thousands upon thousands of dead, all for nothing.

So, to try to outfox the British and the French plantation owners, while securing the colony for republican France, the French government freed *all* the slaves on August 29, 1793, and granted civil and political rights to all black men in the colonies. The French constitutions of 1793 and 1795 both included the abolition of slavery until they were replaced by Napoleon Bonaparte.

What Is Yellow Fever?

So, where does yellow fever come in? After arriving in the West Indies in February 1794, General Charles Grey chose to conquer Martinique, St. Lucia, and Guadeloupe. Troops under the command of General Grey arrived in Saint-Domingue on May 19, 1794. His timing was terrible—it was the rainy season and, therefore, mosquito season. Within two months of arriving in Saint-Domingue, the British had lost 40 officers and 600 men to yellow fever, or "black vomit," as they called it. (It's now believed that black vomit was, in fact, dried blood. Blood in the vomit almost always meant that the infected person was about to die.)

Ultimately, of General Grey's 7,000 men, about 5,000 died of yellow fever while the Royal Navy reported "46 masters and 1,100 men dead, chiefly of yellow fever." British historian Sir John Fortescue wrote, "It is probably beneath the mark to say that 12,000 Englishmen were buried in the West Indies in 1794." These fresh European bodies were no match against mosquitoes—and this was a particularly awful mosquito season.

THE FREE AFRICAN SOCIETY AIDS THE SICK

It's believed that yellow fever came to Philadelphia by ships carrying both white and black refugees from Saint-Domingue. Physician Benjamin Rush (1746–1813) believed that blacks had immunity to the illness and, as such, thought they had an obligation to attend to the afflicted. Rush was an abolitionist. The Free African Society, possibly the first African American benevolent society in the United States, concluded that acting on Rush's plea for help would strike a blow against racism by showing how blacks could be valuable citizens. Led by former slaves Richard Allen (1760–1831) and Absalom Jones (1746–1818), the society demonstrated remarkable courage by nursing the sick and burying the dead. Tragically, Rush was wrong in his estimation that blacks were immune to the fever; they died at a rate almost equal to that of whites, debunking the belief that the Haitians defeated the Europeans because they were immune to yellow fever.

Yellow fever is a hemorrhagic disease, like Ebola. It's caused by a virus transmitted by the *Aedes* mosquito—the same as the one that spreads Zika. In fact, this species of mosquito made landfall in the Caribbean from ships leaving Africa.

Although the vector is the same, the virus is terribly different. When people are living in crowded conditions, like in slave quarters and on sugar plantations (mosquitoes love sugar), the disease can be transmitted from one person to the next by a single mosquito. Even if you swat it and kill it, you may have already been infected.

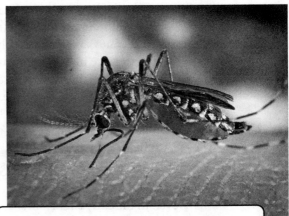

The mosquito species *Aedes aegypti* is a common transmitter of yellow fever, but other mosquitoes in the Aedes genus can also carry it.

In the first stage, the infected person might feel nauseated and tired and have severe muscle aches and joint pains that feel like their bones are breaking. Most of these people will enter a period of remission and feel better. About 15 percent, though, will suddenly take a turn for the worse. This is ironically called "intoxication." The infected start turning yellow because their inflamed liver is trying to release bile, which it what it normally does, but because the liver is inflamed, the channels are narrowed and bile becomes clogged within its normal route into the intestine, where it normally aids digestion. So, instead, bile finds an alternate route: through the bloodstream, where it stains the skin and eyes yellow.

Finally, toxins that the liver would normally expel build up in the body and tamper with the brain. The infected can be anywhere from irritable to insane. Also at this point comes bleeding. You bleed from pretty much any orifice: your mouth, your rectum, your uterus if you're a woman. So, to see somebody who is about to die from yellow fever—the insanity, the black vomit, the bleeding, the yellow skin—is a horrific picture.

Death by the Boatload

As more ships arrived with British troops, more soldiers died of yellow fever. By June 1, 1796—the height of mosquito season—of the thousand men from the 66th regiment, only 198 had *not* been infected with yellow fever; of the thousand men of the 69th regiment, only 515 had *not* been infected with yellow fever. British General Ralph Abercromby predicted that at the current rate of yellow fever infections, all of the men from the two regiments would be dead by November.

As the human and financial costs of the expedition mounted, people in Great Britain demanded a withdrawal from Saint-Domingue, which was devouring money and soldiers while failing to produce much in the way of profit. Military service in Saint-Domingue was seen as a death sentence by the British Army. One British officer wrote of the horror at seeing his friends "drowned in their own blood" while "some died raving Mad." On April 11, 1797, Colonel Thomas Maitland of the 62nd Regiment of Foot landed in Port-au-Prince and wrote in a letter to his brother that British forces in Saint-Domingue had been "annihilated" by yellow fever.

The failed expedition to Saint-Domingue had cost the British treasury four million pounds and 100,000 men either dead or permanently disabled from yellow fever. In the early twenty-first century, historian Robert L. Scheina estimated that the slave rebellion resulted in the deaths of 350,000 Haitians and 50,000 European troops. According to the *Encyclopedia of African American Politics*, "Between 1791 and independence in 1804 nearly 200,000 blacks died, as did thousands of mulattoes and as many as 100,000 French and British soldiers." Yellow fever, not battle, caused most of these deaths. Writer David Geggus points out that at least three out of every five British troops sent to Saint-Domingue died of disease.

This was the only slave uprising that led to the founding of a state that was both free from slavery and ruled by nonwhites and former slaves. It was also the largest slave uprising since Spartacus's revolt against the Roman Republic almost two thousand years earlier.

L'Ouverture used political and military tactics to gain dominance over his rivals. Throughout his years in power, he worked to improve the economy and security of Santo Domingo. He restored the plantation system using paid labor, negotiated trade treaties with the United Kingdom and the United States, and maintained a large and well-disciplined army.

Enter Napoleon

Then came Napoleon. In November 1799, Napoleon Bonaparte gained power in France through a *coup d'état* and passed a new constitution that promised to maintain abolition in the colonies, but he also forbade L'Ouverture from invading Spanish Santo Domingo. A year later, L'Ouverture and his men invaded Santo Domingo anyway, taking possession from the governor, Don Garcia. L'Ouverture brought it under French law, which abolished slavery, and became master of the whole island.

In 1801, L'Ouverture issued a constitution for Saint-Domingue that decreed that he would be governor for life and called for black autonomy and a sovereign black state. In response, Napoleon sought to take back French rule from the Haitians by sending French soldiers and warships to the island, led by his brother-in-law Charles Leclerc. They were under secret instructions to restore slavery, at least in the formerly Spanish-held part of the island. Bonaparte ordered that L'Ouverture was to be treated with respect until the French forces were established; once that was done, L'Ouverture was to be summoned to Le Cap and be arrested; if he failed to show, Leclerc was to wage "a war to the death," and all of L'Ouverture's followers were to be captured, then shot. Once that was completed, slavery would then be ultimately restored. The numerous French soldiers were accompanied by mulatto (a term for mixed race) troops led by Alexandre Pétion and André Rigaud, mulatto leaders who had been defeated by L'Ouverture three years earlier.

All of the French assaults ended in total failure, and after the failure of their last attack, the Haitians charged the French, cutting them down. Leclerc was wounded, and the French lost about 800 men. The final French column to arrive was commanded by General Rochambeau, who brought along heavy artillery that knocked out the Haitian artillery, though his attempt to storm the enemy's position also ended in failure, with about 300 of his men killed. Over the following days, the French kept on bombarding and assaulting the fort, only to be repulsed every time while the Haitians defiantly sang songs of the French Revolution, celebrating the right of all men to be equal and free.

The Haitian psychological warfare was successful, with many French soldiers asking why they were fighting to enslave the Haitians, who were only asserting the rights promised by the Revolution to make all men free. Despite Bonaparte's attempt to keep his plans for slavery secret, it was widely believed by both sides that that was why the French had returned to Haiti, as a sugar plantation could only be profitable

> The Haitian psychological warfare was successful, with many French soldiers asking why they were fighting to enslave the Haitians....

with slave labor. Finally, with food and ammunition running out, Haitian leader Jean-Jacques Dessalines ordered his men to abandon the fort on the night of March 24, 1802, and the Haitians retreated for another day. Even Rochambeau, who hated blacks, admitted in his report: "Their retreat—this miraculous retreat from our trap—was an incredible feat of arms." The French had technically won, but they had lost 2,000 men against an opponent whom they thought to be stupid and cowardly, and it was only shortages of supplies that forced the Haitians to retreat, not because of any military geniuses in the French army.

The French did capture Toussaint L'Ouverture (who would eventually die of pneumonia while imprisoned in the French mountains at Fort-de-Joux), but the expedition as a whole failed because of something even a military expert like Napoleon Bonaparte hadn't thought of: yellow fever. High rates of disease crippled the French army, and Dessalines won a string of victories first against Leclerc—who eventually died of yellow fever—then against Donatien-Marie-Joseph de Vimeur, vicomte de Rochambeau, whom Napoleon had sent to relieve Leclerc with an additional 20,000 men.

In May 1803, with only 8,000 men left standing, Napoleon acknowledged defeat and sent his troops home. The former slaves proclaimed an independent republic that they called Haiti in 1804 with Dessalines—arguably the most successful military commander ever against Napoleon—its first leader. In the rare moment where he felt his reach had exceeded his grasp, Napoleon decided to get out of the colonial game. Where once he had envisioned an empire in North America, in 1803, he sold Louisiana Territory to the United States, instantly doubling its size. The selling price in the Louisiana Purchase was less than three cents per acre, a total of $15 million.

Under Dessalines, Haiti became the first country in the Americas to permanently abolish slavery. He also named himself governor for life while still swearing his loyalty to France. If only the Haitians lived happily ever after.

Haiti's future was destroyed in 1825 when France forced Haiti's people to pay 150 million gold francs in reparations to French ex-slaveholders as a condition of French political recognition and to end the newly formed state's political and economic isolation. In 1838, Haiti pleaded with France to cut its demands to 90 million francs; France agreed, but it would take the first independent black country until 1947 to pay the amount including interest, which is worth about $21 billion today.

Today, Haiti is one of the world's poorest nations; 25 percent of its people live on less than $1.25 per day.

As for yellow fever, it occurs mostly in tropical regions in South America and Africa. In 80 percent of cases, the infection causes very mild symptoms sim-

PLAGUES, PANDEMICS AND VIRUSES

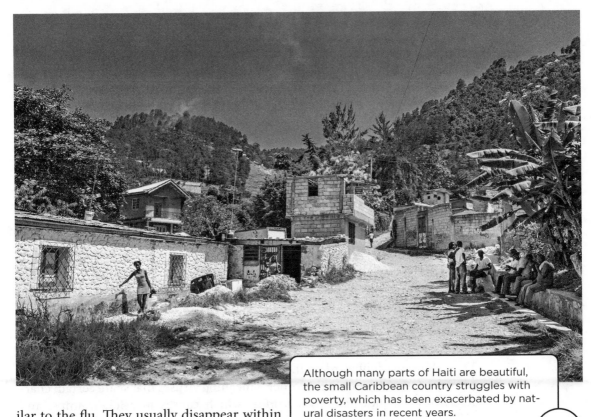

Although many parts of Haiti are beautiful, the small Caribbean country struggles with poverty, which has been exacerbated by natural disasters in recent years.

ilar to the flu. They usually disappear within a few days. In about 20 percent of cases, though, the disease is far more severe, and other symptoms develop: jaundice, kidney disorders, bleeding, convulsions, and coma. Between one-fourth to one-half of these infected patients die. The World Health Organization (WHO) estimates that 30,000 to 60,000 people die of yellow fever each year. Yellow fever is a difficult disease to diagnose, as the symptoms are not enough. A blood sample has to be taken and then tested in a laboratory—and the actual virus still has no actual treatment. Patients can only be helped to overcome the disease by easing the symptoms. Prevention includes spraying insecticides and getting rid of stagnant water, as this is where mosquitoes lay their eggs.

A vaccine was introduced in 1937, and just one dose provides lifelong protection, but it's a tricky vaccine to produce. The virus is first injected into a fertilized chicken egg. The egg is then kept in an incubator for around three days, which is the amount of time it takes for the virus to multiply. Then, the white of the egg, which at this point contains millions of vaccine viruses, is extracted from the egg. The virus is separated and rendered nontoxic. Between one and 300 doses of the vaccine can be obtained from just one egg, a complex and relatively long process. As demand is highly fluctuating, manufacturers do not produce very large quantities. This limited supply is problematic, as the vaccination of millions of people in Angola and Congo is putting considerable pressure on the global stockpile. One possible solution would be to reduce the size of the dose—studies have shown that one-fifth of one dose still provides enough protection—but further studies are required to confirm that this method is truly effective.

Yellow fever erupted during bitter divides over democracy and slavery, and in its wake, it left a changed Caribbean, Europe, and America.

EBOLA

Ebola is a river located in Africa's Democratic Republic of Congo (DRC). In the local Ngbandi language, Ebola was called the *Legbala*, which means "white water." The French, whose language is the official language of the DRC, named it "Ebola"—their adaptation of *Legbala*.

Most people do not know that the Ebola River exists. The Ebola virus, on the other hand, is the stuff of nightmares.

If we reach upward on the Ebola family tree, we find the order *Mononegavirales*. Other viruses in this order—meaning viruses that share certain characteristics—include *Paramyxoviridae*, which causes measles, mumps, and lower-respiratory infections, and *Rhabdoviridae*, which causes rabies. You can think of *Mononegavirales* as the great-grandparent of Ebola and these other viruses as its distant cousins.

After the order comes the even more closely related group called "family." Ebola belongs to the family *Filoviridae*; every virus within this family causes viral hemorrhagic fevers in primates (this means high fevers accompanied by heavy bleeding) and is also found in pigs and bats. *Filoviridae* viruses also replicate in the cytoplasm of a host cell rather than in the nucleus; the nucleus is the more common location for replication. (The smallpox virus and the rabies virus also replicate in cytoplasm.) *Filoviridae* is like the grandparent of Ebola.

Then, just above species on this viral family tree is genus, the Ebola parent. The Ebola genus is *Ebolavirus*. It's divided into six (known) species—think of them as six children—each named for the area where they were first identified:

- *Zaire ebolavirus*—When you think of "Ebola," *Zaire ebolavirus* is the virus you're thinking of. More on that to come.

- *Bundibugyo ebolavirus*—This species was discovered after an outbreak that began on August 1, 2007. It's normally found in Uganda and was first discovered in the Ugandan town of Bundibugyo. It causes the same symptoms as the *Zaire ebolavirus*, but when blood samples from victims were sent to the U.S. Centers for Disease Control and Prevention (CDC), the analysis showed that this was a relative of the other ebolaviruses. A second *B. ebolavirus* outbreak in 2012 was believed to have been caused by eating bushmeat.

Most people do not know that the Ebola River exists. The Ebola virus, on the other hand, is the stuff of nightmares.

- *Reston ebolavirus*—This strain causes Ebola in primates like monkeys but not in humans. The name "Reston" comes from Reston, Virginia, as *Reston ebolavirus* was found in monkeys that Hazelton Laboratories, located in Reston, had imported from the Philippines for research purposes. It's still unclear why the virus was found in primates from the Philippines and not from Africa.

- *Sudan ebolavirus*—The first-ever case of Ebola was reported in June 1976 in South Sudan. The subsequent outbreak infected 284 people and killed 151.

- *Taï Forest ebolavirus*—In 1994, this strain made its one, and so far only, known appearance in the Taï Forest, located in Côte d'Ivoire. Chimpanzees were dying of a hemorrhagic fever, and many tested positive for an ebolavirus infection that was different from those already recorded. One of the scientists performing the necropsies on infected chimpanzees contracted *Taï Forest ebolavirus*. She was transported to Switzerland for treatment and recovered six weeks later; she is the only known human who has been infected by *Taï Forest ebolavirus*.

• *Bombali ebolavirus*, the most recently discovered ebolavirus, was first reported on July 27, 2018, by a research team in the Bombali area of Sierra Leone. *Bombali ebolavirus* was found in the Angolan free-tailed bat and the Little free-tailed bat. In 2019, it also appeared in Angolan free-tailed bats in Kenya and Guinea. *Bombali ebolavirus* can invade human cells, although it has not yet been shown to cause any symptoms.

Of the four that can make humans sick, *Zaire ebolavirus*—the one most commonly known as the "Ebola virus"—is the deadliest; its fatality rate hovers close to 90 percent.

Ebola virus primarily lives and replicates within fruit bats, which means that fruit bats are its most common natural "reservoir." It can live within the bat without killing the bat and spread from the bat to another animal. Scientists believe that humans were first infected with the Ebola virus through handling or eating a fruit bat or

A graphic from a CDC brochure explains how Ebola has transmitted from bats to humans in Africa. After humans contract it, human-to-human transmission is possible.

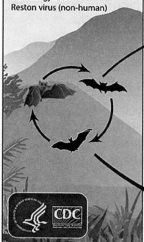

Enzootic Cycle

New evidence strongly implicates bats as the reservoir hosts for ebolaviruses, though the means of local enzootic maintenance and transmission of the virus within bat populations remain unknown.

Ebolaviruses:
Ebola virus (formerly Zaire virus)
Sudan virus
Taï Forest virus
Bundibugyo virus
Reston virus (non-human)

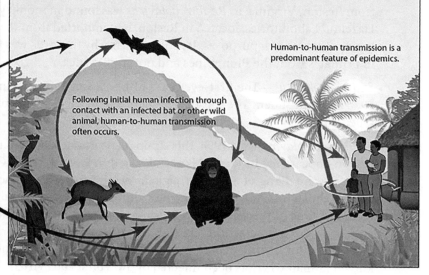

Epizootic Cycle

Epizootics caused by ebolaviruses appear sporadically, producing high mortality among non-human primates and duikers and may precede human outbreaks. Epidemics caused by ebolaviruses produce acute disease among humans, with the exception of Reston virus which does not produce detectable disease in humans. Little is known about how the virus first passes to humans, triggering waves of human-to-human transmission, and an epidemic.

Human-to-human transmission is a predominant feature of epidemics.

Following initial human infection through contact with an infected bat or other wild animal, human-to-human transmission often occurs.

another infected animal. This is called a spillover event—the moment that an animal that is the natural reservoir of a pathogen gives that pathogen to an animal that had never encountered it before. It's also a deadly side effect of humans spreading into territories they'd never been before.

The virus spreads via direct contact (such as through broken skin or mucous membranes in the eyes, nose, or mouth) with:

- Blood or body fluids (urine, saliva, sweat, feces, vomit, breast milk, and semen) of a person who is sick with or has died of Ebola
- Objects (such as clothes, bedding, needles, and medical equipment) contaminated with body fluids from a person who is sick with or has died of Ebola
- Handling or eating infected fruit bats or nonhuman primates like apes and monkeys
- Semen. If a man has recovered from Ebola, his semen can still contain the virus, so someone who has sex with a man who has recovered from Ebola is still at risk of getting it. No evidence exists that Ebola can be spread via sex from a woman to a woman or from a woman to a man.

The period between exposure to an illness and having symptoms is known as the incubation period. A person can only spread Ebola to other people after the incubation period, when they develop signs and symptoms of Ebola.

Transmission between animals and humans is rare, and outbreaks of Ebola virus are often traceable to a case where an individual has handled the carcass of a bat, chimpanzee, or gorilla. The virus then spreads person-to-person, especially within families, in hospitals, and during some funeral rituals where contact among the infected becomes more likely.

Since 1976, 26 Ebola outbreaks have occurred in Africa. The most serious outbreak included 318 people who were infected in 1976 with a fatality rate of 88 percent in the DRC. The last Ebola outbreak began in Guinea in December 2013 and quickly spread to nearby Liberia and Sierra Leone. Within a year, 22,101 suspected cases resulted in a total of 8,818 deaths.

Ebola's First Appearance

A virus is a very small thing: some RNA or DNA and a bit of protein in a hull. It is incapable of doing anything on its own and can only survive and replicate by infecting other cells.

To combat this, we have the immune system. Usually, dendritic cells would activate an army of antiviral cells, support cells, guard cells, and antibody factories that travel to the site of the infection and wipe it out within a matter of days, but when Ebola strikes, it goes straight for the immune system. The first cells it attacks are the dendritic cells, the brains of the immune system.

The first noted infection from *Zaire ebolavirus* happened in August 1976 in Yambuku, a small village in the northern part of

One of the frightening symptoms of Ebola is external bleeding, but this actually only happens in some patients. There are many other complications caused by the virus, as indicated in this graphic.

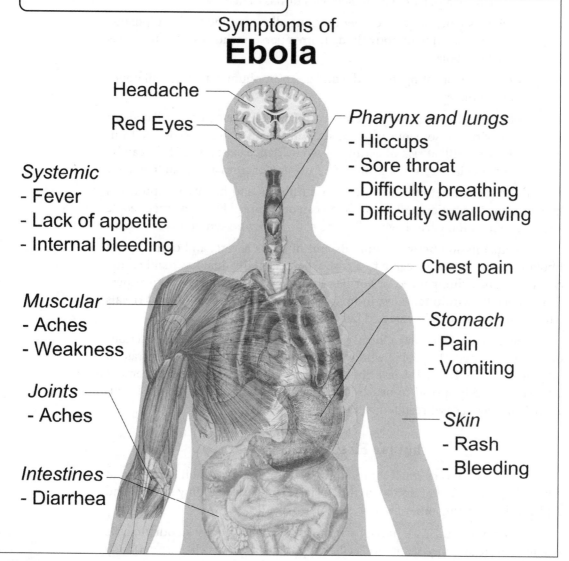

Symptoms of
Ebola

Headache

Red Eyes

Pharynx and lungs
- Hiccups
- Sore throat
- Difficulty breathing
- Difficulty swallowing

Systemic
- Fever
- Lack of appetite
- Internal bleeding

Chest pain

Muscular
- Aches
- Weakness

Stomach
- Pain
- Vomiting

Joints
- Aches

Skin
- Rash
- Bleeding

Intestines
- Diarrhea

the DRC (then known as Zaire). The afflicted was a man named Mabalo Lokela, who was a school headmaster. He began to show symptoms on August 26, after he'd returned from a tour of the Central African Republic with a missionary group; this trip took place from August 12 to 22. Lokela went to the Yambuku Mission Hospital, where he was diagnosed with malaria and given the drug quinine, but he got even worse, and by September 5, he was admitted to Yambuku Mission Hospital again with symptoms that included vomiting, acute diarrhea, chest pains, headache, fever, and, most horrifically, bleeding from all orifices. He died on September 8. Then, his friends and family began to get sick.

After Lokela's body was prepared for burial and then subsequently buried, 21 of his friends and relatives fell seriously ill; only three survived.

Because the Yambuku Mission Hospital had no doctors and only a handful of staff, a cry for help went out on September 12. On September 15, Mgoi Mushola, the first doctor to arrive, wrote a report that became the first description of Ebola. Belgian physician Peter Piot, who would eventually identify the virus, concluded that it was spread by nuns who worked in Yambuku Mission Hospital and had administered injections with unsterilized needles. As a result, dozens of patients who received these injections, as well those those with whom they came into contact, suffered similar symptoms as Mabalo Lokela and died within about a week.

Piot would later write *No Time to Lose: A Life in Pursuit of Deadly Viruses* about Ebola and HIV/AIDS.

The Ebola virus enters the cell by binding onto its receptors. Once inside, it dissolves its outer covering and releases its genetic material, proteins, and enzymes. It takes over the cell, disables its protective mechanism, and reprograms it. The cell now becomes a virus-production machine, using its resources to build more Ebola viruses. Once the cell is saturated, the cell membrane dissolves, and millions of viruses are released into the tissue.

The virus not only prevents the dendritic cell from activating specialized antiviral forces, it manipulates it into sending signals that cause these specialized cells to commit suicide, so the immune system is seriously compromised while the virus multiplies.

Natural killer cells, which would normally destroy our infected cells, also get infected and die before they can stop the disease from spreading. At the same time, Ebola infects macrophages and monocytes—the guard cells of the body. Not only does the virus circumvent their defenses, it also manipulates them into signaling the cells that make up our blood vessels to release fluids into the body. This causes complete mayhem. All over the body, neutrophils are

HOW EBOLA GOT ITS NAME

Late one night, the scientists tracking the virus were debating what to call it. Since it first surfaced in Yambuku, one scientist suggested that it be called the Yambuku virus. However, calling it the Yambuku virus would stigmatize an already stricken village: this had happened before with the town of Lassa, Nigeria, in 1969 for Lassa virus and with Lyme, Connecticut, for Lyme disease.

Karl Johnson, a researcher from the CDC and the leader of the team, suggested naming the virus after a river so as not to put the emphasis on a single place. The first river suggested was the Congo, which is the deepest river in the world and one of the most recognized in Africa, but another virus had gotten there first—the Crimean–Congo hemorrhagic fever virus.

So, the scientists looked at a map for any other rivers near Yambuku. It appeared that the closest river to Yambuku was called Ebola. However, the map was inaccurate, and the Ebola River turned out not to be the closest river to Yambuku. Piot later said, "But in our entirely fatigued state, that's what we ended up calling the virus: Ebola."

activated, awoken by the virus and the macrophages' signals. They begin to do lots of stuff they shouldn't, like signaling the blood vessels to release more fluid, causing internal hemorrhaging.

Another area of the body that Ebola attacks is the liver. Ebola finds it very easy to enter the liver and quickly kills loads of liver cells, causing organ failure and more internal bleeding.

As the virus spreads, it's like bombs exploding everywhere. An incident in one region would be problematic enough, but now it's happening everywhere at once. All the mechanisms the immune system evolved in order to handle infections are now working against you: the virus continues to spread and attack more cells, while the body desperately struggles to stay alive as though its cells were drowning in fluid and viruses.

In a last-ditch effort to stem the tide, the immune system launches what's called a cytokine storm. A cytokine storm is an SOS signal that causes the immune system to launch all of its weapons all at once in a desperate kamikaze attack. Paradoxically, the healthier the immune system, the more damage it can do to itself.

PLAGUES, PANDEMICS AND VIRUSES

This hurts the virus, but it leaves behind tons of collateral damage, especially in the blood vessels. More and more fluid leaves the bloodstream. Blood pours out of your nose and mouth, under your skin, and from your internal organs. You become seriously dehydrated. You just don't have enough blood left to supply your cells with oxygen, and the cells begin to die.

If you reach this point, the chance of you dying is quite high. Currently, six out of ten people who are infected with Ebola die.

During the 1976 epidemic, 318 cases of Ebola were identified in the DRC; of those, 280 died. An additional 284 cases and 151 deaths occurred in nearby Sudan in an unrelated outbreak. Yambuku Mission Hospital eventually closed after eleven of its seventeen staff members died.

Mayinga N'Seka was 22 years old, working at Ngaliema Hospital in Kinshasa City, the capital of the DRC, and was about to travel to Europe to study advanced nursing when she tended to an infected nun who'd been flown in from the Yambuku Mission Hospital. As Peter Piot wrote in *No Time to Lose*:

> Dr. Courteille, the director of Internal Medicine … who was taking care of the nuns and of Mayinga, was careful not to accompany us to the sick nurse's bedside, and it seemed that all the personnel kept a guarded distance from their former colleague. She was very sick, and completely desperate, and convinced she was going to die.
>
> Mayinga had been hospitalized on Friday, October 15, with a high fever and a severe headache. Now, on Monday the 18th, she began bleeding; there were black, sticky stains around her nose, ears, and mouth and blotches under her skin where blood was pooling…. She clung to Pierre Sureau from Institut Pasteur, who soothed her, telling her about [a] serum … that might strengthen her immune system to fight the virus. Sadly the serum didn't work and Mayinga died a few days later.
>
> We drew blood to perform a number of tests that would guide the decision to prescribe supportive treatment for intravascular coagulation, which we thought might be the cause of death in hemorrhagic fever. But none of the technicians or personnel was willing to handle Mayinga's samples for some good reasons, as the hospital lab did not have a containment facility.
>
> I examined her blood, and it was a catastrophe. The platelet count was terrifyingly low. As green and unimaginative as I was, the real lethality of this virus began to sink in, and my hands shook a little

as I handled her blood. Who knew how this virus was transmitted—by insects, or body fluids, or dust.

The Western African Ebola virus epidemic (2013–2016) was the most widespread outbreak of the Ebola virus in history. The first cases were recorded in Guinea in December 2013; later, the disease spread southward to Liberia and then to Sierra Leone. Small outbreaks also occurred in Mali to the north and Nigeria to the east as well as isolated cases in Senegal, which is just north of Guinea, and non-African areas, such as Italy and the United Kingdom.

The number of cases peaked in October 2014 and then began to decline gradually, following the commitment of substantial international resources. By May 2016, the WHO reported that 11,323 people had died, though the WHO also believes that this number is substantially smaller than the real number.

The Kivu Ebola epidemic is the most recent, having first been recorded on August 1, 2018, when it was confirmed that four people had tested positive for the Ebola virus in Kivu, a region in the DRC. By November 2018, the outbreak became the largest in the DRC's history and the second-largest Ebola outbreak in recorded history, behind only the 2013–2016 Western African epidemic. The final death toll was 3,805, and the outbreak was considered finished in April 2020 by the WHO.

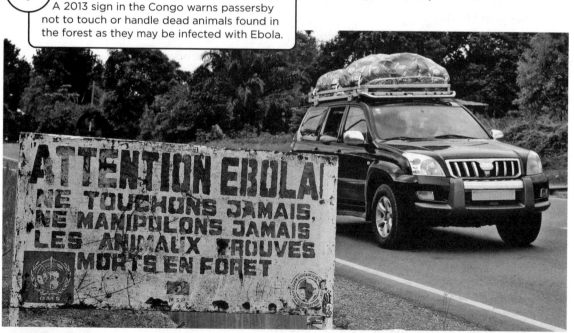

A 2013 sign in the Congo warns passersby not to touch or handle dead animals found in the forest as they may be infected with Ebola.

PLAGUES, PANDEMICS AND VIRUSES

Ebola in the Eyes

The Ebola virus can hide in parts of the body that are called "immuno-logically privileged sites." These are areas where an immune reaction would do more harm than good, like the testes, interior of the eyes, placenta, and cerebrospinal fluid. Whether or not the Ebola virus is present in these body parts and for how long varies from survivor to survivor.

After the Western African Ebola epidemic, almost half of the 15,000-plus survivors developed optical disorders that, left untreated, led to severe eye inflammation, cataracts, and often blindness. In Sierra Leone, an already weak health system was brought to its knees by the outbreak: a country of six million people only had three ophthalmologists.

In February 2015, the outbreak slowed and survival rates improved, but eye complications emerged like a new epidemic. Hundreds of people had visible symptoms, but some also had "quiet" eyes—eyes that were no longer inflamed but, having gone untreated, developed cataracts and retinal and nerve damage. Partners in Health, a global-health nonprofit, stepped in to help coordinate Ebola-survivor eye care in the country.

Ian Crozier was treating Ebola patients at a hospital in Kenema, Sierra Leone, which itself was so riddled with the virus that people were admonished not to touch the walls.

As an article in *The New York Times* described it:

Blood, stool and vomit were ever-present though cleaners mopped with chlorine several times a day. Choruses of delirious patients with bloodshot, eerily vacant eyes would shout "Doctor! Doctor!" over and over. Some were too sick to clean or feed themselves, and there were never enough staff members to tend to them. A patient might lie in one bed and a corpse in the next, waiting to be disinfected, bagged and taken away.

"Those isolation wards are horrible places," Dr. Crozier said.

But there were moments of grace. Mothers whose babies had died would feed children who were orphaned or alone.

"Childless parents took care of parentless children," he said.

Crozier eventually became infected with the Ebola virus and was airlifted to Emory University Hospital in Atlanta, Georgia, specifically into their isolation ward, where he remained for 40 days, the longest stay of any Ebola patient. Crozier is often given the honor of being the sickest Ebola patient ever to survive.

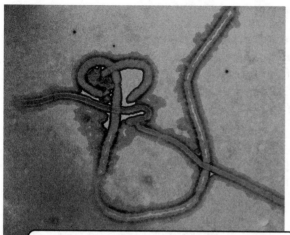

The Ebola virus lives very comfortably in human blood, causing inflamation that leads to a patient's clotting proteins to go into high gear. This can cause blockages, while, at the same time, platelets are low, allowing for more bleeding both internally and, at times, externally.

The *Times* article, dated December 7, 2014, ends with this:

Dr. Crozier hopes to return to West Africa by February or March to help treat more Ebola patients. Survivors are thought to be immune to the strain that infected them, so he figures he has built-in protection.

"There's still a great deal left to be done," he said.

Unfortunately, the virus wasn't done with him. Several months after he was declared free of the virus, Crozier's left eye began to swell, causing him terrible pain and blurred vision. His doctors thought that Crozier's weakened immune system may have left him open to an infection, but after extracting a few drops of fluid from the sore eye, doctors were shocked to find the Ebola virus living comfortably in there.

Though undetectable in Crozier's blood, the virus had been squatting for months in the anterior chamber—the fluid-filled part—of the eye, perhaps even replicating, without spurring an immune response. What triggered a reaction is unknown, but it caused an infection called uveitis. Crozier's blue eye turned green, and the vision in that eye went from blurry to almost nothing until a three-month regimen that included antiviral medication and prednisone began to bring the world back into focus.

Research on where, how long, and at what concentration the virus can survive is ongoing. One of the issues is that so few Ebola victims survive that it's hard to track what happens afterward, but it's estimated that 40 percent of survivors eventually contract uveitis. Luckily, Crozier's sight slowly retuned, and his green eye is now blue again and Ebola free.

ZIKA VIRUS

Flaviviridae is a family of viruses that got its name from the Latin word *flavus*, meaning "yellow," so named because one of the diseases it causes—yellow fever—gives its victims a jaundiced pallor. (As part of the international language of pathogens and their symptoms, the word "jaundice" comes from the French word *jaune*, meaning "yellow.") *Flaviviridae* viruses are mostly spread through mosquitoes; other diseases that come from this family include West Nile virus and Dengue fever, but from 2015 to 2016 a different *Flaviviridae* epidemic frightened the population: the Zika virus.

The Zika virus (ZIKV) was initially found in 1947 from the serum of a sick monkey—called Rhesus 766—that had lived in Uganda's Ziika forest but then became one of many that were unwillingly part of the Rockefeller Foundation's ongoing medical research in the area. *Ziika* is the Lugandan word for "overgrown" (the additional "i" was taken out when naming it), though that moniker no longer applies, as today, the forest is less than one-tenth the size of New York's Central Park due to a highway that cuts through it and an airport built over it. However, in the 1940s, this tropical forest, or jungle, was still dense, hot, and wild, and shortly after its discovery, ZIKV was isolated within *Aedes africanus* mosquitoes, which also live in the same area. Further research determined that both the *Aedes africanus* and the similar *Aedes aegypti* mosquitoes were vectors for ZIKV, passing the virus between monkeys and mice (which were imported to Uganda as part of the testing), causing researchers to believe that the equal-opportunity mosquitoes could also transmit the virus to people.

We don't normally think of appearance when it comes to mosquitoes—we usually just try to kill them—yet mosquitoes do come in different shapes, though they don't vary much in size. No Triassic-esque, gigantic mosquito is lurking deep in the jungle—none that we know of, anyway. However, one way mosquitoes differ from most other creatures is that the female is bigger than the male. She's also the only one that bites in order to draw the blood that feeds her eggs.

Like the rat and the flea (and also the gerbil), *Ae. aegypti* has moved from continent to continent via ships....

The *Ae. africanus* mosquito has distinct, white-and-black stripes along its body that help differentiate it from others. It lives in the African jungles. The *Ae. aegypti* mosquito, which originated in Africa, appears to have had a foothold on the Mediterranean region from the late eighteenth to the mid-twentieth century. It's practically disappeared there but has been tracked to southern Russia, the Republic of Georgia, the southeastern United States, South America, the Middle East, Southeast Asia, the Pacific and Indian Islands, and northern Australia. Like the rat and the flea (and also the gerbil), *Ae. aegypti* has moved from continent to continent via ships, and this method of dispersal, and its widespread colonization and distribution in the tropics, has led to the highly efficient, interhuman transmission of viruses. It is nowadays one of the most widespread mosquito species on Earth.

ZIKV was reported sporadically within Africa and Southeast Asia, but the first outbreak began in Micronesia in 2007 and French Polynesia in 2013. Between 2013 and 2015, an El Niño event occurred, with higher temperatures and torrential rainfall in southern Brazil. Many Brazilians were left homeless due to flooding, but for mosquitoes, these were Eden-like conditions, and their populations exploded. Between 2014 and 2015, an alarming number of patients began coming to Brazilian hospitals with rashes, fevers, and pinkeye, seemingly some sort of mystery infection. Over 6,800 blood samples were tested for various diseases until ZIKV was confirmed to be the one, and unlike the often hideously fatal dengue or yellow fevers, ZIKV patients recovered relatively quickly with no long-term effects. Some doctors said it was like getting the chicken pox or measles—once you had it, you were done with it. The then Brazilian health minister, Dr. Arthur Chioro, told reporters, "Zika virus doesn't worry us, it's a benign disease." He was proven wrong.

A number of babies were soon born in Brazil with tiny heads, a condition called microcephaly. Others looked fine but wailed as though colicky, with a high-pitched scream like they were in pain. Still others seemed unable to gain control of their muscles. Some couldn't focus their eyes; others were deaf. Many profoundly disabled newborns died. None of these infants who were tested had tested positive for ZIKV—but their mothers mentioned that they'd had *doença misteriosa*—Portuguese for "the mystery disease," which is what ZIKV was first called in Brazil—while pregnant. ZIKV was then found in the amniotic fluid of one pregnant mother and in the blood of two stillborn fetuses. Apparently, ZIKV crossed the placental wall and infected the fetus, causing newborn microcephaly. Globally, 2,656 cases of neurological abnormalities were confirmed, 89 percent of which were diagnosed in Brazil.

On February 2, 2016, ZIKV was deemed a Public Health Emergency of International Concern by the WHO after it quickly spread from Brazil, crossing

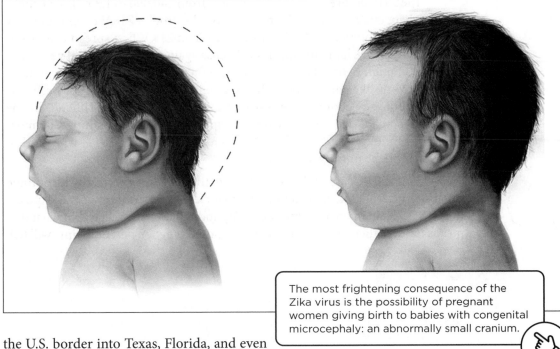

The most frightening consequence of the Zika virus is the possibility of pregnant women giving birth to babies with congenital microcephaly: an abnormally small cranium.

the U.S. border into Texas, Florida, and even Hawaii. The CDC released a domestic travel advisory warning pregnant or planning-to-be-pregnant women to avoid traveling to those areas.

One way that ZIKV greatly differs from other insect-borne diseases like malaria or Lyme disease is that it can also be transmitted sexually, mostly from men to women. The first case of sexually transmitted ZIKV was reported in Colorado in 2008. A woman developed symptoms related to the ZIKV infection, but she hadn't traveled to any region where ZIKV is endemic or normally found. However, she mentioned that she'd had vaginal intercourse with her infected husband after he had returned home from Senegal just before the onset of his symptoms. Since then, the number of sexually transmitted ZIKV cases where ZIKV is not endemic has increased especially because almost 80 percent of ZIKV patients never have any symptoms, and others can spread it after the symptoms have gone. Even pregnant women who have sex with a man who's had ZIKV risk becoming infected and passing the disease on to her baby, so the CDC advises men who have traveled to an area where ZIKV is endemic to either use condoms or not have sex for at least six months after they return. The longest documented interval between a man's onset of symptoms and sexual transmission to a woman is 44 days, but again, that's with an onset of symptoms, so doctors could track Day One to Day Forty-Four. Without symptoms, it's anyone's guess.

The 2015 outbreak infected anywhere from 440,000 to 1.3 million people. So, what happened to Zika? Where did it go? The drop in ZIKV cases is possibly due to the development of herd immunity. When ZIKV first spread from Central Africa, humans had little immune defense against it. Now, several years after the peak, enough people have become immune to the virus that it has, indeed, almost become like chicken pox. "If a large enough proportion of the herd—be it cows or mice or people—are resistant to a disease, it's very difficult for the disease to spread," Dr. Uriel Kitron, an expert in viruses transmitted by mosquitoes at Emory University, told the *Chicago Tribune* in 2017, when ZIKV numbers were beginning to drop.

Even if ZIKV is suddenly eradicated, the ones still affected by it continue to cause concern. Only 6 percent of pregnancies where the mother was exposed to ZIKV resulted in obvious microcephaly and other birth defects, but what that means for the other 94 percent of ZIKV-exposed pregnancies, only time will tell.

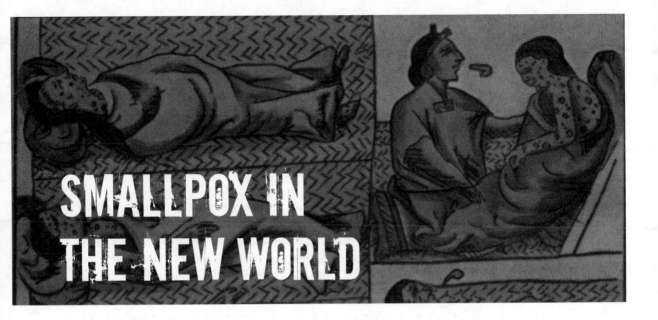

SMALLPOX IN THE NEW WORLD

When European explorers, settlers, and conquerors came to the shores of the Americas, it was the beginning of the end for the civilizations there, including the Inca, Maya, and Aztecs of Central and South America, and the many Indigenous peoples of North America. But it wasn't just guns and cavalry that killed countless native people in the New World. No, the Europeans had a silent partner in their conquests: smallpox.

Many Americans don't know much about the differences between the Maya, Aztec, and Inca civilizations, other than they all once had impressive cities, including pyramids and other great buildings, and that the arrival of the Spanish conquerors ultimately led to their annihilation.

Somewhere betwen 20 to 50 million people are believed to have lived in the Americas shortly before the Europeans' arrival, and almost all of them died of European diseases.

One of the reasons people today don't know the difference between these empires is that their story is often only told as it relates to Europeans, so even in the obliteration of the Aztecs, Maya, and Incas, the Spanish are still in the lead roles, yet these empires were complex and thrived for centuries—though the Maya was the only ancient civilization—before the Spanish conquistadores landed in the New World.

Like the plague, smallpox killed warriors, it killed slaves, and it killed kings, queens, and princesses, and if you happened to survive, you were terribly scarred, emotionally and physically. England's Queen Elizabeth I, who reigned in the sixteenth century, is often shown wearing heavy, white makeup; this was not the fashion of the day but, rather, her best attempt at covering the small-pox-scarred face of a queen.

George Washington survived smallpox as well, having caught the disease in 1751 while in Barbados. He was left only slightly scarred, though he described smallpox as "more destructive to an Army in the Natural way, than the Enemy's Sword."

Variola major and *Variola minor* are the viruses that cause smallpox—or, rather, "caused" because smallpox is the only disease that affects humans that we've successfully wiped off Earth. The last known case was in Somalia in 1977. The infected person was a cook named Ali Maow Maalin. (Maalin recovered but later died in 2013 in Merca, Somalia, from malaria while carrying out polio vaccinations.) Smallpox was officially declared eradicated in 1979.

In terms of size, *Variola* is one of the larger viruses—so gigantic, comparatively speaking, that it can be seen under a regular microscope. *Variola* is shaped like a dumbbell and is covered with two membranes that are themselves covered in tubules. It's highly contagious and spreads through the air in droplets—much the same way you catch a cold or the flu (which are also caused by viruses). Smallpox can also be spread through contact with bedding or clothes that are contaminated with *Variola* that lives in certain bodily fluids, such as the fluids inside a smallpox pustule or scab.

Symptoms usually begin about two weeks after the infection and include exhaustion, high fever, and achiness. Then, it takes a horrific turn, as the skin erupts with sores that spread all over the entire body, oozing pus and disfiguring victims. It's a largely fatal disease that was powerful enough to level empires and redesign the map of the world, and, in the 1980s, it was still being cultivated by the Soviet Union for biological warfare.

Let's back up a minute, though. We're talking about smallpox, but what about chicken pox or even cowpox? What's a pox?

The word "pox" is a plural form of the Old English word "pock," as in "pockmarked," which is precisely what you become when you get the pox. Symptoms don't begin with the initial infection, so at this point, infected people are unaware that they're in an incubation period. They're not even contagious. It's like they're strapped in a roller-coaster, slowly creeping up the tracks. When they become contagious is when lesions develop inside their mouths. Now, the roller-coaster shoots down the slope, the infection is released into the saliva, and it can be spread by coughing or sneezing. Around 24–48 hours after the throat lesions burst, *Variola* aims the next phase of its attack on the skin, and the roller-coaster goes upside down in the loop, where that which can save you,

PLAGUES, PANDEMICS AND VIRUSES

the seat belt of the immune system, has worn thin. You're going to fall.

First, a rash called "macules" appears, usually on the forehead, torso, and extremities. Within a day or so, the macules transform from a rash into raised, blisterlike "papules." Once the papules fill with liquid, they become "vesicles," which then harden into "pustules." As their name suggests, pustules are filled with pus, which is mostly dead white blood cells from our immune system that have accumulated at the site of infection; pustules cover the entire body—even the palms of the hands and the soles of the feet—and harden over the course of a week.

Eventually, the pus leaks out and the pustules scab over, causing scarring and possibly blindness if they settle in the eyes. This is when patients are most infectious since the very scabs contain fragments of the virus bound within a fibrous mesh of skin cells. In fatal cases, death usually occurs from 10 days to two weeks after the onset of the illness, yet the actual cause of death is not clear. One possibility is pneumonia, which can take over the lungs due to a depleted immune system that is vulnerable against countless infections it might've otherwise been able to destroy.

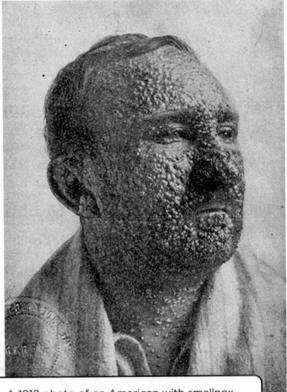

A 1912 photo of an American with smallpox shows how severe the scarring can be. The disease can cause blindness, bone infections, fetal death (in pregnant women), and death.

The Smallpox Family

Taxonomy is a scientific way of classifying all living things from spiders to daffodils. The International Committee on Taxonomy of Viruses (ICTV) are the people who give a virus its name. This is one way to neatly sort out, for example, which order, family, and genus a virus belongs to and arrange it into a kind of pathogenic family tree, which then helps to determine how to fight it. (Note that this naming convention—i.e., order, family, genus—is applied to all living things or, in the case of viruses, semiliving things.)

Based on a range of shared criteria, each is divided into a particular group, then subdivided into a smaller group, then an even smaller one, and so forth. Humans belong to the family *Hominidae*, which includes gorillas, chimpanzees, and orangutans, known as "the great apes." Then, from *Hominidae*, they're subdivided into the genus *Homo*, which includes today's humans as well as Neanderthals, and finally into the species *Homo sapiens*, Latin for "wise man." We are the only *Homo sapiens* on Earth.

Viruses are classified in the same way. The pox virus is the largest and most complex of the viruses that infect mammals, birds, and insects. Its large size, dumbbell-like inner shape, and double rather than single strand of DNA puts it in the genus *Orthopoxvirus*—every virus in this genus has the same traits. These viruses cause fevers and rashes among animals and humans. (Most infections occur in animals and then spread to humans, giving the virus the description "zoonotic.")

What comes after *Orthopoxvirus* is the family *Poxviridae*, which includes the virus that causes smallpox. Humans, vertebrates, and arthropods (i.e., insects, spiders, and crustaceans) can be infected. It replicates in the cytoplasm, the fluid contained within a cell; by comparison, most viruses replicate in a cell's nucleus. This means that a pox virus must come fully equipped with all it needs to replicate since it won't be taking advantage of a host cell's control center.

The genus that comes after *Poxviridae*, called *Orthopox*, specifically targets humans and other mammals—it includes cowpox and monkeypox (but not chicken pox because even though it has "pox" in its name, its virus belongs to

WHITE POX KILLING CORAL REEFS

Sea creatures can die from pathogens as well. Human waste has caused what's known as "white pox" in coral reefs, specifically in the Florida Keys and the Caribbean. "This is quite an unusual discovery. It is the first time ever that a human disease has been shown to kill an invertebrate," said University of Georgia professor James Porter, one of the study researchers. "This is unusual because we humans get disease from wildlife, and this is the other way around." Most wastewater isn't filtered in these areas but disposed of in septic systems on land, allowing contaminants to leak into the ocean. The bacteria *Serratia marcescens* causes intestinal problems in humans, which can lead to larger than usual amounts of unfiltered feces and urine in the water, which then carry the bacteria to the coral. It causes irregular white patches or blotches that result from the loss of coral, and the coral ultimately dies.

the family *Herpesviridae*, not *Poxviridae*). *Variola major* and *Variola minor* are the species of virus that infect humans, with the former being more virulent than the latter.

    Variola replicates much the same as other viruses. It binds to a receptor on the cell's outer membrane, then is drawn into the cell, where an enzyme called uncoatase "unwraps" the virus's membrane and allows its DNA to enter the cell's cytoplasm. This is where infection begins. The DNA then replicates with the help of proteins called Guaneri bodies. About 10,000 viruses are produced from each infected cell. Even though *Variola* is large and complex as far as viruses go, replication is relatively quick—about 12 hours—until the host cell dies and the viruses are released. (Some, like the virus that causes Dengue fever, can take more than a day.)

> Even though *Variola* is large and complex as far as viruses go, replication is relatively quick ... until the host cell dies and the viruses are released.

Farming Leads to Infection

    In the interest of increasing agriculture and farm development, humans have tried over centuries to domesticate countless animals. Through trial and error, they learned that the best animals to domesticate usually have certain characteristics: they reproduce at a young age, give birth to at least one or two offspring a year, and don't cost a lot to feed. They should also have a social hierarchy. Imagine a typical video game where you're fighting the head bad guy or boss. Once the boss is killed, all its followers usually die as well. Although not as dramatic in the wild, if you're able to control the boss, or alpha male and female, you're able to control the entire herd.

    Another critical trait is that the animal needs to be able to work for humans. Just as some people cannot work in an office cubicle, some animals just are not wired to live on a farm. Horses can be domesticated, but no one has been able to domesticate their cousin, the zebra. Zebras have a combination of unpredictability and skittishness that can lead to getting kicked in the head—which is why you normally don't see people riding zebras.

So, which animals make the cut? Aside from horses, people have also successfully domesticated chickens, pigs, goats, cows, and donkeys—these were among the livestock that Europeans brought with them, along with wheat and barley, when they traveled to the New World.

Interestingly, none of the livestock that the Europeans introduced to the New World were native to Europe. They originated at the Fertile Crescent, the part of the Middle East where agriculture began. Once people were able to cultivate grain and domesticate animals, they—along with their grain and livestock—moved into North Africa and Europe. By the sixteenth century, the time of the conquistadores, domesticated animals that had originated in the Fertile Crescent dominated European farms.

The Aztecs

The Aztecs didn't call themselves "Aztecs." They were "Mexica" (meh-SHEE-ca). "Aztec" was a name given to them based on their legendary homeland, Aztlán, and it's the one we use today.

We know very little about the Aztecs before their civilization took hold; in 1430, their *Tlatoani* (meaning "emperor" or "king"), named Itzcoatl, demanded that all historical manuscripts, known as codices, be burned. Consequently, Itzcoatl then created a new mythological Aztec history, one that worshipped Huitzilopochtli, the god of the sun and the patron of the largest pre-Columbian city-state, Tenochtitlán.

Huitzilopochtli's name is commonly translated as "southern hummingbird," a docile-sounding sobriquet that belied his stature as a warrior god. Priests who

---

THE SERPENT WALL OF TENOCHTITLÁN

The Templo Mayor was Tenochtitlán's most important building, measuring 1,200 feet on each side and surrounded by a wall covered in carvings of snakes, known as the *coatepantli* or "Serpent Wall." The north (right) side was dedicated to Tlaloc, the god of rain. It was painted with blue stripes and marked the summer solstice, the time of growth. The south (left) side was dedicated to Huitzilopochtli, the god of war. It was painted red and marked the winter solstice, the time of war.

---

interpreted Huitzilopochtli's signs brought the Aztecs south from their legendary home, Aztlán, to
their new home in today's Mexico. (Where Aztlán
was located is still debated: Oregon, California,
and northern Mexico, among several other territories, have been put forth as possible locations.)
This was a journey that supposedly took hundreds
of years and crossed thousands of miles.

By the beginning of the 1400s, the Aztec
Empire was an alliance of three city-states: Tenochtitlán, Texcoco, and Tlacopan (though
Tenochtitlán became the dominant city-state).
This alliance controlled most of northern and
central Mexico and included territory as far
away as Guatemala and Honduras—80,000
square miles that they were able to acquire as
fierce warriors. The Aztec military, which included men from allied and conquered territories, were divided into elite groups, like the Eagle and Jaguar warriors, and swept aside their rivals as though flicking off bugs.

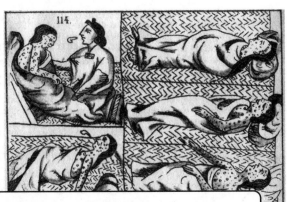

Native Americans were killed off en masse
not so much by swords and guns of the Europeans but by diseases such as smallpox. This
sixteenth-century illustration shows Aztecs
dying of the disease.

Aztec warriors wore padded, cotton armor, held a shield covered in animal hide, and carried weapons like sharp, obsidian sword-clubs and bows and
arrows. The Eagle and Jaguar warriors wore spectacular feathers and animal
skins and headdresses to signify their elite rank. Battles were concentrated in
or around major cities, and when these fell, the victors claimed the surrounding
territory. Regular tributes were extracted, and captives were taken back to Tenochtitlán for ritual sacrifice.

Not only the political and religious capital, Tenochtitlán was the center of
trade and commerce, overflowing with gold, greenstone, turquoise, cotton, cacao
beans, tobacco, tools, weapons, and slaves. Its people created magnificent architecture and artwork, like the Templo Mayor pyramid, which is what many people think
of when they think of the Aztecs. Dominating the city was the huge sacred precinct,
with its temples and monumental ball court. The Aztecs also provided Tenochtitlán
with an impressive irrigation system, including large canals that bisected the city,
which was itself surrounded by flooded fields that greatly increased the amount of
food they produced. Beautiful flower gardens also boomed around the city.

The Spanish arrived in 1519. Within two years, 3.2 million Aztecs would
be dead, along with their entire civilization. No rebuilding could occur, as happened in Europe after the Black Death, and no shifting of religion or economics.
It was finished.

A Tale of Two Conquistadores

Hernán Cortés de Monroy y Pizarro Altamirano, also known as Hernando Cortés, was born in 1495 in Medellín, part of what was the Kingdom of Castille (now western Spain). His family's pedigree was more impressive than its wealth, and since this was a time of great adventure on the high seas, the haughty and mischievous Cortés dreamed of leaving Medellín—and his impending future as a civil servant—to join his kinsmen in exploring the New World. Cortés would eventually conquer the Aztecs.

His maternal grandmother, Leonor Sánchez Pizarro Altamirano, was the first cousin of Gonazalo Pizarro y Rodriguez. Gonazalo's son was conquistador Francisco Pizarro. (This meant that Cortés and Francisco Pizarro were second cousins, once removed.)

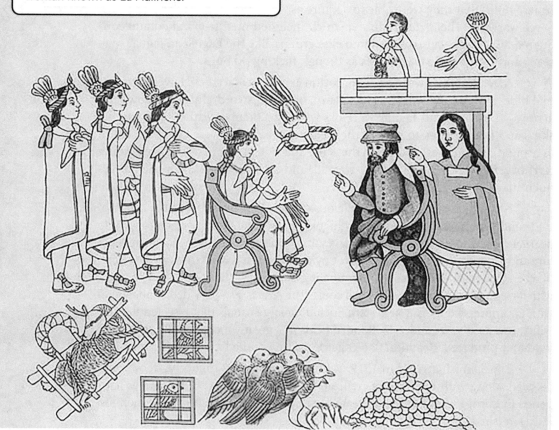

A c. 1550 illustration showing Hernán Cortés meeting the Aztec leader Moctezuma. With Cortés is his interpreter, the native woman known as La Malinche.

Like Cortés, Pizarro came from Castille, but unlike Cortés, no one is positive when he was born (historians date it to sometime between 1471 and 1476). His father was a soldier, and his mother was a servant; Pizarro was illegitimate and grew up poor and uneducated. He was illiterate. He spent his youth as a swineherd in a nondescript town called Trujillo. He would eventually conquer the Incas.

In 1504, Cortés left Spain for the island of Hispanola (which is now split into Haiti and the Dominican Republic). For 15 years, he rose through the ranks of the Spanish political machine, played a large role in the conquest of Cuba, and became *alcalde*, or mayor, of Santiago, Cuba. Cortés also became a rich man, thanks to his mines, cattle, and slaves.

However, as in Medellín, Cortés's wanderlust came roaring back—especially after he heard about the enormous quantity of gold and riches, all for the taking, on the mainland of the New World. In 1518, he left to see Mexico, accompanied by 11 ships and 500 men, on an expedition paid for by the Cuban governor and Cortés's brother-in-law, Diego Velázquez. Cortés's orders were only to establish a trade agreement with the Natives, then return to Cuba, so that Velázquez and his men could take over the mainland. This would ensure that the riches and legends would go to Velázquez. Cortés, nobody's fool, founded Villa Rica de la Vera Cruz, or Veracruz (meaning "true cross"), on May 18, 1519, as soon as he and his men made landfall. It was the first Spanish town in what is now Mexico. Cortés named himself ruler and ignored Velázquez's authority. The building of Veracruz was helped by the Totonac, whom Cortés had won over by imprisoning the men who collected Totonac taxes on behalf of Aztec emperor Moctezuma.

The Spanish then marched inland toward the Aztec Empire, guided by a fellow Spaniard who had stayed behind during an earlier expedition and now acted as translator. Cortés and his men defeated the Tlaxcala, who had been fighting the Aztecs for the last 100 years. Now, Cortés had 500 Spanish soldiers and an army of 3,000 Tlaxcala with him as he entered the Aztec holy city of Cholula in October 1519, where he slaughtered 3,000 people and leveled the city.

Cortés then marched victoriously into Tenochtitlán, the Aztec capital. Tenochtitlán was indeed a sight to behold, with its pyramids, canals, and gold. This was a city larger than any other European city except perhaps Constantinople.

Aztec emperor Moctezuma and his chiefs, bedecked with gold, feathers, and jewels, invited Cortés to join him as an honored guest in his palace. Cortés, of course, accepted, and Moctezuma had the royal palace of Axayácatl prepared for him. While in the palace, the conquistadores found the secret room where Moctezuma kept the treasure he had inherited from his father. According to

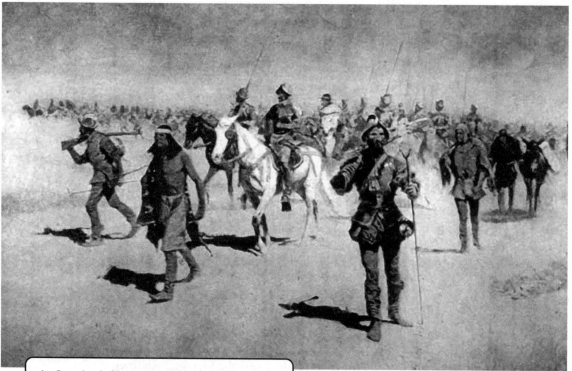

As Spaniards like Juan Vázquez de Coronado explored, conquered, and settled the new world, they brought horses, livestock, and disease with them (from a 1905 painting by Frederic Remington).

one Spaniard, the treasure consisted of a "quantity of golden objects—jewels and plates and ingots.... The sight of all that wealth dumbfounded me."

Cortés, along with five of his captains, convinced Moctezuma to "come quietly with us to our quarters, and make no protest.... If you cry out, or raise any commotion, you will immediately be killed." So, just like that, Moctezuma was a prisoner, though still led as a puppet ruler, with Cortés pulling the strings.

Cortés sent expeditions to find out just where all the gold was. Moctezuma had to pay a tribute to the Spanish king, which included his father's treasure. (The Spanish would melt these treasures down into coins, destroying what must have been incredible works of art.) Finally, Moctezuma let the Catholic conquistadores build an altar on their temple next to the Aztec gods.

Then, word made it to Cortés that Velázquez's soldiers had landed at Veracruz with orders to drag him back in chains. According to accounts, at least one of Velázquez's soldiers had smallpox. (The introduction of smallpox had been attributed to an African slave named Francisco Eguía, but this is now

PLAGUES, PANDEMICS AND VIRUSES

heavily disputed. It's quite difficult—and, back then, arguably impossible—to trace an epidemic to one person, especially because others were asymptomatic. It was easier just to blame a slave.)

Immunity

As mentioned, domesticated animals like horses, pigs, and chickens were native to the Middle East and dominated the landscape of Europe. These animals helped us develop agriculture, but they also carried diseases which jumped from them to us, including smallpox, influenza, and measles. The only domesticated animals of Mesoamerica were the llama and the alpaca. By the 1500s, generations of Europeans had developed an immune system that was able to cope with many of these illnesses. (Europeans at the time still died of smallpox, measles, and the flu, but not in the millions like the Native Americans did.)

Even though the Aztecs and the Spanish were all human beings, their bodies were not the same, given the vastly different worlds they and their ancestors had become acclimated to. The immune system of a European was far different from that of a Maya, an Inca, or an Aztec—or, for that matter, any Native American. It recognized these diseases that caught the Native immune system by surprise and overwhelmed it until population after population died.

The Europeans who made landfall and were infected with diseases either had them in a dormant state, were actively infected but had no symptoms, or only had mild symptoms because their immune system was getting rid of the disease. They therefore often unknowingly passed the diseases to Natives, starting epidemics. The trade of Native American captives and the continued use of commercial trade routes led to the usual horrific outcomes.

EVOLUTION OF INCA LUNGS

The Inca Empire included populations that extended through the Andes Mountains, and those who had lived there for generations had developed an anatomy that allowed them to breathe in high altitudes, which have less oxygen. Compared to the Spanish, the Andres-dwelling Incas had almost one-third larger lung capacity, slower heart rates, four pints more blood volume, and double the amount of hemoglobin—a protein that carries oxygen from the lungs to the rest of the body.

Cortés rushed back to Veracruz and defeated his would-be captors, convincing the survivors to travel with him to the city of gold. He then returned to find the Aztecs engaged in an enormous rebellion against the Spanish. Cortés and his men turned and fled.

However, what neither Cortés nor the natives realized was that smallpox had now taken hold in the New World and traveled with the Spanish to Tenochtitlán, where it was about to wipe out large swaths of the Western Hemisphere. By 1519, it had spread roughly 150 miles north from Veracruz to Tenochtitlán. It killed many of its victims outright, particularly infants and young children. Many other adults were incapacitated by the disease because they were either sick themselves, caring for sick family members, or simply lost the will to resist the Spaniards. Consequently, no one was left to harvest crops, which caused widespread famine, further weakening their immune systems. In many cases, everyone in a house died. With no time to bury so many people, homes were

TYPHOID MARY

Mary Mallon was born in Ireland in 1869 and came to the United States in around 1883, finding work as a cook. In 1900, she worked in Mamaroneck, New York, where, within two weeks of the start of her employment, residents developed typhoid fever. In 1901, she moved to New York City, where members of the next family for whom she worked developed fevers and diarrhea, and the laundry maid died. Mallon then went to work for a lawyer and left after seven of the eight people in the house got sick.

A typhoid researcher named George Soper tried to find a common thread within all the families. He believed it was the cook, Mary Mallon, even though she herself was never sick. The New York City health inspector determined she was a carrier, and Mallon was held in isolation for three years. Mallon was called "Typhoid Mary" in a 1908 issue of the *Journal of the American Medical Association*. The name stuck. After returning to life as a cook at the Sloane Hospital for Women in New York City, 25 people there were infected, and two died. Mallon spent the rest of her life in quarantine at the Riverside Hospital in the Bronx. On November 11, 1938, she died of pneumonia at the age of 69. Supposedly, an autopsy uncovered live typhoid bacteria in her gallbladder, though George Soper wrote, "There was no autopsy." Mallon's body was cremated, and her ashes were buried at St. Raymond's Cemetery in the Bronx.

simply demolished over the bodies. (Also, a series of epidemics occurred over the subsequent 50 years, which killed even more than the first epidemic. The Aztecs called it *cocoliztli*, which may have been typhoid fever. "Nobody had the health or strength to help the diseased or bury the dead," one Franciscan friar wrote in 1577. "In the cities and large towns, big ditches were dug, and from morning to sunset the priests did nothing else but carry the dead bodies and throw them into the ditches.")

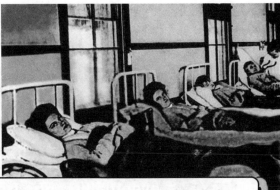

"Typhoid" Mary Mallon is shown here in the foreground in her hospital bed. Doctors showed she was personally responsible for spreading the disease to dozens of people.

By the time Cortés and the Spanish had returned to Tenochtitlán with 8,000 Tlaxcala, their foreign diseases had already done considerable damage. Moctezuma would eventually be killed, with accounts varying from him being stoned to death by his angry former followers to the Spanish killing him. His brother, Cuitláhuac, took over as emperor, but he soon died of smallpox. Now, the Aztecs lacked stable leadership and were in a state called *interregnum*—Latin for "inter-reign," or a time between rulers. This is a time when societies are the most unbalanced, and, actually, the Aztecs would never have another ruler.

Aztec sources agree that Cuitláhuac died from a terrible pestilence—reported variously as *cocoliztli* (illness, pestilence, smallpox), *huey zahuatl* (leprosy), or *totomonaliztli* (blisters). These terms describe the symptoms but not the diseases. Since smallpox had never existed before, they had no word for it. (Smallpox is the disease cited as the one that most leveled the New World empires, but the Europeans also brought with them plague, chicken pox, cholera, diphtheria, the flu, malaria, measles, scarlet fever, sexually transmitted infections, typhoid, typhus, tuberculosis, pertussis, and the common cold.)

The Aubin Codex, a pictorial record of Aztec history, starts with the Aztecs' departure from Aztlán and extends to Cuitláhuac's death after the arrival of the Spanish. The pictograph, which shows Cuitláhuac's death, depicts his enshrouded corpse covered with tiny circles, the symbol for smallpox, according to the late Mexican historian Orozco y Berra.

Cortés's victory at Tenochtitlán set in motion the rapid collapse of the Aztec Empire. Smallpox continued to ravage the indigenous population and cripple their capacity to resist the Spanish—and, in truth, they had little way to fight back. While the Spanish had gunpowder and steel, the indigenous tribes only had the clubs, darts, and arrows.

About 200,000 Aztecs died trying to save their city until Cortés and disease strangled the life out of it.

Mortality estimates would eventually range from one-quarter to one-half of the population of central Mexico. In 1541, a Spanish monk named Fray Toribio de Benavente Motolinía published the *History of the Indians of New Spain*, a sympathetic account of the people he ministered to in the name of the Catholic Church. In the first chapter of *History*, Motolinía used the biblical allegory of the 10 plagues to help the reader understand the ravages that destroyed an entire people. The account begins with the smallpox that erupted in Tenochtitlán in 1520. His account has been used by many to explain the origins of the first "virgin soil" epidemic to destroy sixteenth-century Central America. (The "Captain Narváez" referred to was a soldier sent by Cuban governor Velázquez to stop Cortés.)

> **Mortality estimates would eventually range from one-quarter to one-half of the population of central Mexico.**

The first was a plague of smallpox, and it began in this manner. When Hernando Cortés was captain and governor, at the time that Captain Pánfilo de Narváez landed in this country, there was in one of his ships a negro stricken with smallpox, a disease which had never been seen here. At this time New Spain was extremely full of people, and when the smallpox began to attack the Indians it became so great a pestilence among them throughout the land that in most provinces more than half the population died; in others the proportion was little less. For as the Indians did not know the remedy for the disease and were very much in the habit of bathing frequently, whether well or ill, and continued to do so even when suffering from smallpox, they died in heaps, like bedbugs. Many others died of starvation, because, as they were all taken sick at once, they could not care for each other, nor was there anyone to give them bread or anything else. In many places it happened that everyone in a house died, and, as it was impossible to bury the great number of dead, they pulled down the houses over them in order to check the stench that rose from the dead bodies so that their homes became their tombs. This disease was called by the Indians "the great leprosy" because the victims were so covered with pustules that they looked like lepers. Even today one can see obvious evidences of it in some individuals who escaped death, for they were left covered with pockmarks.

Tenochtitlán had been almost totally destroyed using the manpower of the Tlaxcalans plus Spanish weaponry and germs, and once it finally fell, the Spanish continued to decimate it like a rabid pack of wolves. Tenochtitlán is now Mexico City. The surviving Aztecs were banished to live among their enemies in Tlatelolco. As a result of Cortés's success, King Charles I of Spain appointed him as governor of New Spain.

Pizarro and the Incas

Francisco Pizarro was roughly 20 years older than his cousin Hernándo Cortés, but since he'd come from much less, his career as a sailor and conquistador may have been driven more by need than want. Regardless, he was proficient at both. He was named *alcalde* of Panama City.

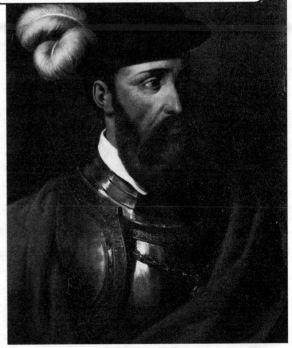

A cousin of Hernándo Cortés, Francisco Pizarro conquered what is now modern-day Peru, land of the Incas.

Pizarro's band comprised mercenaries and adventurers—similar to what Pizarro himself had been as a youth—but by middle age, Pizarro was a wealthy man; where Cortés had made his fortune in the Caribbean, Pizarro had made his in Central America. Now, Pizarro and his men were heading south, with a lust for wealth driving them further into the unknown, which consisted of topography designed to conquer *them*: mountains, desert, and rain forest. However, rather than turning back once the Andes Mountains came into view, Pizarro and his men became the first Europeans to scale them—no mean feat considering that the Andes has the second-highest elevation in the world and is the longest contiguous mountain range in the world, cutting through today's Colombia, Ecuador, Peru, Bolivia, Chile, and Argentina.

The region was cold, seemingly endless. The altitude made it difficult to breathe; the Spanish weren't used to conditions like these. Even though at this time, Spain controlled nearly one-third of Europe, they had nothing like the Andes there.

Pizarro and his men didn't wander forever, though—eventually, they crossed into the Inca Empire.

Those who spoke Quechua, the Incas' main language, named their empire Tawantinsuyu: *tawa* meaning "four"; *ntin*, a suffix denoting a group, so *Tawantin* means "group of four"; and *suyu*, meaning "regions." Taken together, the Inca Empire was "the land of four regions."

Unlike most civilizations that extend east and west, the Inca Empire ran north and south. Geographically, it was unique but complicated. Cast a straight line from east to west through Eurasia, and you'll have a population of people and animals on the same latitude, dealing with similar climate and food.

Now, cast a longitudinal line from north to south through the Inca civilization, and you'll see a vast range of climate and food. This made it more challenging to travel and to trade materials and knowledge. So, for all the Inca might within their numbers, their geography hindered them in developing a system of writing or new technologies. This did not mean they were a backward society, however. As anthropologist Gordon McEwan wrote in his 2006 book, *The Incas: A New Perspective*:

> The Incas lacked the use of wheeled vehicles. They lacked animals to ride and draft animals that could pull wagons and plows.... [They] lacked the knowledge of iron and steel.... Above all, they lacked a system of writing.... Despite these supposed handicaps, the Incas were still able to construct one of the greatest imperial states in human history.

A civilization without wheels was able to build stunning temples, set up stepped irrigation within its mountains, and develop a system of communication that wasn't writing, but it was so complex that we still cannot "translate" it today.

The word "translate" is in quotes because it's not like translating Russian into English or, at its most basic level, words into words. It's translating knots into words. *Quipu* (KEE-pu) comprised one major textile cord, or top cord, with countless numbers of subsequent, multicolored textile cords radiating from it. Tied within each of these were knots that may have been used for calculations in a manner similar to an abacus; however, we don't know the specifics because even after hundreds of years, we've had luckless attempts to decipher their meaning. They might be epic stories, or they might be songs, but for now, they are mute, as no one has managed to make them "speak" (though some strides have been made in applying meaning to the color of textiles). The Spanish burned *quipu* and outlawed new ones on the grounds that they were being used to worship pagan gods, among other transgressions. About 1,000 remain today.

What we do know is that the Incas were masters of weaving—practically composers. They built ships out of rope. They engineered extensive suspension bridges made out of grass that were reinforced every year and spanned canyons.

Conversely, the small number of Spaniards were deep in their territory, but they had swords and guns. They came from an east-to-west civilization that benefited from all those things the north-to-south Incas did not— trade, connections, interaction with other civilizations. This led to an exchange of not only goods but germs. By the sixteenth century, Pizarro's ancestors had survived any number of diseases, not to mention most probably the Black Death, and had gifted him and other Europeans with a robust immune system.

The four regions of the Inca Empire are shown here. The native name for the empire is Tawantinsuyu, which means "the land of four regions."

The reign of the Incas was brief compared to a civilization like the Maya— it began in the thirteenth century and ended in 1532—but it spanned a territory larger than that of the Aztecs and Maya—it was the largest in the Western Hemisphere—with a population of 10 to 15 million people. In addition to bridges and ships, the Incas built massive temples, administrative centers, and an extensive road and canal system. Terraces and irrigation works were carved into mountains, and a multitude of crops were grown at all different elevations, which the Incas did in an inhospitable land without the aforementioned perks that other grand civilizations enjoyed, including wheels, horses, iron, or a written language.

Because the empire stretched roughly 2,500 miles and included an enormous variety of cultures, religions, languages, and climate, the Incas allowed territories to be governed under local leaders, yet all answered to the emperor. The long-reigning Emperor Huayna Capac had just died of what could have been the measles, smallpox, or influenza, which was also beginning to kill off enormous numbers of his people. These European diseases had reached the Incas before the Europeans had, in part because of a well-engineered road system.

Before he died, Huayna Capac named one of his sons as successor, not knowing that this son was already dead. Power was then handed over to another son, Huáscar, though this may have been a bad idea, as Huáscar was the type of person who would steal other men's wives and execute them if they objected. However, this account, it should be noted, came from Atahualpa, Huáscar's brother and the man who wanted to be emperor. Atahualpa waged a treacherous civil war against his brother and won—but not before tearing the empire apart and not long before Pizarro arrived.

On November 15, 1532, Pizarro and his men—about 170 of them—met Atahualpa in the valley of Cajamarca. They brought documents from the Spanish king saying that the Inca Empire was now Christian land that belonged to Spain—though the expedition wasn't really about land per se. It was about gold—each conquistador was promised a share of the riches and had visions of Aztec-ish loot dancing in their heads. For Pizarro—already a rich man, though always looking to get richer—it was also about making his mark on the world, like his cousin Hernando Cortés had done. The document went on to declare that Pizarro would be the Spanish governor.

Atahualpa didn't know this, but just 500 miles north, Central America and the Caribbean were being colonized by the Spanish—"colonized" meaning burned, wrecked, and destroyed....

Atahualpa had been waiting for the Spaniards; he'd been told they were approaching, and rather than have them killed, he wanted to see them, perhaps partly out of curiosity, perhaps partly out of strategy.

Atahualpa didn't know this, but just 500 miles north, Central America and the Caribbean were being colonized by the Spanish—"colonized" meaning burned, wrecked, and destroyed, with the

PLAGUES, PANDEMICS AND VIRUSES

Native people dead or dying of disease and a European world rising from the ashes. Spain had recently united after seven centuries of Muslim occupation. A rural country, its conquistadores came from small towns and villages like Trujillo, home of Pizarro, yet they were master horsemen who used this skill in the New World like part of a Spanish cavalry. The sight of a horse to a Native American—remember, this was a new animal to them—could be terrifying, especially if it was charging.

However, even if Atahualpa had been aware of this, they certainly had nothing to fear—men with four-legged creatures be darned; only a handful of them were around compared to between 40,000 and 80,000 Incas (based on conquistador estimates). Encamped along the heights of Cajamarca with a large force of troops who'd just won the war against Huáscar, the Incas felt they had little to fear from the Spanish.

Atahualpa left the armed warriors who had accompanied him about half a mile outside of Cajamarca. His immediate party still had more than 7,000 members but were unarmed except for small battle-axes that were for show rather than battle. Atahualpa's attendants wore gold and silver headdresses, and the main party was preceded by a group who sang while sweeping the roadway in front of Atahualpa. At sunset, 80 high-ranking men wearing royal blue carried Atlahuapa in a litter covered with parrot feathers and silver. Atahualpa's intention was to impress the small Spanish force—this fierce warrior had not anticipated an ambush.

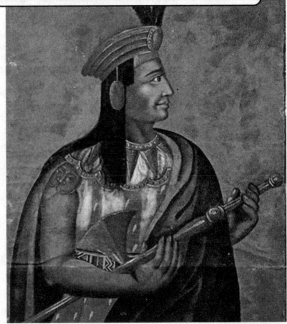

Incan emperor Atahualpa was the last of his race to lead his people before the Spanish defeated them. His predecessor, Huayna Capac, had died a few years before from smallpox.

Meanwhile, the Spanish infantry and cavalry were hidden in nearby buildings and alleyways, awaiting the signal to charge—Pizarro had ordered his men to remain silent and hidden until the guns were fired. During the hours of waiting, tension rose among the greatly outnumbered Spanish, and Francisco Pizarro's cousin, Pedro Pizarro, wrote that many of the conquistadores soiled themselves "out of pure terror."

Upon entering the square, the group who sang and swept split their ranks to allow Atahualpa's litter to be carried to the center, where all stopped. An Inca holding a banner approached the building where the artillery was concealed, while Atahualpa, surprised at seeing no Spanish, called out to them.

Tito Cusi, an Inca ruler, was the source of *An Inca Account of the Conquest of Peru*, his version of the Spanish invasion, which he told in 1570 to Spanish missionary Fray Marcos Garcia. According to Cusi, when his father, Atahualpa's brother, first heard about the Spaniards' arrival:

> He was beside himself and said, "How dare those people intrude into my country without my authorization and permission? Who are these people and what are their ways?" The messengers answered, "Lord, these people cannot but be gods, for they claim to have come by the wind. They are bearded people, very beautiful and white. They eat out of silver plates. Even their sheep, who carry them, are large and wear silver shoes. They throw thunder like the sky.... Moreover, we have witnessed with our own eyes that they talk to white cloths [paper] by themselves and that they call some of us by our names without having been informed by anyone and only looking into the sheets, which they hold in front of them.... Who could people of this manner and fortune be but gods?"

Cusi recounted that at Cajamarca, Pizarro and Hernando de Soto met Atahualpa at the town center, where the Inca emperor offered them a gold chalice with *chicha*, beer made from fermented corn. Pizarro poured the drink onto the ground and then gave Atahualpa a letter, which he said was written by God and the Spanish king. Offended by Pizarro's disrespectful manner, especially in the midst of such opulence, Atahualpa threw the "letter or whatever it was" on the ground, stood, and yelled, "If you disrespect me, I will also disrespect you!" and yelled that he would kill them, at which point Pizarro gave the signal to attack.

The Spaniards ran out into the square, unleashing gunfire at the unarmed Incas and surging forward as a single force. The effect was devastating, and the shocked and unarmed Incas offered little resistance. The cavalry charged on horseback against the Inca forces, and in combination with gunfire (and these were not even guns that worked well, often misfiring or breaking), the noise, gun smoke, and charging horses terrified the Incas.

The first target of the Spanish attack was Atahualpa and his top commanders. Pizarro rushed at the emperor on horseback, but Atahualpa remained motionless. The Spanish severed the limbs of those carrying his litter so they could reach him, but they were astounded that the attendants ignored their wounds and used their remaining hands to hold it up until several were killed outright and the litter fell. Atahualpa, however, remained on it—perhaps staying true to the Inca philosophy that a warrior never backs down. His attendants rushed to place themselves between their emperor and the Spanish, knowing they were about to be killed. While Pizarro's men were cutting down Atahualpa's attendants, Pizarro rode to where a Spanish soldier had finally pulled Atahualpa from his litter. One soldier attempted to kill Atahualpa, but Pizarro blocked the attack since Atahualpa was worth more alive than dead, and Pizarro was slashed on the hand as a consequence. That would be the closest any Spaniard would get to a casualty.

The main Inca force, which had retained their weapons but remained about half a mile away in a meadow outside Cajamarca, scattered in the melee as survivors tore away from the square and headed right toward them. The stampede had even broken down a 15-foot length of wall in the process. These Incas were veterans, warriors who far outnumbered the Spanish. However, the shock of the ambush amid the spiritual significance of losing their emperor and most of his commanders within minutes shattered Inca morale, throwing their ranks into chaos and leading to a massive rout by the Spanish. No evidence exists that any of the main Inca force attempted to engage the Spaniards in Cajamarca after the initial ambush.

In the first 10 minutes of the Battle of Cajamarca, 7,000 Incas died. The number of Spanish casualties was zero. Atahualpa was imprisoned by the Spanish and a handful of Native allies—with help from one cannon and many swords, guns, and horses.

Pizarro declared that he would release the emperor if the Incas could fill a room in Cajamarca's temple with gold and silver. They did, and then Atahualpa was executed. The money was shared between Pizarro and his other men.

The conquistadores were awed by the empire they'd just destroyed. Cuzco, the capital, was laid out in the form of a puma and was dominated by fine buildings and palaces, the richest of all being a gold-covered and emerald-studded complex that included a temple to the Inca sun god, Inti. Pizarro himself said that Cuzco was so beautiful, "it would be remarkable, even in Spain."

Some of the Incas who'd survived the previous civil war, Spanish overthrow, and smallpox decided to move and relocated to a new capital, Vilcabamba, where they held out

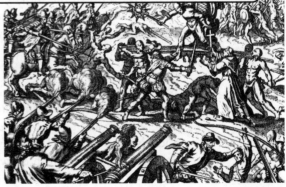

More of a massacre than a battle, the Spanish, under Pizarro's leadership, killed seven thousand Incas at Cajamarca, captured their emperor, and then executed him.

TB AND NATIVE AMERICANS

Tuberculosis appears to have been present among Native populations before the European arrival, as lesions were found in prehistoric Mesoamerican mummies; after isolating the lesions and analyzing the DNA, microbiologists discovered it was tubercular bacteria. It may have come from bison, or different species or subspecies may have existed between the hemispheres.

for 40 years, but by 1572, the Spaniards had completely taken over, and they had nowhere else to hide.

Disease took care of the rest of the Incas. Smallpox killed half of the Inca population during the first epidemic. A typhus outbreak occurred in 1546, influenza and smallpox in 1558, smallpox again in 1589, diphtheria in 1614, and measles in 1618.

Incidentally, on September 16, 1542, almost nine years after conquering the Incas, Pizarro was killed by a rival, Diego de Almagro II, who was then tried and executed near Cuzco, Peru.

What We Lost

What legacy came from this? In contrast to the subsequent African slave trade, which consisted largely of adult males, indigenous American enslavement in North and South America under the Spanish and the English consisted primarily of women and children. According to Andres Resendez, author of *The Other Slavery: The Uncovered Story of Indian Enslavement in America*, "If we were to add up all the Indian slaves taken in the New World from the time of Columbus to the end of the nineteenth century, the figure would run somewhere between 2.5 and 5 million Native slaves."

During this period, more than 2,500 Natives were shipped to the Iberian Peninsula as slaves. By the mid-1550s, Spanish queen Isabella officially declared Native American slavery illegal, but it continued in Spanish colonies via a loophole called the *encomienda* system. The Spanish crown provided an *encomienda*, or "grant," to a Spanish *encomendero*, or "colonizer," held in perpetuity by him and his descendants. The Natives, who were now essentially considered slaves belonging to the Spanish crown, were forced to work for these *encomenderos*. In addition, a requirement for conquerors to receive their grants was that they

PLAGUES, PANDEMICS AND VIRUSES

had to convert the Natives to Christianity and make Spanish their primary language. Natives were subjected to torture and possibly death if they resisted. The *encomienda* system, because it was tied to the indigenous people, also facilitated intermarriage of the indigenous people, who were usually women, with non-indigenous spouses, who were usually Spanish or Creole men, and set the stage for the rise of the mixed-blood, or *mestizaje*, caste system by the 1700s. Mixed-blood offspring couldn't legally be subject to the *encomienda* slave system because they were mixed and no longer "Native." Therefore, the *encomienda* system led to the rise of the Mestizo identity and the renunciation of their indigenous past. The *encomienda* system was finally outlawed in 1542.

The Maya

The Yucatán Peninsula juts out of northeastern Central America, with the Gulf of Mexico at its north and west and the Caribbean Sea to the east. It is part of present-day Belize, Guatemala, and Honduras and is 76,300 square miles in size—roughly the size of South Dakota. It was once home to the Maya. They were known for their art, architecture, complex astronomical calendar, and written language that has been the most translated of all pre-Columbian Mesoamerican languages. They were the New World's most advanced civilization. Though we think of the Maya, Incas, and Aztecs as ancient, only the Maya bears that crown.

Despite the centuries through which it persisted, though, the Maya had undergone a colossal change long before the Spanish arrived. No one is sure why mainly because the Spanish destroyed most of the Maya writings, and much of what did survive disappeared over time.

What we do know is that in the eighth and ninth centuries, trade declined and intense conflicts began. By 850 C.E., large-scale architectural development, like the stepped temples that were integral to the Maya people, had all but stopped. Today, many Maya ruins are still surrounded by the jungle; it's a site rife with archaeological discoveries. The secrets of former Aztec capital Tenochtitlán are now hidden beneath the pavement of Mexico City, but the more remote places, like Maya's great city, Chichen Itza, having once been forgotten, lay untouched.

It was a lawyer from New Jersey and a draftsman from London who uncovered the Maya. John Lloyd Stephens and Frederick Catherwood were two explorers who documented Maya ruins from Copán in Honduras up to Chichen Itza in Mexico. The fascinating stories written by Stephens in his *Incidents of Travel in Central America, Chiapas and Yucatan* and *Incidents of Travel in Yu-*

PLAGUE IN A CLASSIC SCI-FI NOVEL

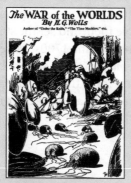

Martians are defeated by microbes in H. G. Wells's *The War of the Worlds*.

In 1897, British writer H. G. Wells published *War of the Worlds*, a science fiction tale about Martians overtaking the world. Wells said that he wrote the book after a talk with his brother about the genocide of native Tasmanians by the British.

The native Tasmanians were distantly related to indigenous Australians, though they had been separated from each other for around 8,000 years. When the British began their colonization of Tasmania in 1803, the population of indigenous people was about 7,000–8,000, many of whom were already dying from diseases thought to have been contracted from earlier contact with European sailors, explorers, and seal hunters. In addition, many women were left infertile by venereal diseases. In 1830, British pastor George Robinson moved the remaining 100 Tasmanians—who referred to themselves as *Palawi*—to nearby Flinders Island. The idea was to save the few who were left, but most who moved there died of disease regardless. The remaining 14 were then resettled in southern Tasmania: "14 persons, all adults, aboriginals of Tasmania, who are the sole surviving remnant of ten tribes," according to an 1861 article in the British newspaper *The Times*. "Nine of these persons are women and five are men. There are among them four married couples, and four of the men and five of the women are under 45 years of age, but no children have been born to them for years. It is considered difficult to account for this…. Besides these 14 persons there is a native woman who is married to a white man, and who has a son, a fine healthy-looking child…." The article, titled "Decay of Race," adds that, after first asking to "leave to go," the survivors were generally healthy and still made hunting trips to the bush, and were now "fed, housed and clothed at public expense" and "much addicted to drinking."

At the end of *War of the Worlds*, after destroying much of Earth, the Martians suddenly die of an Earth-borne pathogen for which they have no immunity. Sadly, the opposite was the case in Tasmania. Fanny Cochrane Smith, believed to be the last full-blooded Tasmanian, died in 1905.

catan as well as Catherwood's own book of lithographs, *Views of Ancient Monuments in Central America, Chiapas and Yucatan*, propelled the Maya out of obscurity and captured the imaginations of those as far away as Europe—only 150 years after the empire had been decimated by Europeans.

The Story of the Maya

The first Maya civilizations have been carbon dated back to c. 3000 B.C.E. in what's known today as Belize. The Maya then were mostly farmers who grew crops like corn, beans, and squash and hunted and fished alongside their neighbors and trading partners, the Olmecs.

The Maya society as we began to know it started in c. 1000 B.C.E. Now more than just hunters, the Maya were building canals and irrigation systems that made extensive trade viable. Teotihuacán was one of the largest and most sophisticated cities of the preindustrial world. By 600 B.C.E., the Maya had developed complex social, political, and cultural systems, based largely in the city of Kaminaljuyu in today's Guatemala.

This worked great until something went wrong. The "Classic Maya collapse"—meaning the end of the Classic Maya civilization—dates between 250 and 900 C.E. It was a long, slow decline, whose causes may have partly been due to a long-term drought. Tree ring and lake sediment records indicate that some of the most severe and prolonged droughts to hit Mesoamerica occurred between 650 and 1000, particularly between 700 and 800, a period of time that coincides with end of the Classic Maya period. In *The Great Maya Droughts*, archaeologist Richardson Gill analyzed an array of climatic, historical, geologic, and archaeological data and concluded that a prolonged series of droughts likely caused the Classic Maya collapse. With this drought brought excessive warfare for dwindling resources, foreign invasions, and less trade. The theory also exists that the collapse was caused by the devastation of its agriculture by the 535 C.E. eruption of the Ilopango volcano.

The Mayans once had a great civilization—as evidenced by the fabulous ruins one can still see in Mexico—that likely fell into ruin by drought, war, diminishing resources, and disease.

Also, their extensive construction may have disrupted the homes of parasites and insect-borne diseases that led to dysentery-type diseases, especially among the very young. This also took place long before the Spanish arrived.

Although "collapse" connotes a complete demise, the Maya continued. They moved from their base in the southern Lowlands up to the

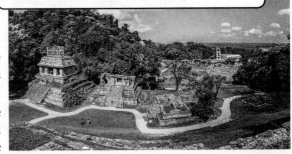

THE ANNALS OF THE CAKCHIQUELS

The *Annals of the Cakchiquels* is a Maya manuscript written in the Kaqchikel language between 1571 and 1604 and is a significant example of Native American literature not only due to its way of conveying how its people saw their world but because it still exists. It contains mythology and historical information as it pertains to the Kaqchikel ruling class of the Maya who lived in what is now Guatemala.

The authors describe hearing of a plague that arrived in the Aztec capital city of Tenochtitlán in the fall of 1520, which may have been smallpox. The *Annals* also contain an account of a second epidemic that began in 1559:

> First there was a cough, then the blood was corrupted, and the urine became yellow. The number of deaths at this time was truly terrible. The Chief Vakaki Ahmak died, and we ourselves were plunged in great darkness and great grief, our fathers and ancestors having contracted the plague, O my children.

> Great was the stench of the dead. After our fathers and grandfathers succumbed, half of the people fled to the fields. The dogs and vultures devoured the bodies. The mortality was terrible. Your grandfathers died, and with them died the son of the king and his brothers and kinsmen. So it was that we became orphans, oh, my sons! So we became when we were young. All of us were thus. We were born to die!

> In the sixth month after the arrival of the Lord President in Pangán, the plague which had lashed the people long ago began here. Little by little it arrived here. In truth a fearful death fell on our heads by the will of our powerful God. Many families [succumbed] to the plague. Now the people were overcome by intense cold and fever, blood came out of their noses, then came a cough growing worse and worse, the neck was twisted, and small and large sores broke out on them. The disease attacked everyone here. On the day of Circumcision [January 1, 1560], a Monday, while I was writing, I was attacked by the epidemic.

PLAGUES, PANDEMICS AND VIRUSES

northern Yucatán. This brought a change in architectural and artistic styles and fewer examples of pictographic writing. It was also the beginning of the great city, Chichen Itza, where a united Maya created a new empire.

The Defeat of the Maya

On July 30, 1502, Christopher Columbus arrived at one of the Bay Islands off the coast of Honduras. He sent his brother Bartholomew out as a scout. As Bartholomew and his men went exploring, a large trading canoe approached. Bartholomew Columbus boarded the canoe and found that it was a Maya trading vessel from Yucatán, carrying well-dressed Maya and a rich cargo. The Europeans looted whatever took their interest from among the cargo and seized the elderly captain to serve as an interpreter; the canoe was then allowed to continue on its way. This was the first recorded contact between Europeans and the Maya and would lead to a long series of battles where no one truly ended up the victor.

Francisco de Montejo was born in 1479 in Salamanca, Spain. A successful conquistador, in 1527, Montejo was named by the Spanish king as capitan general of Yucatán, where the Maya lived. Since he had such a title, Montejo then attempted to conquer the Yucatán along the east coast. He arrived in Valladolid with 400 soldiers but no interpreter and was misled by the seemingly docile nature of the Maya. Montejo was not prepared for all that he was about to encounter.

The Spaniards suffered greatly due to the rough terrain and lack of water. Often, they found the villages deserted or hostile. Amid their travels, they were ambushed by Natives armed with arrows, lances, swords, and shields made of very large tortoise shells adorned with snail shells and antlers. The Spaniards found themselves at a disadvantage, being unable to use their horses properly on account of the uneven ground, though the Spaniards greatly kept up the fight. Only after a second day of fighting did the Natives retreat, leaving 1,200 of their men dead. This was in the last weeks of 1527.

Two years later, still driven by thoughts of gold and precious jewels, Montejo decided to try conquering Yucatán from the west, which he pursued until 1535, when his forces were driven out. The sole chaplain on the expedition, Francisco Hernandez, later attributed the failure to the lack of priests.

In 1542, after repeated battles, Francisco de Montejo the Younger (son of Francisco de Montejo) achieved the surrender of the western Yucatán Peninsula and founded today's Meridia. Lord Naabon Cupul reluctantly allowed him to settle the Spanish town of Ciudad Real at Chichen Itza. After six months of Spanish rule, Naabon Cupul was killed during a failed attempt to kill Montejo the Younger.

EL DORADO

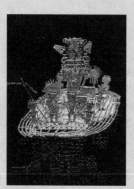

El Dorado, "the golden one," was the term used by the Spanish to describe a mythical tribal chief of Colombia's Musica people, who, as an initiation rite, covered himself with gold dust and submerged himself in Lake Guatavita. Over time, the legend of El Dorado grew from being a man to a city to a kingdom and then finally to an empire.

In hot pursuit of a myth, conquistadores roamed in what is today Colombia, Venezuela, and parts of Guyana and northern Brazil for the city and its fabulous king. Consequently, much of northern South America, including the Amazon River, was mapped. The constant push into Maya territory was partly because they hadn't found El Dorado, though conquistadores were sure they would, but by the beginning of the nineteenth century, most people dismissed the existence of the empire as a myth.

A vessel (pictured) shows a golden figure on a golden raft representing the ceremony of covering the body of a dead ruler in gold dust.

The death of their lord only served to inflame the anger of the Maya, and in mid-1543, they laid siege to the small Spanish garrison at Chichen Itza. Montejo the Younger abandoned Ciudad Real by night, and he and his men fled west.

The primary goal of the conquistadores was to locate vast quantities of gold and silver. Trace amounts of these metals were found that had been transported to the Maya kingdom via their various trade routes from Colombia and Ecuador, but the Spanish did not find the riches that they had hoped for.

The Spanish colonization entailed forced labor and mandatory conversion to Christianity. The Maya who refused to give up their religion were arrested and tortured for heresy. Maya artifacts were destroyed, and all but a few of their sacred texts were burned. Disease killed off many others. However, because the Maya lands weren't anywhere near as attractive or lucrative as the Aztec lands, which were filled with gold, they were not as decimated. Their lack of "wealth" from a European perspective saved what few territories existed.

Also, unlike the Aztec and Inca empires, the Maya had no single political center that, once overthrown, would bring about their end. Instead, the Spanish had to subdue independent Maya city-states almost one by one—many of which kept up a fierce resistance—for little revenue in return.

The last Maya territories (and the last holdouts from Spanish control in the Americas)—Tayasal and Zacpeten—remained independent until they were finally subdued by the Spanish in 1697.

Today, many Maya are full-blooded Natives and often speak Spanish as a second language. In some parts of the Maya territories, use of the 260-day Maya calendar and Maya agricultural practices continue, keeping their languages and traditions alive.

North America

The Lakota called smallpox "the running face sickness." Indigenous people of North America were just as susceptible to European diseases as those in Mexico and South America, though a comparable empire didn't necessarily exist, like the Aztec, to give a kind of context to the genocide, so sometimes it all gets fused together.

The disease trajectory through the New World is not easily tracked; countless outbreaks were only sporadically recorded. (This lack of effectively recording illnesses and mortalities came into play more than 500 years later during the COVID-19 pandemic.) Smallpox was lethal to these Native Americans, bringing widespread epidemics and often affecting the same tribes over and over again. In addition to biological differences, cultural norms of the

ARRIVAL OF HORSES IN THE AMERICAS

Before the arrival of the Spaniards, Natives had never seen horses. They were not indigenous to North or South America, so the idea that the Natives who lived in the Plains had long been great horsemen is not true. They did take to riding the horse, but it was no earlier than the mid-1600s. From a trade center in Santa Fe, New Mexico, the use of horses spread slowly north. The Comanche are believed to be among the first Native groups to master horsemanship. By 1742, the Crow and Blackfoot tribes had achieved the same skills. The horse eventually became an integral part of the lives and culture of Native Americans, especially the Plains Indians, like those in Nebraska, Oklahoma, and the Dakotas, who used them for travel, warfare, and hunting bison.

Natives made them more susceptible. The emphasis they placed on visiting the sick to comfort and heal them worked against the population, and again, with no knowledge of germ theory—even the Europeans were still sticking to the theory of humors at the time—the Native Americans had no conception of isolation. Many societies believed that disease was caused by sorcery or vulnerability due to a lack of protection by the spirits.

As far as sickness, not all groups were affected in the same way. The more nomadic, the lower the mortality. The buffalo hunters of the North American Plains had less mortality from disease early on because they were frequently on the move, whereas other groups who were more sedentary disappeared completely. The Pueblo of today's southwestern United States declined but not in enormous numbers and not until the late seventeenth or early eighteenth century. The Spanish had explored the southwest United States in the sixteenth century and settled in the seventeenth century, but the most successful Native revolt in North America happened in New Mexico in 1680, when the Pueblo kicked the Spanish out.

Smallpox Blankets

Over the decades, history students have been taught that in their hunger to destroy the Natives, colonists "gifted" them with blankets full of smallpox. This use of smallpox as a biological weapon against Native Americans was first reported by William Trent, a nineteenth-century trader and militia captain, but for all the outrage the account has stirred up over the years, no clear verdict has been reached on whether or not the biological attack even happened.

In the late spring of 1763, the Delaware, Shawnee, and Mingo warriors laid siege to Fort Pitt in present-day Pittsburgh. The fort's commander, Captain Simeon Ecuyer, reported in a June 16, 1763, letter to his superior, Colonel Henry Bouquet, that the situation was dire, as local traders and colonists were taking refuge inside the fort's walls. Ecuyer wasn't just afraid of Native Americans. The fort's hospital had smallpox patients, and Ecuyer feared a smallpox epidemic striking within the fort.

Trent wrote in his diary that on June 23, 1763, two Delaware emissaries had visited Fort Pitt and tried to persuade the British to abandon it. Unsuccessful, they asked for provisions and liquor. The British complied and also reportedly gave them gifts—two blankets and a handkerchief that had come from the smallpox ward. Trent wrote, "I hope it will have the desired effect."

Historian Philip Ranlet of Hunter College casts doubt on the incident. "There is no evidence that the scheme worked," Ranlet says. "The infection on

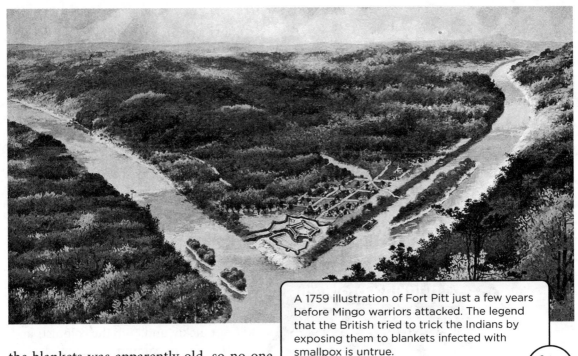

A 1759 illustration of Fort Pitt just a few years before Mingo warriors attacked. The legend that the British tried to trick the Indians by exposing them to blankets infected with smallpox is untrue.

the blankets was apparently old, so no one could catch smallpox from the blankets. Besides, the Indians just had smallpox—the smallpox that reached Fort Pitt had come from Indians—and anyone susceptible to smallpox had already had it."

The most important indication that the plan was a dud, Ranlet says, "is that Trent would have bragged in his journal if the scheme had worked. He is silent as to what happened."

Even if it didn't work, the fact that British officers were willing to contemplate using smallpox against the Natives was a sign of how they felt about them. Paul Kelton, a historian at Stony Brook University, told *History.com*, "Even for that time period, it violated civilized notions of war," and he noted that they knew the disease "would kill [Native] women and children, not just warriors."

The Legacy of Disease

In pre-Columbian times, many tribes made fermented drinks, though the alcohol content was much lower than what people drink today. The rate of excessive alcohol use within the indigenous communities is still unknown, but it's believed that drinking alcohol may have been mainly used for ceremonial and spiritual purposes.

PLAGUES, PANDEMICS AND VIRUSES

Historical research has shown that the damage the Europeans inflicted on the Native populations, coupled with the ... introduction to alcohol, may have contributed to their initial drinking problems.

However, among early European colonists, alcohol was consumed on a regular basis, often as a substitute for contaminated water or to treat various medical ailments. Europeans made highly alcoholic distilled spirits and viewed drinking as socially acceptable.

Historical research has shown that the damage the Europeans inflicted on the Native populations, coupled with the indigenous communities' sudden introduction to alcohol, may have contributed to their initial drinking problems. Native demand for alcohol increased quickly, and both the colonists and the Native community used alcohol for trade and money. Booze played a pivotal role in the shaping of early America.

The passage of alcoholism between families through the generations may also be a leading factor for continued substance-abuse problems in the modern Native community. Young Native Americans are likely to have first been exposed to substance use by their parents or from another relative—so drinking and drug use is often normal. Other environmental issues, such as earlier age of onset use, exposure to trauma, and acculturation hardship, also contribute to the inherent risk.

Other issues are at play. Today, Native Americans have higher rates of tobacco use than white, Asian, or black communities. Native American men are about as likely to be moderate to heavy drinkers as white men, but about 5 to 15 percent more likely to be moderate to heavy drinkers than black or Asian men. Native Americans have far greater rates of obesity and are also less likely to engage in regular physical activity than white adults. In sum, Native Americans and Alaska Natives face high rates of health disparity compared to other ethnic groups.

Resurrection

Despite this, it's easy to use data to find the low points to discover what needs to be improved. It's not always easy to quantify art, music, or literature as success. Joy Harjo is a poet, musician, playwright, and author as well as being a member of the Mvskoke tribe and has the distinction of being the first Native American U.S. poet laureate.

At an exhibit at New York's Metropolitan Museum of Art, a sign reads: "The Metropolitan Museum of Art is situated on the Lenape island of Manhahtaan (Mannahatta) in Lenapehoking, the Lenape homeland." It continues: "We pay respect to the Lenape peoples–past, present, and future–and their continuing presence in the homeland and throughout the Lenape diaspora." An exhibit that was part of the American wing features artwork made by Native artists, including one piece by Standing Bear entitled "Battle of Little Bighorn," showing the famous 1876 battle between the U.S. Army and Native armies. It also contains a shaman's amulet from Alaska, masks from the northwest coast, clothing from the Arctic, and moccasins from Alabama. "These aren't extinct cultures; many cultures are still continuing, like with traditional beadwork and basketmaking," said Sylvia Yount, curator of the American wing. "We are doing programming with contemporary artists and tribal leaders to make sure dialogues are visible." In addition, Plains Indian drawings detailing massacres, battles, hunting, and religious practices are featured alongside contemporary art by Wendy Red Star, a multimedia artist. One review of her work stated, "Wendy Red Star, Crow Indian cultural activist and performance artist, offers an alternative view, focusing on performances and artworks that contest the images of the vanishing dark-skinned Indian."

A $15 million memorial honoring Native American and Alaska Native veterans is in Washington, D.C.

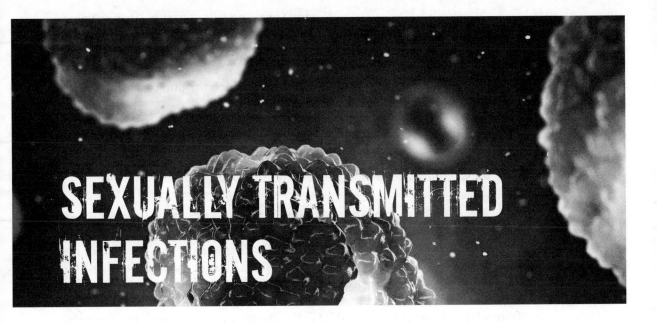

SEXUALLY TRANSMITTED INFECTIONS

Your parents had sex. Your grandparents had sex. People are having sex right now.

Even when one reaches a certain age, the desire to get it on doesn't go away: the elderly do it, too, but just as people don't necessarily think about drug abuse among the aged, they also don't think about sexual intercourse among the aged—and neither do the aged themselves, as if both sides just don't want to deal with "it." Doctors don't think to test for it, and their patients aren't going to mention it.

Baby boomers are now becoming grandmas and grandpas, but they grew up during a time with a less inhibited view toward sex and a more open view toward self-fulfillment; where sex was concerned, about the most frightening part was getting pregnant, and if you were gay, even that wasn't an issue.

Since baby boomers are no longer getting pregnant and sexually transmitted infections (STIs) are usually thought of as an unpleasantness only the young need to worry about, it would seem like sex for older people is no big deal. People are retiring, have time on their hands … and get into trouble like teenagers because that way of thinking has turned nursing homes and retirement communities into hotbeds for diseases like gonorrhea, syphilis, chlamydia, herpes, hepatitis, and HIV/AIDS. People may get older, but STIs do not.

Even the Bible makes reference to venereal diseases, which it calls "issues." While little is written about medicinal care, prevention came in the manner of threats. Moses cursed those who disobeyed him, and therefore God, with the "ulcer of Egypt." From Deuteronomy 28:27: "The Lord strike thee with the ulcer of Egypt, and the part of thy body, by which the dung is cast out, with the scab and with the itch, so that thou canst not be healed."

Whether you're a grandparent reading this book, a teenager, or a person of any age, sex education is critical in keeping you healthy, even if part of that education includes the fact that multiple sexual partners means that condoms are a must, no matter how old you are. Here are a few reasons why.

HERPES SIMPLEX 1 AND 2

Herpes. Most of the time when the herpes simplex virus (HSV) infects someone, no symptoms occur. This increases the chance of it spreading from one person to another, so it silently, stealthily, moves through a population. In this case, herpes will either show up above the waist (generally from a type of herpes called HSV1) in the mouth and tongue or below the waist in the genitals (generally from HSV2).

Herpes is transmitted through sex or childbirth, as babies can get neonatal herpes during delivery when they come into contact with vaginal secretions. Women should take extreme caution during pregnancy, as neonatal herpes can cause lesions on the newborn's skin, eyes, or mucus membranes or cause infections of the central nervous system that can lead to seizures. If untreated, these symptoms can become more serious and develop into sepsis, organ failure, and death, which is especially terrifying because about 70 percent of affected babies are born to mothers without HSV2 symptoms.

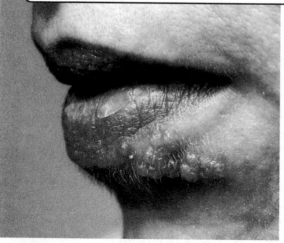

Cold sores on or around the lip are one indication of a herpes infection.

HIV—the virus that causes AIDS—infects a person by binding to cells in the immune system; the rabies virus infects a person or animal by binding to cells in the nervous system. HSV1 and HSV2 infect a person by entering through the mucosa—which covers the parts of the body that come into contact with the outside world—and binds to the mucosa's epithelial cells. Epithelial cells are part of our immune system's first line of defense against pathogens.

Herpes is most contagious when lesions are present, but it can also spread through what's called "asymptomatic shedding," or times when the virus is transmitted in saliva or genital secretions when no sores are present.

Once inside an epithelial cell, the virus starts the lytic cycle, when its DNA gets translated by enzymes that help to form viral proteins. These proteins are then packaged into new herpes viruses, which then leave the cell to infect neighboring epithelial cells. However, HSV1 and HSV2, like rabies, are known as "neurotropic viruses," meaning they infect the cells of the nervous system, specifically the sensory motor neurons of the face (the trigeminal ganglia) and genitals (the sacral ganglia), which are ultimately where the herpes virus settles in.

This virus settles in for life: herpes has no cure, and once an infection starts, it cannot be stopped. If you contract herpes, you will always have herpes. You won't always have breakouts, but the virus will never leave your system. (The virus that causes chicken pox is not from the same family as pox viruses, as the name would suggest, but from the herpes family of viruses, and, like herpes, once you have chicken pox, you will always have it in your system. That doesn't mean you'll get chicken pox again—you most probably won't—but you may get a painful rash outbreak called shingles that results from the same virus and tends to affect people 50 and older. If someone who's never had the chicken pox is around someone with shingles, they themselves won't get shingles, but they might get the chicken pox.)

HSV1 and HSV2 are clever as far as viruses go. They don't destroy the sensory neurons in the way the rabies virus takes over the entire nervous system and eventually kills the host. Instead, they use the trigeminal and/or sacral ganglia ("ganglia" are groups of neuron cell bodies) to make themselves at home. (In rare cases, HSV can cause neurological damage, like meningitis or encephalitis. This happens when some of the viruses escape into the bloodstream and reach the brain. Also rare is when HSV1 causes an outbreak in the genital area and HSV2 in the mouth area.)

These viruses can stay dormant in our nerve cells for long periods of time, which means that you may not get a breakout as soon as you're infected. Indeed, it can be a long time before you do show symptoms of herpes, so, for example, those with genital herpes may have no idea they're infected and therefore pass it on to a sexual partner, but at some point, the virus in a neuron reactivates, making copies of itself and sending them back down the axon, where they infect epithelial cells and blister the skin. This is what's called the reactivated or recurrent infection. Though our immune system can stop the epithelial breakout, HSV will still be hiding out in the sensory ganglia.

This may be repeated throughout a person's lifetime. The process can be triggered by stress or a viral illness like a cold, though nothing is definite. Because the virus first reactivates in the neuron, people with herpes may have a tingling or pain called a "prodrome" (from the Greek word *prodromos*, meaning

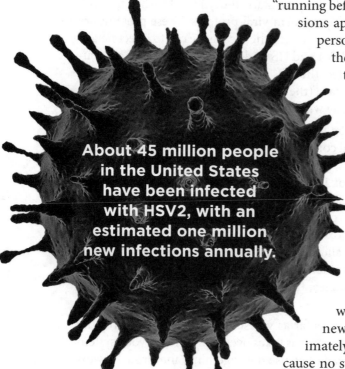

About 45 million people in the United States have been infected with HSV2, with an estimated one million new infections annually.

"running before") a day or two before skin lesions appear. This is good because the person can start treatment to mitigate the outbreak, usually with oral antiviral medications. On women, these blisters can be on the vulva's inner lips (labia minora), outer lips (labia majora), or cervix, and on men, they're on the shaft of the penis.

On the positive side, recurrent episodes are usually less severe than the first.

About 45 million people in the United States have been infected with HSV2, with an estimated one million new infections annually. Approximately 85–90 percent of infections cause no symptoms and therefore remain undiagnosed. The number of HSV2 cases corresponds with statistics like the number of sexual partners, the length of time a person has been sexually active, race, gender, and the presence of other STIs. Although we have adopted safer sex methods because of AIDS, they have fallen as fears of HIV have fallen; consequently, studies in the United States have shown that the frequency of HSV2 infections is rising.

GONORRHEA

Gonorrhea is caused by a bacteria called *Neisseria gonorrhoeae*. Although not a virus like herpes, it has similarities—for example, it's transmitted by sex and/or childbirth. It's also known as "the clap," possibly from the Old French word for brothel (*clapier*).

If a woman infects a man with gonorrhea, *N. gonorrhoeae* will travel up the urethra within the penis and latch on to its walls—walls that are lined with epithelial cells. This leads to an immune reaction, where the white blood cells reach the urethra and attack the bacteria, causing inflammation. Symptoms include pain during urination or overall burning in the genitalia. This is referred

170

to as urethritis. If the bacteria spread up to the prostate, you can get prostatitis. (The prostate, along with the nearby seminal vesicles, produces much of the fluid that makes up a man's ejaculate.)

An unpleasant side effect is that the white blood cells, dead epithelial cells, and bacteria will slough off through the penis in the form of pus, or, even worse, they won't slough off and a backup of pus in the urethra will occur, called an abscess. If antibiotics don't help this, a doctor will have to drain the pus himself or herself. To do this, he or she may thread an instrument up the urethra to puncture and drain the abscess, or they may insert a hollow needle in the perineal area between the scrotum and anus and suck up the pus through the needle.

Also, *N. gonorrhoeae* can infect the epithelial cells that line the anus or rectum, causing pustules in one of the places you least want them.

Gonorrhea in women presents as pustules, and urethritis can happen in women as well as vaginitis. Also, women can have pain during sex due to cervicitis, an inflammation caused by *N. gonorrhoeae* in the cervix. It can even reach the fallopian tubes and cause an infection within the entire pelvic cavity.

Gonorrhea also travels through the bloodstream and reaches your joints, and while white blood cells are just doing their job chasing after *N. gonorrhoeae*, their war on gonorrhea can cause joint inflammation and arthritis.

Like herpes, gonorrhea can spread to the central nervous system, affecting the lining around the spinal cord and brain. An infection of this lining, or meninges, is meningitis. Unfortunately, this is more common in small children than in adults, which is why *N. gonorrhoeae* is one of the infections pregnant women are screened for before they give birth. In fact, women and infants are much more likely to be affected than men by gonorrhea because an early infection tends to be more asymptomatic; they're also more likely to develop additional problems directly related to gonorrhea like fallopian tube scarring, infertility, and pelvic inflammatory diseases.

What's frightening about gonorrhea isn't just its ability to infect the parts of our bodies we hold dear—our brains and genitals—but that

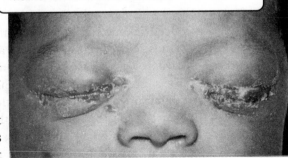

Pregnant women who contract gonorrhea can pass the disease on to their children, which is what happened with this infant who has microbial keratitis around the eyes, something that occurs in about 28 percent of mother-to-child transmissions.

> Today, we're down to one form of treatment for gonorrhea: an injection of ceftriaxone combined with an oral dose of azithromycin. That's all that now stands between us and untreatable gonorrhea....

N. gonorrhoeae has grown resistant to almost every drug historically used to treat it. This was first noticed in the 1980s, when penicillin and tetracycline became powerless against it. They're now no longer prescribed to treat gonorrhea at all. In the 1990s, they were replaced by fluoroquinolones, but by the 2000s, resistance to fluoroquinolones steadily began until it was no longer prescribed for patients in Asia and the Pacific Islands; then, it was no longer prescribed in California; then, it was no longer prescribed for men who had homosexual sex; and then, eventually, it was no longer prescribed for anyone with gonorrhea in the United States. Gonorrhea infects close to 80 million people around the world each year, and that number has been rising partly because of decreasing condom use as HIV/AIDS fears have waned and also because of poor detection rates, failed treatments, and increased travel, causing people to carry drug-resistant strains from one country to another, according to the WHO.

Some countries have been particularly hard hit with drug-resistant strains of gonorrhea in recent years, most notably India, China, Indonesia, parts of South America, Canada, and the United States (a lack of consistent data means that little is known about strains in Africa or the Middle East).

Today, we're down to one form of treatment for gonorrhea: an injection of ceftriaxone combined with an oral dose of azithromycin. That's all that now stands between us and untreatable gonorrhea, and even that treatment won't last forever because gonorrhea is constantly evolving through a process called horizontal gene transfer. Plasmids, which are small, circular DNA molecules containing a bacterium's genetic material, can easily be transferred from one bacterial species to another. In the case of gonorrhea, should an *N. gonorrhoeae* plasmid contain antibiotic-resistant genes, the *N. gonorrhoeae* acquiring it will become resistant to antibiotics, too.

CHLAMYDIA

Gonorrhea is the second-most-common STI in the world. It's often paired with the most common: chlamydia. *Chlamydia trachomis* is so named because of the eye infection—trachoma—that accompanies it. Like gonorrhea, chlamydia is spread through sex and/or childbirth, but it's also spread through direct contact, though *C. trachomis* can only live outside of the body for about a minute—so, for example, scratching an infected area like the genitalia and then immediately touching another part of the body, like the eye, can spread the infection.

When *C. trachomis* enters the vagina or urethra, it behaves the same as *N. gonorrhoeae*, traveling up toward the cervix or prostate. Interestingly, *C. trachomis* is an intracellular bacterium, meaning that it likes to live within a host's cell, in this case an epithelial cell, and, as with gonorrhea, the symptoms arise from our immune system attacking the infection; because the infection is within our own cells, the immune system has to kill our cells. This causes swelling, burning, and also pain during sex, and again, women infected with chlamydia are in danger of pelvic inflammatory diseases and infertility.

Back to direct eye contact: *C. trachomis* infects the conjunctiva, the red segment on the inside of the eyelid. This will lead to bumps that accumulate and scratch the eye, causing irritation and what's known as conjunctivitis. If it spreads over the pupil, it causes a film: trachoma. Trachoma is responsible for the blindness or visual impairment of about 1.9 million people around the world. Blindness from trachoma is irreversible.

SYPHILIS

O Syphilis! O peste cruelle!
Que ses ravages sont affreux!
Que de cons désolés par ell
Et que de fouteurs malheureux!
C'est là le mal de l'opulence.
Le mal français par excellence.
Le mal commun dans tout pays,
Le mal des prudes, des coquettes,
De duchesses et des soubrettes,
Des portefaix et des marquis.

Loosely translated, this means, "You could be rich, you could be poor, but syphilis will get you no matter who you are."

PLAGUES, PANDEMICS AND VIRUSES

173

Treponema paladin is a corkscrew-shaped virus that causes syphilis. It is extremely sensitive to oxygen and is one of only two organisms in medical microbiology that cannot be grown in a lab (the other being the virus that causes leprosy). Humans are its only reservoir, meaning that we are the only living organisms on Earth that get syphilis.

The prominent theory maintains that syphilis is a New World disease brought back by Christopher Columbus and other European voyagers. Just as the Europeans introduced illnesses like smallpox to the indigenous Americans, so did indigenous Americans introduce syphilis to Europeans. Columbus's first voyages to the Americas occurred three years before the first recorded European outbreak of syphilis: 1494–1495 in Naples, Italy, during a French invasion. Because it was spread by French troops, syphilis was called the "French disease." It was not until 1530 that the word "syphilis" was first used by Italian physician and poet Girolamo Fracastro.

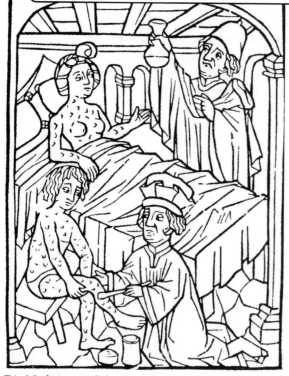

A 1498 medical illustration depicting patients with syphilis. While many Native Americans died of diseases brought to the New World by Europeans, many believe that syphilis was one plague that took the opposite route.

In 2011, the *Yearbook of Physical Anthropology*, an annual supplement of the *American Journal of Physical Anthropology*, stated that the "skeletal data bolsters the case that syphilis did not exist in Europe before Columbus set sail." Radiocarbon dating of skeletons has revealed definitive cases of syphilis in indigenous Americans during the pre-Columbian period and confirmed that the disease existed in the Americas for at least a millennium.

All cases of Old World syphilis overlap the year 1493, the date of Columbus's return. These results, the lack of syphilitic evidence in huge, pre-Columbian European and North African samples, and the sudden appearance of syphilis in many of the same samples after 1493 all indicate that syphilis has existed since ancient times in the New World but appeared in Europe and North Africa only after Columbus's return voyage.

In Aztec mythology, the god Nanahuatzin became the sun by throwing himself into the Spirit Fire, died, and was reborn as Tonatiuh, the sun, giving light and life to the world.

Nanahuatzin also means "full of sores" or "little, pustule-covered one." He's represented as a man deformed by syphilis, with sores on his arms and deformed feet, which may have driven him to throw himself into a fire in the first place.

Syphilis began to infect Europe in the late 1400s, and by the mid-1700s, France in particular was obsessed with the disease. Condoms grew more popular, with entire stores dedicated to selling all types from linen to animal bladders. They were sold at pubs, barbershops, markets, and even the theater. The first recorded inspection of condom quality is found in the memoirs of famed Venetian playboy Giacomo Casanova, who would test for holes by inflating them before use.

French writer Voltaire's most popular novel, *Candide*, includes a character, Pangloss, who had lost his nose to syphilis. This was meant to be a slap in the face (literally) to Pangloss's unending and quite irritating optimism. (On syphilis, Voltaire once noted: "Depend on it when 30,000 men engaged in pitch battle against an equal number of the enemy, about 20,000 on each side have the pox.") In 1792's *Les Liaisons dangereuses*, or *Dangerous Liaisons*, writer Pierre Choderlos de Laclos condemned the antagonist, the former ravishing beauty Madame de Merteuil, to a life of disfigurement from syphilis. Since this took place on the eve of the French Revolution, it represented what he felt the rich truly looked like. (Interestingly, two film versions of the book were produced at the same time—neither end with Madame de Merteuil becoming disfigured from syphilis; she was just made irrelevant—or was possibly killed—by those in the French Revolution.)

Even the Church got involved; the lieutenant general of the Paris police forced local priests to address venereal issues in God's house.

GOODYEAR AND THE CONDOM

Charles Goodyear—after whom the Goodyear Tire and Rubber Company is named—significantly changed the condom with the advent of rubber vulcanization during the Industrial Revolution. Sulfur and natural rubber were heated together to form a more malleable and durable material with higher elasticity and strength. By 1860, condoms were produced on a large scale; the major benefit was that they were cheaper and could be reused. Rubber condoms were originally made to size—bespoke, as it were. This is the dawn of condoms becoming rubbers. It's not known if Goodyear himself wore condoms, though since he was married and had five children, it's possible that he did not.

It was only a matter of time before STIs became the fault of women. According to 1747's *James's Medical Dictionary*, the conclusion was that it was women's organs that carried the virus. Historian Eric Maria Benabou noted, "From there came the notion of women's corruption and major responsibility in the disease." Men were categorized as the innocent victims of dangerous prostitutes.

Other innocent victims of syphilis included babies born to syphilitic mothers and children who were raped by syphilitic men....

Other innocent victims of syphilis included babies born to syphilitic mothers and children who were raped by syphilitic men who were told that that having sex with a virgin would rid them of the disease; obviously, an element of pedophilia was tied into this. Vaugirard Hospital for Syphilitic Infants was built in 1790 with, for its time, state-of-the-art research and medical equipment; the idea was not only to help these tragic cases but also forestall depopulation that would be caused by syphilis.

Also in 1790, a Dr. Lecointe published *La sante de Mars*, or *The Health of Mars*, which not only railed against prostitutes corrupting good men—often soldiers—and leaving them barren but also against France's general moral health, with the outcome again being depopulation. "How many brave soldiers are lost to this dreaded disease?" he asked. "Paris contains 40,000 courtesans who do nothing but distract young men from their duties. What has happened to good families, to morals, to Nature?" Dr. Lecointe's prescription was to regulate prostitution because "why should the strongest, most valiant soldiers not produce equally robust children?" In this reproductive utopia, sons would become the next generation of soldiers, and the daughters would become the next generation of prostitutes.

It wasn't until 1837 that American-born French doctor Philippe Ricord separated syphilis from gonorrhea as two distinct venereal diseases; this explained why, for instance, mercury treatments cured syphilis but did nothing against gonorrhea. Both viruses were isolated in 1879 and 1905. In 1906, blood testing started the diagnoses of these separate STIs.

The Language of Syphilis

Writing a book is "a horrible, exhausting struggle, like a long bout of some painful illness," author George Orwell once said. Indeed, many writers have struggled with a host of diseases and conditions: three of the four Brontë sisters *and* their brother died of tuberculosis; blindness struck the seventeenth-century poet John Milton; and depression has been a writer's miserable companion for centuries, the lone friend of those who take up the pen as a solitary occupation.

In his book *Shakespeare's Tremor and Orwell's Cough: The Medical Lives of Famous Writers*, Dr. John J. Ross of Boston's Brigham and Women's Hospital took a look at how disease may have infected not only the body but also the words of the world's most beloved authors. In particular, Dr. Ross focuses on playwright William Shakespeare and syphilis—Shakespeare's obsession with it and, as the title suggests, the possibility that Shakespeare had it.

In *Measure for Measure*, three citizens of Vienna openly discuss venereal disease. One of them, Lucio, upon seeing a brothel madam approaching, says, "I have purchased … many diseases under her roof." *Measure for Measure* premiered in 1604, the year after the government closed London's brothels.

The standard treatment for syphilis during Shakespeare's time—the Elizabethan Era— was mercury; as the saying goes, "a night with Venus, a lifetime with Mercury." Mercury's more alarming side effects included uncontrollable drooling, gum disease, terrible mood changes, and tremors. The Bard was supposedly promiscuous and was reported to be part of a love triangle where all three contracted syphilis.

Dr. Ross observed:

Shakespeare was more preoccupied than his contemporaries with sexually transmitted diseases. For example, I can find only 6 lines referring to venereal infection in the 7 plays of Christopher Mar-

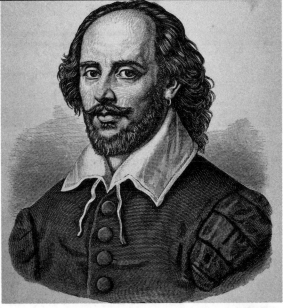

The renowned English playwright and poet William Shakespeare seemed to be fascinated by STIs, mentioning them dozens of times in several of his works.

lowe. However, 55 lines in *Measure for Measure*, 61 lines in *Troilus and Cressida*, and 67 lines in *Timon of Athens* allude to venereal disease. Shakespeare's references to syphilis are often odd and misplaced, leading Anthony Burgess to characterize Shakespeare as having a "gratuitous venereal obsession." Several critics have suggested that Shakespeare himself had syphilis.

"A pox o' your throat, you bawling, blasphemous, incharitable dog!" was one of the many colorful insults that Shakespeare was famous for peppering throughout his work; this one is from *The Tempest*. The "pox" of this play doesn't mean smallpox, which wasn't understood to be a chronic disease until later in the fifteenth century, but syphilis. Syphilis/pox fills Shakespeare's plays:

- "A pox of the devil" (*Henry V*)
- "The vengeance on the whole camp! or, rather the Neapolitan bo-neache!" (*Troilus and Cressida*)
- "All the contagion of the south light on thee...." (*Coriolanus*)
- "Coin words till their decay against those measles, Which we disdain should tetter us, yet sought the very way to catch them." (*Coriolanus*)
- "But yet thou art my flesh, my daughter. Or rather a disease that's in my flesh which I must needs call mine: thou art a boil, A plague sore, an embossed carbuncle." (*King Lear*)
- "A pox of that jest! and be-shrew all shrows!" (*Love's Labour's Lost*)
- "Now a pox upon her green-sickness." (*Pericles*)

Basically, it was a pox on whatever one ridiculed, disdained, or damned.

Syphilis was more severe in Shakespeare's time than it is today. French historian Claude Quétel, in his *History of Syphilis*, notes that all the original works that cover syphilis agree on the principal characteristics of what was then a new disease: high contagiousness, chancres, and aches and pains in the head and bones followed by a reddish rash. Then, after a brief respite, tumors start to appear at random in muscles or bones, eating away at the nose, lips, palate, larynx, and genitals.

Syphilis Treatment

Syphilis is found worldwide. The French called it the Neapolitan disease, and the English, Germans, and Italians called it the French disease. The Russians blamed the Poles; the Poles blamed the Germans; the Dutch blamed the Belgians; the Portuguese blamed the Spanish; and both India and Japan blamed the Portuguese.

In America, it's the third-most-common STI. Overall, fewer cases have occurred since doctors began treating it with penicillin, though there have been slight upticks corresponding to changing sexual behaviors. The introduction of the birth control pill was one of them. Another was an increase in prostitution and drug use in the 1990s. Another uptick occurred recently: since 2012, more than 50,000 new infections are being treated per year. The reason for that is unknown so far, but it could be a resistance to penicillin and/or the opioid crisis.

In America, it's the third-most-common STI. Overall, fewer cases have occurred since doctors began treating it with penicillin, though there have been slight upticks corresponding to changing sexual behaviors.

Three stages of infection occur:

- Primary syphilis: The beginning phase where painless sores called chancres appear around the mouth or genitalia.

- Secondary syphilis: Rashes appear on the body.

- Tertiary syphilis: Various organs, like the brain, spinal cord, heart, liver, and testicles, are affected.

Penicillin treatment works during the primary and early secondary stages of syphilis. For tertiary syphilis, three times the dose of penicillin is needed. Syphilis that has reached the brain and spinal cord—known as neurosyphilis—is a life-threatening complication of syphilis. How well a patient recovers depends on how severe the neurosyphilis is before treatment. Treatment involves an antibiotic penicillin that is either injected several times a day for 10 to 14 days or given orally four times a day combined with daily muscle injections, with both taken for 10 to 14 days.

Treatment also includes mandatory follow-up blood tests at 3, 6, 12, 24, and 36 months to make sure the infection is gone as well as spinal taps every 6 months.

The Tuskegee Experiment

Between 1932 and 1972, the venereal disease section of the U.S. Public Health Service, in conjunction with Tuskegee University, a historically black college in Alabama, conducted the "Tuskegee Study of Untreated Syphilis in the Negro Male." It was unethical, it was racist, and it was funded by the U.S. government. In this study, 600 poor, black farmers were lied to and told that they'd be receiving free health care if they participated in clinical testing. In reality, the purpose of this study was to observe the path of untreated syphilis. Since syphilis cannot be created in labs and does not infect animals, black men—and their families—were used as lab rats.

Of the 600 men, 399 already had syphilis; 201 were deliberately infected with it. The men were told that the study was only going to last six months, but it actually lasted 40 years, even after funding ended. None of the men infected were ever told that they had syphilis, and none were ever treated for it. According to the Centers for Disease Control and Prevention, the men were told that they were being treated for "bad blood," which could've meant anything.

The study continued until 1972, when Peter Buxton, then an employee of the U.S. Public Health Service, reported his findings to the Associated Press. He was fired four months later. The resulting victims of the study were not just the 600 men but the 40 wives who contracted the disease and the 19 children born to the infected women.

After World War II, the horror of Nazi medical abuses led to the Nuremberg Code, which protected the rights of research subjects. In other words, a research subject needed to be told the scope of the study and then give what's called "informed consent." What the U.S. Public Health Service had gotten at Tuskegee was uninformed consent, as the participants were flat-out lied to. This was specified in 1964 by the WHO; however, no one reevaluated the Tuskegee Study according to the new standards and in light of treatment—penicillin—that had become available. When interviewed for a 1992 episode of ABC's *Prime Time Live*, Dr. Sidney Olansky, Public Health Service director of the study from 1950 to 1957, admitted that "the fact that they were illiterate was helpful, too, because they couldn't read the newspapers. If they were [lit-

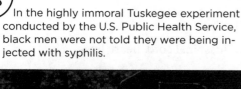

In the highly immoral Tuskegee experiment conducted by the U.S. Public Health Service, black men were not told they were being injected with syphilis.

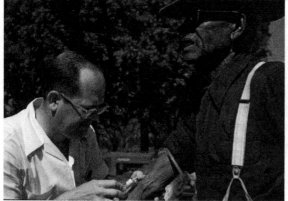

erate], as things moved on they might have been reading newspapers and seen what was going on."

The result of the Tuskegee experiment was more distrust of the government among the black community. In the early years of the HIV/AIDS crisis, persistent rumors spread that the government deliberately caused HIV/AIDS by introducing the virus to the black community either as some kind of experiment or to decimate the black population altogether. This mistrust in the government and the health system continues today.

> A class-action lawsuit filed by the NAACP cost the U.S. government $10 million to pay the victims and their descendants....

A class-action lawsuit filed by the NAACP cost the U.S. government $10 million to pay the victims and their descendants and forced the government to provide free medical treatment to surviving victims and surviving infected family members. Additionally, Congress assembled a commission that created regulations deterring such abuses in the future. A collection of materials compiled to investigate the study is held at the National Library of Medicine in Bethesda, Maryland.

HIV/AIDS

Chances are that you've never seen a virus under a microscope, but if you have seen one online or in a book, it's not hard to be surprised by the beauty of some of them. A human immunodeficiency virus (HIV) looks the way it does not to attract other viruses but to attach to an immune system cell and use it as a host to make more viruses. If HIV were formed differently, it wouldn't be able to attach to an immune system cell and replicate and, therefore, would die out. However, it just so happens that in order to make this attachment come together, a work of art evolved. Go look in a furniture store, and chances are that you'll see home decor that resembles a virus. Ironic, then, that such an elegantly arranged particle has killed more than 25 million people.

HIV causes acquired immunodeficiency syndrome (AIDS). Remember our acquired immunity? The name "Acquired Immunodeficiency Syndrome" doesn't mean that you've acquired a deficient immune system; it means that your acquired immune system has become deficient and its numbers are falling. As its name states, AIDS is not a disease (as it's often called) but a syndrome—a group of symptoms that occur at the same time. It's the last stage of an HIV infection. Most who reach this point have such a weakened immune system that they're left defenseless from illnesses and die from what's known as "opportunistic infections"—infections that a healthy immune system could wage war against but that a compromised one simply cannot. More AIDS victims die of cancer than of any other illness.

Only two people have ever been cured of AIDS—male patients in 2008 and 2017 who received bone marrow transplants, although no one is certain how they were 100 percent cured. The average lifespan for HIV/AIDS patients is ten years if they receive no treatment.

The fact that we discovered that HIV causes AIDS so soon after AIDS was first recognized is due to much greater medical knowledge and technology than our forefathers had. Think back to the plagues of the 500s, the 1300s, and the 1600s—they were all following a medical be-

A graph showing how a typical HIV infection runs its course from initial exposure to death. The body's defensive lymphcites gradually decrease, leaving the body increasingly vulnerable to potentially fatal diseases.

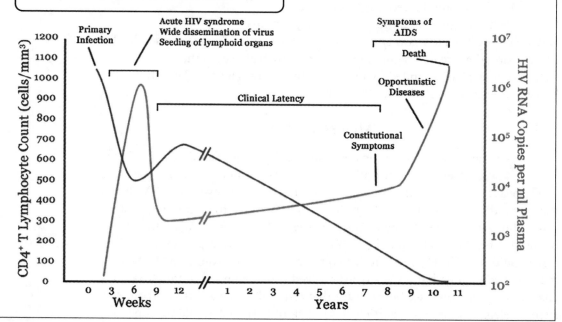

PLAGUES, PANDEMICS AND VIRUSES

lief system formulated in around 150 B.C.E. AIDS was first given its name in 1982 by the CDC; people with HIV were able to be treated before the virus progressed to AIDS by 1995.

However, parallels do exist between plague and AIDS (which was given the nickname "the gay plague" in the 1980s). This largely had to do with a misunderstanding of how it was spread. Since so many illnesses are spread through the air, it was assumed that HIV and even AIDS were contagious in the same way. This led to widespread confusion, violence, and isolation—all of these reactions based on fear.

Because gay men were the most visible AIDS victims, many viewed this as God's punishment for their sinful ways (also hearkening back to the aforementioned plagues as God's punishment). Never mind that babies caught HIV from infected mothers or that 90 percent of hemophiliacs caught HIV from blood transfusions before HIV screening was developed—these were innocent victims caught in the middle of a war between God and man because some men loved men.

So, let's pretend we're educating the American public around, say, 1985, as to what HIV is, what AIDS is, how to contract it, and how to avoid it.

We'll start again with the definition of a virus because HIV is a bit different from other viruses. Usually, a virus attaches to a host cell's receptors, enters the host cell, and hijacks its biological mechanisms, so instead of the host cell making new cells, the virus uses the cell's DNA to make more viruses. These new viruses will eventually burst through the cell wall, kill the cell, and find new cells to bind to. The process is then repeated billions of times over. The common cold forms this way.

HIV is known as a "retrovirus" because it reverses—"retro"—the direction of the normal gene-copying process through an enzyme called "reverse transcriptase." Its genetic material does not contain the DNA double helix; it contains a single strand of RNA. Therefore, an extra step is needed to transform RNA into DNA and build new viruses. (DNA dictates what the cell is going to do and how it's going to do it.)

Remember helper T cells? They're the cells in our acquired immune system that sound the alarm to attract additional white blood cells to an infection site and also release chemicals that stimulate other white blood cells to multiply. They're also the primary target of HIV.

The design of the proteins covering HIV fit the design of the receptors covering a helper T cell. Because of this, the HIV proteins can bind to these receptors, then pierce the cell membrane, injecting HIV into the helper T cell.

The enzymes and RNA are then released into the cell and, using the enzymes along with the host's own molecules, reverse transcriptase gets to work. The single strand of RNA is converted into a single strand of DNA, then that new single strand of DNA is reverse transcribed to create a double strand of DNA. (This process leads to many typos—transcriptase is a bad proofreader—but these typos help HIV to constantly mutate, thus preventing an effective vaccine from being created.)

By now, another enzyme, called integrase, grabs that double strand of DNA and carries it into the host cell's nucleus. The integrase finds the host's chromosome and cuts a nick into it, allowing the viral DNA to insert itself into the host's DNA. (This is how integrase gets its name—it integrates the viral DNA into the host DNA.) From this moment on, the victim has a lifelong infection.

The structure of the HIV virus.

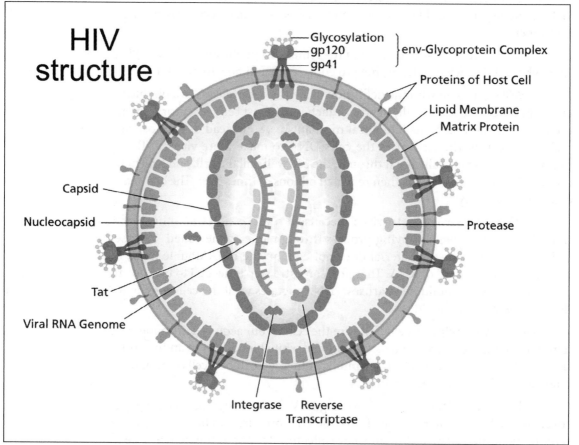

HIV structure

- Glycosylation
- gp120
- gp41
} env-Glycoprotein Complex

Proteins of Host Cell

Lipid Membrane

Matrix Protein

Capsid

Nucleocapsid

Protease

Tat

Viral RNA Genome

Integrase   Reverse Transcriptase

PLAGUES, PANDEMICS AND VIRUSES

Inside the host's cell are enzymes that direct the normal route of transcription: DNA to RNA. Now that the viral DNA is the host's DNA, the enzyme is converting *viral* DNA into viral RNA.

So, what's the point of turning DNA back into RNA? First, the RNA has to become DNA in order to attach to the DNA of the host's cell and become part of that cell's genetic makeup, but it then has to turn back into RNA so that its ingredients can be recreated over and over again in new viruses.

Within the host's cytoplasm—that liquid area between the cell membrane and the nucleus—are particles called ribosomes. The viral RNA enters the cytoplasm and attaches to a ribosome. Through a process called translation, the ribosome reads the RNA and creates proteins, just as it's supposed to do—except now, they're the proteins that are ingredients of HIV, such as reverse transcriptase and integrase, so the host cell—which had once been an essential part of our immune system—is now a virus factory.

Ribosomes also build capsids that enclose the HIV materials; these materials within the capsid assemble into what are called "immature viruses." They push their way through the host's cell membrane, a process called "budding," which causes it to bulge, then break off and enclose the virus, releasing the retroviruses into the body. The host cell dies along with as many as two billion other host cells each day.

After a series of chemical reactions, the immature cells will mature and repeat the cycle, beginning to break down a person's immune system.

Depending on the type of HIV and its mutations, it can either kill macrophages or travel on them to helper T cells, causing certain death for the T cells. Eventually, the victim will be completely vulnerable to infections. A healthy T cell count is anywhere between 500–1,500 cells per cubic millimeter of blood. Someone with HIV has about 150 cells per cubic millimeter of blood.

Despite this whirlwind of activity going on within an infected person, HIV leaves no trace, or symptoms, for great lengths of time. It's almost like a hunter stalking its prey—which is why one person can infect many over the course of several years without knowing they're sick. Meanwhile, their entire immune system is under attack, leaving all cells vulnerable.

The virus has to do more than get into our bodies and replicate. It has to get out of our bodies so it can infect someone else, after which they can infect someone else. HIV does not live long outside the body, which is why it doesn't spread through the air like a cold or even the plague. Instead, it breaches our defenses through the fluid route—blood, semen, vaginal fluid, and even breast milk. (The only bodily fluids that don't spread HIV are saliva and tears due to their high salt content.)

So, sharing hypodermic needles, vaginal birth, and breastfeeding are among the ways that HIV can be transmitted from one person to another—not hugging, touching, drinking from the same straw, or sharing clothes.

However, sexual activity is the best way for an opportunistic virus to travel from one person to another—and it's not just AIDS that's plagued people who have sex, whether gay or straight. More than 50 sexually transmitted infections, or STIs, exist, including syphilis, herpes, chlamydia, and gonorrhea. Some can be embarrassing and are incurable, like herpes, but herpes won't kill you. Others, like syphilis, can—but none inflict the kind of damage wrought by AIDS.

When AIDS made headlines in the early 1980s, it was at first called GRID, or

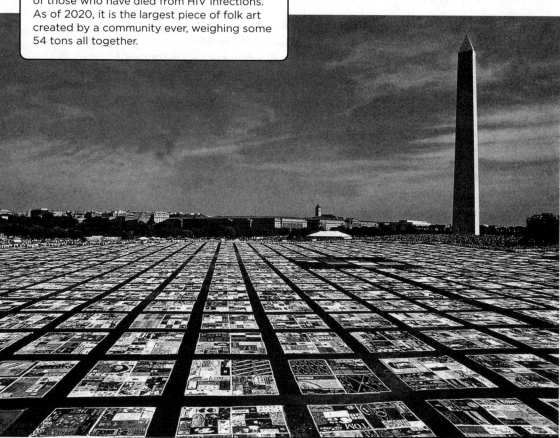

The AIDS Memorial Quilt (shown here on display in Washington, D.C.) honors the lives of those who have died from HIV infections. As of 2020, it is the largest piece of folk art created by a community ever, weighing some 54 tons all together.

"gay-related immune deficiency." Though this term was never officially used in the medical community and was also soon changed to AIDS to reflect all AIDS victims, calling it GRID showed how it was considered a disease that targeted only gay men and, even more specifically, promiscuous gay men.

(Remember—AIDS is not a disease. As mentioned before, it's a syndrome. HIV is not a disease; it's a virus. So, the term "gay disease" is wrong on both counts.)

This is where HIV and the plague diverge. Although the Church originally tried to blame the disease on people's sinful nature—it was an answer that made sense and kept them off the hook—even the Church changed its tune after priests started dying just as frequently as farmers. Meanwhile, culturally, it's been frowned upon to blame the victim, so unless you went out, sought someone with plague, and did your best to contract it, you wouldn't be blamed—or, indeed, hated—for getting sick.

Despite that, gay men, sick or not, were blamed for spreading AIDS. It was an illness written off as something that struck only gays and drug addicts: the outcasts. If you weren't a gay man or an IV drug user, you had nothing to worry about. Meanwhile, those who were dying were blamed for dying.

Simian immunodeficiency virus (SIV) is a virus related to HIV and is present in a variety of ape and monkey species, including chimpanzees, mandrills, colobus monkeys, guenons, and this rhesus macaque (pictured), among others. It is believed that HIV/AIDS may be a mutation of SIV/SAIDS.

Where Did AIDS Begin?

AIDS originated in primates that live in the African jungles. Even before AIDS, experts warned that frequent human and monkey contact could cause dire problems, though they couldn't predict how dire. Why did they think this? Think back to the European farmers who caught the pox from livestock. If these zoological diseases could happen on farms, they could also happen in the jungle.

Research now estimates that HIV emerged in West Africa sometime around the 1940s, perhaps as early as the 1920s. One of the major factors in the spread of HIV was deforestation, which displaced numerous African tribes. People were forced to move deeper into

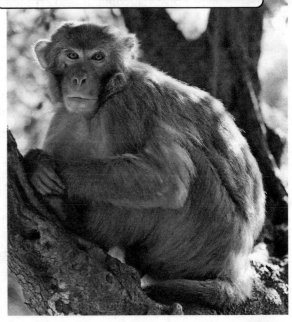

PLAGUES, PANDEMICS AND VIRUSES

the bush and encounter primates they had no experience with or immunity from. (Habitat displacement, whether it be bats, apes, or people, plays a pivotal role when it comes to spreading diseases.)

As these tribal populations grew, they began to keep primates as pets and for meat, thus beginning HIV's jump from animal to human.

We now know that HIV is related to the simian immunodeficiency virus, or SIV. We've only had to face HIV for several decades; SIV—also a retrovirus—has existed in monkeys and apes for at least 32,000 years. This length of time has given some of these primates immunity to SIV, though primates that don't normally come into contact with SIV have not developed an immunity and can contract SIV and develop Simian AIDS, or SAIDS.

Another reason why it's a bad idea to eat wild animals—wild animals also eat wild animals. A chimpanzee, though mostly vegetarian, will hunt and eat monkeys, and if it catches SIV, it's most likely caused by eating a monkey that had it. This led to a recombination of SIV within the chimpanzee, then eventually SAIDS within the chimpanzee population. Another recombination led to HIV/AIDS after humans ate infected chimpanzee meat.

However, it wasn't people dying in Africa from AIDS that made the world take note; it was young, healthy men in New York City in the early 1980s who were dying in droves from what had been a rare form of cancer called Kaposi's sarcoma. It also erupted throughout gay communities in San Francisco, heralding what would soon become the worldwide pandemic that is still with us today.

Kaposi's sarcoma is caused by human herpes virus 8, or HHV8, and can occur on the skin or within the mouth, respiratory system, or gastrointestinal system. Nearly one-third of those who were victims of the first major wave of AIDS also developed Kaposi's sarcoma. This once rare cancer became so common that it was given the name "AIDS rash."

GEOGRAPHIC ORIGINS OF HIV

In October 2016, the journal *Nature* reported that the strain of HIV responsible for almost all AIDS cases in the United States was carried from the Democratic Republic of Congo to Haiti in around 1967, spread from there to New York City in around 1971, and then from New York City to San Francisco in around 1976.

Conspiracy theorists went wild when the disease made headlines. Was it a right-wing plot? A left-wing plot? Was it some form of biological warfare accidentally let loose? Also, don't forget the ever-present wrath of God.

Public officials ignored it. Treatment was stalled because of stigma and fear. Some who did speak out demanded quarantines in order to separate the "innocent" victims from the homosexuals and drug addicts. What else was stalled? Care, research, and compassion.

How Patient O Became Patient 0

In 1981, a young scientist named William Darrow from the CDC was tasked with discovering what had caused this possible pandemic. Some doctors thought it came from inhaled drugs called "poppers." *The New York Times* reported that it might be "overexposure to sperm," but Darrow had heard a rumor that several of the first AIDS casualties had been lovers. Could this be some kind of sexually transmitted disease?

HIV is not transmitted just by sexual contact but also by drug use. The common practice among users of heroin of sharing needles offered the perfect way for the virus to leap from person to person.

Darrow became part doctor, part detective, part investigative reporter—interviewing scores of gay men about their sex lives. On one particular day, three men who didn't know each other mentioned the same lover.

He was a French Canadian flight attendant named Gaëtan Dugas. He fit the profile perfectly: a gay man with movie-star looks who traveled for a living (reminiscent of how plagues were spread from port to port) and who, by his own admission, had had more than 750 sexual partners over the previous three years.

He was also the perfect villain: promiscuous and unashamed; foreign; beautiful. The kind of man many loved to hate. The *New York Post* even damned him with the headline "The Man Who Gave Us AIDS."

Dugas, of his own free will, visited the CDC in Atlanta, Georgia, to provide blood samples and the names of more than 70 sexual partners. He even volunteered at a nonprofit to help others who had HIV. Dugas died of AIDS-related complications in 1984 at the age of 31. Here, it was thought, must be the person who spread AIDS worldwide.

Analysis now shows that the strain of HIV in Dugas's blood, taken a year before his death, was a kind that had already been infecting men in New York City long before Dugas began visiting gay bars there in 1974. Also, his original designation was not "Patient 0" but "Patient O"—the "O" stood for "Outside Southern California," where the research began. It was misread, and the name stuck.

And the Band Played On

In 1987, Randy Shilts, a *San Francisco Chronicle* reporter, wrote *And the Band Played On: Politics, People, and the AIDS Epidemic*, a chronicle of the early days of AIDS research and discovery. The idea for the book came to Shilts—who was gay—after he heard esteemed journalist Bill Kurtis make a joke at an awards ceremony in San Francisco: "What's the toughest part about getting AIDS? Convincing your wife you're Haitian."

(In fact, the earliest AIDS victims were dubbed members of the "4-H Club": homosexuals, hemophiliacs, heroin addicts, and Haitians.)

According to Shilts, "Bill Kurtis felt that he could go in front of a journalists' group in San Francisco and make AIDS jokes. First of all, he could assume that nobody there would be gay and, if they were gay … [wouldn't] take offense at that…. [T]hat summed up the whole problem of dealing with AIDS in the media. Obviously, the reason I covered AIDS from the start was that, to me, it was never something that happened to those other people."

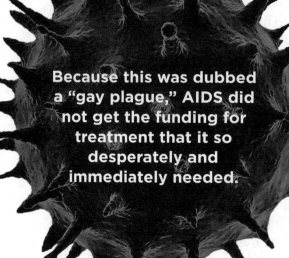

> Because this was dubbed a "gay plague," AIDS did not get the funding for treatment that it so desperately and immediately needed.

In 1970s San Francisco, it was not uncommon for gay men to have multiple sexual partners on a weekly basis. That added up to more than 1,000 per year. Because this was dubbed a "gay plague," AIDS did not get the funding for treatment that it so desperately and immediately needed. If it had, who knows how many millions of people would have gone on to live longer lives without infecting others?

Indeed, this was a time when mass media was shaping what we thought about everything from politics to war to ring around the collar—and AIDS was no different. Whereas plagues were in a time and place before TV, radio, or film coverage—and details were often maddeningly vague—AIDS was the top story in global national news; Randy Shilts was profiled on *60 Minutes* (and was introduced as "Randy Shilts, a gay" by reporter Harry Reasoner); and scores of men walking arm and arm in places like San Francisco were shown to an often revolted audience.

However, three people changed the way people viewed AIDS: one was a famous Hollywood heartthrob, one was a kid from Indiana, and one was an all-star basketball player. Their backgrounds are vastly different, but they're united by an illness that defined the rest of their lives and their legacies.

A Movie Star Is Gay

Rock Hudson was a dashing and charismatic actor who was largely famous in the 1950s and 1960s. The definition of tall, dark, and handsome, yet also with a glint in his eye, Hudson starred opposite Elizabeth Taylor in the box-office smash *Giant* and was often paired with good-girl Doris Day in a series of madcap comedies that ended with the two of them living happily ever after.

That was Tinseltown. In real life, Rock Hudson was gay, though in many ways, it wasn't difficult for Hudson to act the part of a straight man; few people thought a manly man like Rock Hudson would be having sex with men. After all, he had a manly man name: Rock. (His real name was Roy Scherer Jr.)

It's a common misconception that in the days before social media, enormous secrets like Hudson's would be kept under wraps as a kind of honor code among celebs. *Confidential Magazine*, a once famous Hollywood tabloid, threatened to publish a story about Hudson's homosexuality, effectively blackmailing him into revealing lurid secrets about other stars in exchange for their silence. Hudson then made haste to the altar, where he married his agent's secretary, Phyllis Gates, in 1955. The marriage lasted three years and produced no children.

Rock Hudson's closeted life continued for decades. Then, everything changed in 1985. On July 17, Hudson collapsed shortly after checking into Paris's Ritz Hotel; as this coincided with a time when AIDS was on everyone's minds, those who had known the truth about Hudson's sexuality began speculating out loud that perhaps he had AIDS. First, Hudson's flack blamed it on liver cancer. Then, anorexia. Eventually, denials soon gave way to a public admission of the truth: Rock Hudson was gay, and he was dying of AIDS.

Though Hudson certainly didn't want to be the poster boy for AIDS, the fact that a "normal" person could get AIDS, not just Gaëtan Dugas, began to

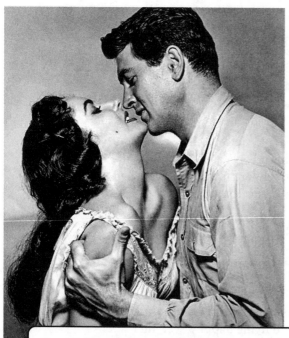

Heartthrob actor Rock Hudson (shown here with Elizabeth Taylor in the 1956 film *Giant,* for which he won an Oscar) surprised many fans when it was revealed he was gay (although this was common knowledge in the film industry) and had HIV, which led to his death in 1985.

change the public's perception of AIDS victims ever so slightly. In *And the Band Played On,* Randy Shilts wrote, "It was commonly accepted" that two phases of AIDS existed in the United States: "There was AIDS before Rock Hudson and AIDS after." It also helped lead to more donations to fund research for a cure. *People* magazine reported: "Since Hudson made his announcement, more than $1.8 million in private contributions (more than double the amount collected in 1984) has been raised to support AIDS research and to care for AIDS victims … Congress set aside $221 million to develop a cure for AIDS."

Not everyone suddenly changed their tune, though. Rock Hudson was a longtime friend of Ronald and Nancy Reagan, who were the president and first lady of the United States when Hudson got sick. (Ronald Reagan, before he became president, was an actor as well.) While Hudson lay dying in a Paris hospital, his publicist, Dale Olson, reached out to the White House with the message that "only one hospital in the world can offer necessary medical treatment to save the life of Rock Hudson or at least alleviate his illness." Olson was referring to a French military hospital that Hudson was denied access to because he was American—but, surely, an intervention from the Reagans would bypass medical and diplomatic red tape.

It was First Lady Nancy Reagan who turned down the request. Rock Hudson died on October 2, 1985, at the age of 59. Millions would die after him.

Ryan White

Ryan White was a typical 1980s kid—he lived in Indiana, had a paper route, and went to middle school. The one major difference was that White was a hemophiliac, which meant that his blood lacked the ability to clot, so even the smallest injury could lead to massive bleeding.

To combat this, White had weekly blood transfusions where he was given medication called factor VII, which is culled from the plasma of nonhemophiliac blood donors. Unfortunately, in the early 1980s, blood donors were not screened for HIV. Between 1979 and 1984, nearly 90 percent of hemophiliacs treated with blood-clotting factors like factor VII became infected with HIV and/or hepatitis C through blood transfusions.

In 1984, White became severely ill with pneumonia; during a lung biopsy, he was diagnosed with AIDS. So, not only did White have hemophilia, he now had a syndrome that would eventually cause his death. White was given six months to live; he had just turned 13.

Miraculously, over the course of several months, White's health began to improve to the point where he felt well enough to return to school, but another battle was about to begin: this was for his dignity as a kid who only wanted to go to school.

A year before Ryan's diagnosis, *The Journal of the American Medical Association* sent out a press release declaring, "Evidence suggests household contact may transmit AIDS." While most people in White's school district probably didn't read the press release, their fears echoed it. As seen with diseases like the plague, when people don't know where a disease comes from and how it spreads, it's fear that often takes over. For certain people, fear can make them unable to even get out of bed. For others, it can cause anger and violence. Central Indiana was now forced to grapple with AIDS, and many were not ready.

People on White's paper route cancelled their deliveries rather than risk getting AIDS. A cashier threw his mother's change at her rather than hand it to her. The family's tires were slashed, White's school superintendent and principal barred him from attending school, and he had to listen to classes over the phone. Eventually, the Indiana Board of Education and the county health officers deemed that White was not a danger to his classmates and allowed him to come back to school, but there,

> *The Journal of the American Medical Association* sent out a press release declaring, "Evidence suggests household contact may transmit AIDS."

he was greeted with reporters and protestors and had to be escorted by his step-father. Inside school was no easier, as his classmates called him a "faggot" and threatened to kill him. The school forced White to eat alone with disposable utensils, use a separate bathroom, and refrain from taking gym class. All this, and he still had to have weekly blood transfusions, which was what put him into this situation to begin with.

Parents took their children out of school, though many did keep their children enrolled despite the perceived threat. However, after an unknown assailant shot a bullet through a window of White's house, the family moved from Kokomo, Indiana, to Cicero, Indiana—and, therefore, White had to attend a new school, where he was greeted with handshakes from the superintendent, principal, and classmates. Not everyone greeted White so warmly, but time and education had made Cicero a much more welcoming place for White and his family.

So, it was the plight of a young boy as an innocent victim within the AIDS crisis—he was not a drug addict nor a promiscuous flight attendant nor a famous actor who'd perpetuated a ruse for decades—that propelled Ryan White into the spotlight. As an accidental advocate for HIV/AIDS, White was suddenly seen with A-list celebrities like Elton John, got a kiss from his celebrity crush, Alyssa Milano, and received a Mustang from Michael Jackson. In January 1989, ABC aired *The Ryan White Story* in which White had a cameo.

Though it was AIDS that gave Ryan White the opportunity to meet celebrities, speak at the President's Commission on the HIV Epidemic, get a brand-new car, and befriend other children with AIDS, White maintained that he would trade it all so as not to have a terminal illness. A little more than a year after *The Ryan White Story* aired, the real Ryan White was admitted to the Riley Hospital for Children in Indianapolis, Indiana, with a severe respiratory tract infection. Elton John was one of the people at his bedside. He died on April 8, 1990, at the age of 18—more than five years after he was given six months to live.

Even though Ronald Reagan didn't acknowledge Rock Hudson's death in 1985, by 1990, the now former president wrote a tribute to White, which was printed in *The Washington Post*: "We owe it to Ryan to make sure that the fear and ignorance that chased him from his home and his school will be eliminated. We owe it to Ryan to open our hearts and our minds to those with AIDS. We owe it to Ryan to be compassionate, caring and tolerant toward those with AIDS, their families and friends. It's the disease that's frightening, not the people who have it."

On August 18, 1990, the Ryan White CARE Act was authorized by Congress and is the largest federally funded program in the United States for people living with HIV/AIDS. In 1991, the first year that funds were appropriated, around $220 million was spent; by the early 2000s, the number had increased almost tenfold. The act was reauthorized in 1996, 2000, 2006, and 2009. The program provides care for around 500,000 people a year and, in 2004, provided funds to 2,567 organizations. The Ryan White programs also fund local and state primary medical care providers, support services and health-care-provider training programs, and provide technical assistance to such organizations. In 2013, the Ryan White CARE Act expired, though the program remains as Congress continues to appropriate funding.

Magic Johnson

Earvin "Magic" Johnson Jr. was born in Lansing, Michigan, to parents who both played basketball. As the number-one draft pick by the Los Angeles Lakers in 1979, he became one of the NBA's greatest players of all time, living up to the nickname he'd been given as a teen.

Then, in 1991, while still at the height of his career and after he'd won this third MVP award, Johnson held a press conference, where he announced his immediate retirement. The reason? He was HIV positive.

So, Magic Johnson was a heroin addict? Gay? A gay heroin addict? Johnson said he was none of these, but he admitted that he'd had "harems of women" whom he'd slept with during his time with the NBA even though he was recently married and had a young child. (Neither his wife nor son tested positive for HIV.) Johnson wanted to tell the public that he was retiring because of HIV—and not a reason concocted by his public relations team—because he believed that the public should know that heterosexual, non-IV drug users could get the virus, too … and, essentially, if Magic Johnson could get it, so could anyone. Also, he wanted to teach others not to "discriminate against people who have HIV and AIDS."

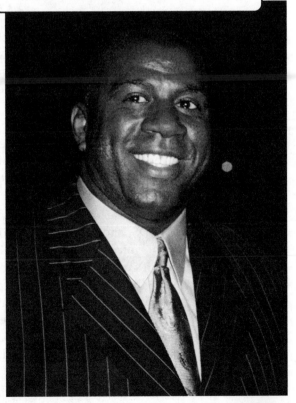

Famous former basketball player Earvin "Magic" Johnson found out he had HIV in 1991 but has survived thanks to proper medical care. He established the Magic Johnson Foundation to increase awareness and fund research for HIV/AIDS.

The presidential response this time, from George H. W. Bush, was, "For me, Magic is a hero."

In 1992, Johnson joined the National Commission on AIDS, a committee appointed by members of Congress and the Bush Sr. Administration. Johnson left after eight months, saying that the White House had "utterly ignored" the commission's recommendations of universal health care and the expansion of Medicaid to cover all low-income people with AIDS—issues the United States is still dealing with now.

Johnson is the head of the Magic Johnson Foundation, a charity organization that began after Johnson retired. According to its website, the "I Stand with Magic" campaign has provided free HIV/AIDS testing to more than 38,000 Americans in sixteen major cities and educated nearly 280,000 people about HIV, risk factors associated with the disease, and the importance of HIV testing. Since 2003, its partnership with AIDS Healthcare Clinics has tested over 3,750 adults and identified positive results for over 1,000 people tested. The foundation also supports at-risk children.

AIDS Is Still Here

AIDS catapulted its victims and loved ones into action. It gave them a voice. It forced public policy to change. It altered the mindset of blaming the victim for getting sick. It also galvanized the LGBTQ+ movement because they knew they were fighting for their lives in the face of a government who wanted to turn its back on them.

Though we have come a long way in developing treatment for a virus that's still relatively new, one of the reasons AIDS is still so deadly is its relative youth. It's only about 70 years old, which isn't quite long enough for a human being to develop or inherit an immunity and also not enough time for AIDS to evolve into a less virulent strain.

Close to 35 million people are HIV positive, 25 million people have died of AIDS, and more than 2 million children have AIDS. About 70 percent of people infected with HIV live in sub-Saharan Africa. AIDS has devastated Africa. It's reduced the life expectancy down to where it had been in the 1880s. More than 100 years of medical progress in Africa has been wiped out in less than a decade. Seven sub-Saharan countries now have a life expectancy of less than 40 years; Botswana's life expectancy went from 72 to 39 years. (It has recovered to 69.4 years in 2020.) More children die of AIDS in Botswana than all other types of death combined.

Malaria, which has also killed millions of Africans, is spread by mosquitoes. Given that HIV is a virus that's contracted through internal contact, it would stand to reason that mosquitoes would be the perfect vector for HIV—like fleas with the plague. Fortunately, HIV can't replicate within a mosquito, and the virus subsequently dies. But malaria is a huge help to HIV because someone with malaria has a large number of helper T cells to fight it off. Remember, it's these T cells that are attacked by HIV, so someone with malaria who then becomes infected with HIV faces horrific health repercussions. HIV helps malaria as well. HIV's attack on the immune system increases the risk of catching malaria because you now have an increasingly worn-down immune system.

War, poverty, lack of education, and famine are friends of HIV as well. These issues, along with casual sex and spreading needles, take precedence over HIV/AIDS education and safe practices. So much for calling it "the gay plague"—today, nearly half of new AIDS cases are among people who identify as heterosexuals, and more than half of them are women. The most prevalent way AIDS is spread in Africa and the United States is prostitution.

Young, black women are particularly at risk. Although they account for just 7 per-

> The good news is that cases of AIDS are going down, as are deaths. More and more people are surviving because of better medications. However, the virus is not gone, nor will it ever be, so it is best to remain cognizant of risky behaviors that can expose you to HIV.

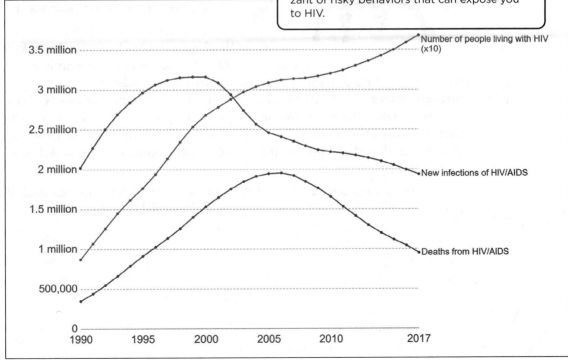

cent of the U.S. population, they comprise 50 percent of AIDS cases—and those are just the ones that are reported.

The best drugs available to combat HIV before it develops into AIDS are called azidothymidine, or AZT, and highly active retroviral therapy, or HAART. These must be taken every day for the rest of the victim's life, no matter how healthy they feel. Survival also comes with a huge price tag—HAART alone costs about $10,000 per year. Imagine trying to afford that in the Western world. Now, imagine trying to afford that in a developing country where you can't even get clean water.

So much for calling it "the gay plague"—today, nearly half of new AIDS cases are among people who identify as heterosexuals....

Vaccines are usually derived from parts of dead microbes or live microbes taken from a weakened strain. When injected, the immune system does what it's programmed to do: destroy the invader and remember it through memory T- and B cells in case of repeat invasion. But because HIV can rapidly mutate—thanks to frequent typos during reverse transcriptase—attempts to create vaccines with HIV segments have been unsuccessful. However, we have developed vaccines against the simian and feline versions of AIDS, so hope still exists.

The fact remains, though, that millions of people have already died of AIDS, and millions more people are going to die of AIDS in the future.

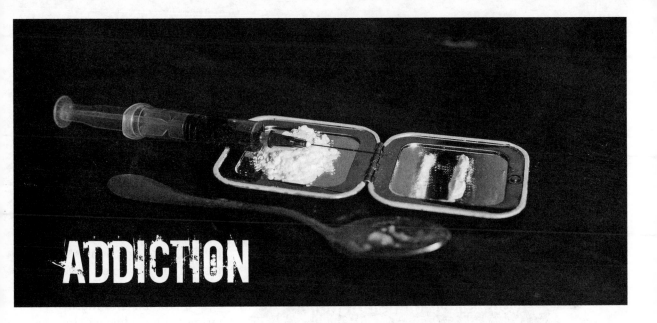

ADDICTION

Is addiction a disease? This is a question that's been asked and answered in a myriad of different ways for decades. In the strictest sense, addiction does not fit the pathogen-plus-host model. No cocaine virus or gambling bacterium exists, yet the host is often as powerless to addiction as they would be if stricken with *Y. pestis*.

Addiction may not have a pathogen, but it does have a chemical equation. Our brains come equipped with a reward system, something that makes us feel good when, for example, we get an A on a test, get married, or buy a house. This euphoria doesn't last forever, but we scarcely know when it ends, such is its mild dissipation.

However, when an addict's euphoria comes to an end, their whole body goes into an apocalyptic-size panic. Trembling, nausea, hallucinations, sweating, diarrhea, depression, anxiety—it's all there in droves, and for alcoholics or pill addicts, the electromagnetic system in the brain can often go wild, causing hysteria, seizures, and death.

It's as if nature did not intend for us to feel *this* good. The feeling is beyond natural, beyond anything our reward system can muster on its own. Addicts keep pushing the boundaries that nature set up—feel-good checkpoints that brain chemicals shouldn't be allowed to pass.

Addiction and the AIDS epidemic have a lot in common: both are cloaked in shame, silence, and blame. Nearly every family is in some way affected by addiction, yet it's still met with derision. In addition, the addict will generally feel that they aren't worthy of help, even if they want it. Brief moments of sobriety are too painful. It's a giant cocktail, so to speak, of scorn from without and within.

Left untreated, addiction has dire consequences—jails, institutions, or death. Decades of scientific research have shown that this is a chronic medical issue because, whether you believe that addiction is a disease or a choice, one thing is for certain: It damages the brain. The mechanisms behind addiction are the prefrontal cortex, which is the part responsible for things like judgment and decision making—what motivates our behavior. Then, the next part is the striatum, which puts you into action—it makes you pursue goals, desires, and wants. Finally comes the midbrain, which makes dopamine, which works with the striatum to get you to focus on your goal. In addiction, you get a large amount of dopamine coming toward the striatum from cigarettes, alcohol, gambling, sex—or whatever your drug of choice is.

A connection also exists between the striatum and the prefrontal cortex in order to control our behavior. We do this all the time, usually with some bal-

> **Decades of scientific research have shown that this is a chronic medical issue because, whether you believe that addiction is a disease or a choice, ... it damages the brain.**

ALCOHOL TOLERANCE

Tolerance builds up after repeated alcohol use but not after repeated alcohol withdrawal. Alcohol withdrawal gets worse over time. Repeated withdrawals can go from terrible headaches and anxiety to hallucinations—both visual and auditory—seizures, insanity, and death. Known as delirium tremens, or DTs (*delirium* is Latin for "going off the furrow," which is a metaphor for going off track while plowing), nicknames include the shakes, barrel fever, blue horrors, bottleache, drunken horrors, elephants, gallon distemper, quart mania, and pink spiders.

ance between impulse and control. ("I want that $5,000 sofa … but I guess I shouldn't put it on my MasterCard.") In addiction, though, the fibers that connect the striatum and the prefrontal cortex wear down, so less communication occurs between them, which results in less impulse control when it comes to that drug of choice. ("It's just a credit card; I'll pay the sofa off.") Indeed, the number of connections decreases over time.

Once the addict quits their drug of choice, however, these connections grow back, especially those between the striatum and prefrontal cortex—helping the addict to act less impulsively when it comes to reaching for that bottle, those pills—or that sofa.

Two schools of thought exist when it comes to an addiction: 1) it's a brain disease; and 2) it's learned behavior, just like we learn to play the piano.

Regardless of whether or not it's a disease, addiction does "infect" its victims and those who come into contact with them. Families are destroyed, work performance suffers, and driving while impaired kills almost 30 people in the United States every day. Addiction behaves just like a virus that goes from person to person—the behaviors may be different, but they're all symptoms of the same problem.

ALCOHOLISM

A blood test can tell whether or not a person has alcohol in their system, but no blood test exists for alcoholism.

No single gene is responsible for alcoholism; hundreds of genes are in a person's DNA that may amplify the risk of developing an alcohol-use disorder. Identifying these genes is difficult because each plays a small role in a much larger picture, but studies have shown that certain combinations of genes have a strong relationship to alcoholism.

Genetics are responsible for about 50 percent of the risk a person has for developing alcoholism. This means that while genes play a role, they're not the only factor that determines whether or not a person will become an alcoholic. Behavioral genes are also passed down that

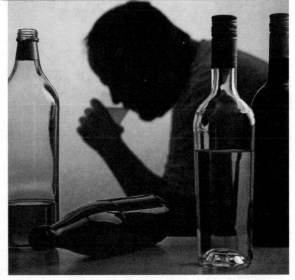

Is alcoholism a disease? A behavior? Both? Studies indicate that genetics could influence whether or not someone has alcoholic tendencies by 50 percent.

could influence a propensity for alcoholism. Mental illnesses, such as depression and schizophrenia, are more common in people with a family history of these disorders. People with mental illness have a higher risk of turning to substance abuse as a way of self-medicating.

Some of the genes that can play a role in alcoholism include those that impact how we metabolize alcohol. For example, many people who are Asian have a genetic variant that changes the way they metabolize alcohol; they may not experience the characteristic euphoric feelings that others do. This leads them to avoid alcohol in many cases, reducing their likelihood of becoming an alcoholic.

Drunk History

The *Epic of Gilgamesh* is perhaps the oldest written story that we have. It is an epic poem retelling the exploits of a king who reigned over the Sumerian city-state of Uruk—now part of Iraq—in around 2700 B.C.E.

The poem includes a character, Enkidu, who is taught how to eat and drink like a man by a prostitute named Shanhat:

Enkidu knew nothing about eating bread for food,
And of drinking beer he had not been taught.
The harlot spoke to Enkidu, saying:
"Eat the food, Enkidu, it is the way one lives.
Drink the beer, as is the custom of the land."
Enkidu ate the food until he was sated,
He drank the beer—seven jugs! and became expansive and sang
  with joy!

The world's oldest brewery, dating back 5,000 years, was found in ancient Egypt. It could produce up to 300 gallons of beer per day. As their civilization developed along the Nile River, Egyptians faced the same challenges of alcohol that people do today, like excessive drinking and the associated problem of workplace absenteeism.

The ancient Romans were famous for their potent potables. Bacchus was a Roman god who brought about peace and serenity through wine. Wine would be served all day long at parties, paired with multiple-course meals. To the Romans, wine was as necessary as our daily bread and was also the great equalizer—it was given to the wealthy, peasants, slaves, and women. Not surprisingly, given their feelings about the Germanic people, Romans were not fans of beer. Roman historian Tacitus wrote, "To drink, the Teutons have a horrible brew fermented from barley or wheat, a brew which has only a very far removed similarity to wine," while Roman emperor Julian composed a poem claiming that

two Dionysuses should exist—one for wine and one for beer—since, according
to him, wine was the nectar of the gods and beer smelled like goat.

> Who and from where are you Dionysus?
> Since by the true Bacchus,
> I do not recognize you; I know only the son of Zeus.
> While he smells like nectar, you smell like a goat.
> Can it be then that the Celts because of lack of grapes
> Made you from cereals? Therefore one should call you
> Demetrius, not Dionysus, rather wheat born and Bromus,
> Not Bromius.

Dipsomania

Alcoholism was first given the name "dipsomania" in 1819 by German
physician C. W. Hufeland, a term used by psychoanalysts as renowned as Sigmund Freud.

However, the defining of habitual drunkenness, as it was then known,
and its adverse consequences were not well established medically until the eighteenth century. The term "alcoholism" was first used in 1849 by Swedish physician Magnus Huss to describe the systematic adverse effects of alcohol.

In his 1892 book *Clinical Lectures on Mental Diseases*, writer T. S. Clous-
ton tells the story of a man referred to as F. D., "an educated, professional man

---

FREUD'S ADDICTION

Sigmund Freud knew a thing or two about addiction aside from studying it in his patients. He began using cocaine in 1884, and while
alcohol did little for him, Freud was bowled over by cocaine's therapeutic
properties—he used it on and off for about ten years. What Freud was
utterly powerless against, though, was nicotine. Freud smoked about 20
cigars a day, and if he couldn't have one, he would become terribly agi-
tated. One of the most famous pictures of him, taken in around 1921,
shows him holding a cigar. After a doctor diagnosed Freud as having jaw
cancer, Freud was unable to stop smoking even though his doctors told
him it would kill him. His brain had become wired so as to prefer death
over quitting smoking. Freud died in 1939 from an intentional morphine
overdose to stop the agony of his cancer.

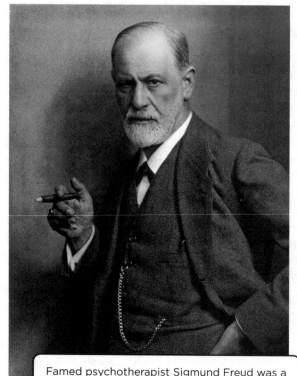

Famed psychotherapist Sigmund Freud was a cocaine user, but he was even more addicted to using tobacco.

… who had worked very hard and was very successful":

He had taken too little holiday, and unfortunately, from the mistaken idea of its real use, had committed the common but terrible mistake of trusting to alcohol to restore his weariness, keep himself up to his work, and produce sleep. It seemed to do this at first. But he soon could not work nor sleep without it, and it lost its power, so he had to take more of it, and oftener. At last he got absolutely dependent on it.… [H]e took still bigger doses, and had an attack of acute alcoholism. After this he pulled up, but only for a time … in six months he was as bad as ever, and had severe alcoholic convulsions. This occurred again and again and he became temporarily maniacal.… He died, after a few years, demented … and with the degenerated brain neurine that usually follows the continuous use of alcohol.

In 1920, the effects of alcohol abuse and chronic drunkenness boosted support for the prohibition of alcohol in the United States, resulting in a constitutional ban on the production, importation, transportation, and sale of alcoholic beverages that lasted until 1933; this policy made celebrities out of gangsters like Al Capone but also resulted in the decline of death rates from cirrhosis—scarring of the liver frequently caused by excessive drinking—and alcoholism. In 2005, alcohol dependence and abuse were estimated to cost the U.S. economy approximately $220 billion per year, more than cancer and obesity.

That $220 billion includes medical costs from injuries on the job, money lost from taking days off, money lost from losing jobs, the cost of rehab facilities, car accidents, domestic violence, fetal alcohol syndrome, and general criminal behavior, just to name a few.

Estimates of the global costs of alcohol abuse, collected by the World Health Organization, vary from 1 to 6 percent of a country's GDP. In addition to the United States's $220 billion, one Australian estimate was that alcohol's social costs were 24 percent of all the country's drug abuse costs; a similar Canadian study concluded that their alcohol's share was 41 percent. A 2001 study in the United Kingdom totaled the cost of all forms of alcohol misuse to be £18.5–20 billion.

The idea of "hitting rock bottom" means different things to different people, but it largely refers to the point where the user either has to give up drinking or die. This is usually after the person has experienced so much loss that even drinking doesn't dull the pain, yet the idea of not drinking is so terrifying that it's almost impossible to comprehend: it's as if the world would stop spinning.

The concept of powerlessness over alcohol (and alcoholics) is promoted by 12-step recovery groups such as Alcoholics Anonymous (AA) and Al-Anon—the first group is for alcoholics and the second is for those who have a loved one who's an alcoholic. Sometimes, people belong to both groups.

In May 2013, the American Psychiatric Association issued the fifth edition of the *Dia-*

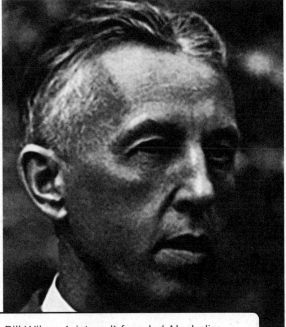

Bill Wilson (pictured) founded Alcoholics Anonymous with Dr. Bob Smith and Sister Ignatia of the Sisters of Charity of Saint Augustine.

THE FOUNDING OF ALCOHOLICS ANONYMOUS

Bill Wilson (aka Bill W.) was a stockbroker who, after hitting rock bottom, had started to recover with the help of a precursor to Alcoholics Anonymous (AA) called the Oxford Group. When a business trip to Akron, Ohio, went badly, the newly sober Wilson, desperate to stay that way though ferociously tempted otherwise, went through a phone book and called the phone numbers in a church directory, looking for alcoholics to talk to, until he was eventually put in touch with a fellow struggling alcoholic, Dr. Bob Smith. Wilson talked to Dr. Bob, as he became known, about his desire to relapse, and he didn't drink that night or at any other time. Dr. Bob relapsed the following month and was helped by Wilson, taking his last drink on June 10, 1935, to stop withdrawal symptoms before performing surgery. That date is considered by recovering alcoholics in AA to be the date AA began.

gnostic and Statistical Manual of Mental Disorders (DSM-5). In this edition, alcohol-use disorder (AUD) can be categorized as mild, moderate, or severe. The diagnosis is based on 11 criteria. The severity of the disorder depends on the number of criteria the individual meets. From 0 to 1, the person does not have an AUD. From 2 to 3, the diagnosis is mild; from 4 to 5, moderate; and 6 or more, severe.

- Missing work or school
- Drinking in hazardous situations
- Drinking despite social or personal problems
- Craving for alcohol
- Buildup of tolerance
- Withdrawals when trying to quit
- Drinking more than intended
- Trying to quit without success
- Increased alcohol-seeking behavior
- Interference with important activities
- Continued use despite health problems

One criteria not mentioned is blackouts. Blackouts occur when someone becomes so drunk that they do not remember events that happened while they were drinking. These can range from the embarrassing and silly to committing murder in a blackout, not remembering it, then going to prison for a murder they don't remember committing.

THE CRACK EPIDEMIC

The name "crack" first appeared in *The New York Times* on November 17, 1985. In an article titled "Program for Cocaine-Abuse Under Way," reporter Donna Boundy quoted Ellen Morehouse, the director of outpatient adolescent services at a program called The Recovery Center: "'Last year one-third of the students seen in the Student Assistance programs reported having tried cocaine,' she said. 'That was considerably more than we'd seen in other years.' Three teen-agers have sought this treatment already this year, she continued, for cocaine dependence resulting from the use of a new form of the drug called 'crack,' or rock-like pieces of prepared 'freebase' (concentrated) cocaine."

It oddly sounds like a more innocent time—a time when a reporter had to describe what crack was and put it in quotes. Now, the crack epidemic—so named because it spread like an epidemic—goes hand in hand with memories of 1980s urban decay for those who lived through it and YouTube videos for anyone who didn't. A year after Donna Boundy's article came out, more than 1,000 articles on crack were written: it got famous.

The crack epidemic didn't begin in a squatter house on the edge of town; it began with drug kingpins faced with daunting economics. In the early 1980s, so much cocaine was coming into Miami from the Caribbean that its price plummeted. In economic terms, this is called negative inflation, or deflation; more product was being produced than the demand required. (Yes, economics applies to the drug trade as well.) This is where crack came in. Suppliers converted cocaine—a powder—into a solid, smokeable form and sold it in smaller quantities with a potency, or purity, that made the demand soar. Also, it was easier to slip it by the Coast Guard and the Navy. As early as 1981, people were starting to smoke crack beginning in the Caribbean and extending all the way to California.

The term "purity" is ironically often used to describe illegal drugs, especially cocaine. The more actual cocaine that is being sold to a user, the purer it is because when a user buys cocaine, they're not buying only cocaine.

A supplier gets a brick of pure coke, which will get diluted enough so that the supplier will end up with two bricks—they'll have added ingredients to increase the yield. If you've ever heard of cutting coke, it means adding agents like baking soda, laundry powder, laxatives, or even other drugs like novocaine into the mix. The cutting starts with the supplier, then recurs again and again through the ranks until it reaches the dealer on the street. In some cases, a user is barely left with anything more than baking soda.

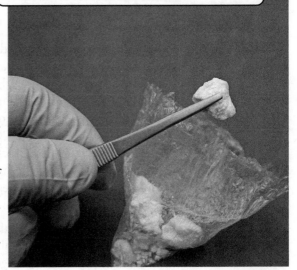

Crack is a form of cocaine that has been condensed from powder to solid to make it more potent and even more addictive than regular coke.

Crack had higher purity than street powder; this was because a supplier didn't have to sell as much product. A smaller amount of crack got you way higher than the equivalent amount of powdered cocaine. In 1984, powdered cocaine was sold on the street with an average of 55 percent purity for $100 per gram. One gram with that level of purity would get a casual user high but not addicted. Meanwhile, crack had an average purity level of more than 80 percent for the same price. Additionally, in cities like Baltimore, Chicago, Detroit, Los Angeles, New York, and Philadelphia, you could get a dose for $2.50—so if you were a drug addict, which would you choose?

Here's the answer: In 1985, crack-related hospital cases rose by 12 percent, from 23,500 to 26,300. In 1986, they rose by 110 percent, from 26,300 to 55,200. Between 1984 and 1987 they rose to 94,000.

Also, instead of being snorted, crack, which is smoked, gives the user an even greater high (in about 8 seconds), which means an even faster crash (after about 5–10 minutes), an even greater need to hit that high again, and an even faster rate of addiction. Perversely, diluted cocaine helps both the supplier and the user—the supplier has more to sell, and the user doesn't hit the unbelievable and deadly high that comes from pure cocaine. The crash after pure cocaine is enough to drive someone literally insane with the need for more. Those feel-good boundaries that our brain put in place are now smashed to smithereens and using has become the single most important goal in your life—more important than your job, your partner, and your kids. Your job, your great love, your whole reason for living, is getting high. (Having said that, it should be noted that not everyone who smokes crack ends up addicted—everyone's brains and physiology are different—but the need to get high specifically with crack has seen a disproportionate amount of people destroy their lives.)

The crack epidemic grew multiple tendrils: crackheads, baseheads, and crack houses that looked bombed out; rampant crime; and addicts who walked around like zombies who itched. (One side effect of crack was hallucinations of insects crawling all over your body.)

Crack Babies

Crack babies also existed. A crack baby was a child born to a mother who used crack while pregnant. Because, as mentioned, crack was more important to an addict than anything else, the addicted mother's brain put using before the health of her baby or, indeed, herself. Photos and reports of crack babies were at the forefront of news stories about the crack epidemic. Headlines like "Cocaine: A Vicious Assault on a Child," "Crack's Toll Among Babies: A Joyless View," and "Studies: Future Bleak for Crack Babies" were the norm. Smoking crack while pregnant was considered a far more deviant moral issue than smoking cigarettes or drinking while pregnant. Pregnant women who used illegal drugs commonly lost custody of their children, and, in the 1990s, many were prosecuted and jailed.

The other tendrils from the epidemic, like increasing violent crime in poor American neighborhoods, resulted in an equally violent backlash in the form of stricter criminal penalties, longer prison sentences, and racial profiling. Those convicted in federal court of possessing five grams of crack received a *minimum* mandatory sentence of five years in federal prison. That same sentence was given to someone convicted of possessing 500 grams of powdered cocaine. Prison sentences for crack were even worse than those for heroin. The majority of crack sentences were ten to 20 years, while those related to heroin were five to ten years.

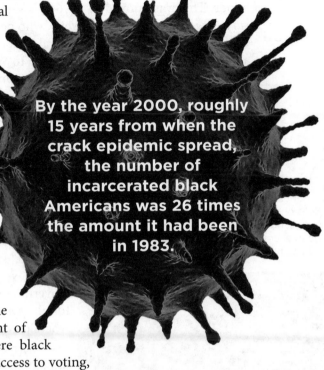

By the year 2000, roughly 15 years from when the crack epidemic spread, the number of incarcerated black Americans was 26 times the amount it had been in 1983. By 2012, almost 30 years from when the crack epidemic spread, 88 percent of those imprisoned from crack were black Americans. These people had lost access to voting, housing, and employment, and the stigma of being arrested for crack meant that job opportunities were severely limited once the sentence was over. Setbacks that were virtually impossible to overcome led to increased crime in poor black communities, especially for those who couldn't get jobs because they'd been arrested for using or selling crack.

Since black Americans were the demographic who most used crack, this gave the government *carte blanche* to create laws specific to crack since they couldn't create laws that were specific to race. It was an effective way to imprison black people without having to do the same to white people. It also furthered the myth that the black community was riddled with drugs and poverty and, even worse, was full of people who didn't work and lived off of welfare and food stamps. It was a criminalizing of urban black people, especially men.

Conspiracy Theories

The crack epidemic furthered the black community's mistrust of law enforcement, the medical community (which had already taken a hit because of the Tuskegee experiment), and the government as a whole. Rumors spread that the government had intentionally brought crack into black neighborhoods. This was buoyed in 1996 by a series of articles in San Jose's *The Mercury News* by reporter Gary Webb, who described a drug triangle in the 1980s connecting CIA officials in Central America, a San Francisco drug ring, and a Los Angeles drug dealer. According to Webb, the CIA used the profits from selling crack to an "expendable" black population to fund the agency's covert ops in Central America. The CIA's clandestine past made these articles an easy sell. African American leaders like Congresswoman Maxine Waters pointed to Webb's articles as proof of a plot to destroy black America. While speaking at a Baltimore Urban League dinner in 1997, Waters declared, "It doesn't matter whether [the CIA] delivered the kilo of cocaine themselves or turned their back on it to let somebody else do it…. They're guilty just the same."

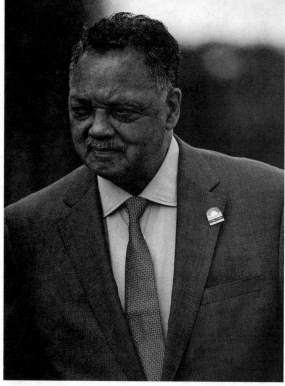

Baptist minister and activist Jesse Jackson Sr. is one African American leader who has suggested the crack cocaine epidemic has been encouraged by the U.S. government as a way to hurt the black community in America.

"What makes it so believable to me is that there is just abounding circumstantial evidence," said Reverend Jesse Jackson. "There is the weight of a lot of experiences with our Government operating in adverse or conspiratorial ways against black people. The context is what's driving the story."

African Americans who were not household names thought the reporting was credible. An October 31, 1996, edition of *The New York Times* ran an article titled "Though Evidence Is Thin, Tale of C.I.A. and Drugs Has a Life of Its Own" that quoted Don Middleton, then a 33-year-old jazz musician: "The established press ignored the story until they found out that black folks weren't going to just let this one be swept under the rug…. The white press is pointing fingers at the black community, saying we're paranoid and quick to see conspiracy at every turn of the corner. Where have they been for the last 30 years? Can I just mention the Tuskegee syphilis study, Cointelpro, Watergate, Iran-Contra. Hello, America?"

Beverly Carr, then a resident of south-central Los Angeles, said, "Everybody my age or older has always known that something like this was going on…. They're targeting the young black men. It's just ruining a whole generation."

As time passed, though, the veracity of Webb's articles was questioned. Fellow journalists and Webb's own editor accused him of creating a massive conspiracy for his own professional gain. Webb later confessed that no hard evidence existed that the CIA or any of its agent employees carried out or profited from drug trafficking.

Despite this, the story of the CIA bringing crack into the inner city had kept its hold. In response to the public outcry following Webb's articles—collectively titled "Dark Alliance"—the CIA conducted an internal investigation of its role in Central America related to the drug trade. Frederick Hitz, the CIA inspector general—an independent role filled by presidential nomination and confirmed by the Senate—led the investigation. In October 1998, the CIA released a declassified version of Hitz's report that cleared the CIA of complicity with the inner-city crack cocaine trade, but the report said that the CIA, in a number of cases, didn't bother to look into allegations about narcotics, and it describes how little or no direction was given to CIA operatives when confronted by the rampant drug trafficking in Central America in the 1980s.

The CIA's Central American operations weren't funded by the inner-city drug trade, but they did little to nothing to curtail it.

Gary Webb committed suicide on December 10, 2004, at the age of 49, but after a local newspaper reported that Webb had two gunshot wounds to the head—something that seemed impossible for a suicide—another conspiracy theory began. When queried by local reporters, Sacramento County coroner Robert Lyons replied, "It's unusual in a suicide case to have two shots, but it has been done in the past, and it is in fact a distinct possibility." The media noted widespread rumors that Webb had been killed as retribution for his "Dark Alliance" series, but Webb's ex-wife, Susan Bell, told reporters that she believed that he had died by his own hand. "The way he was acting it would be hard for me to believe it was anything but suicide." According to Bell, Webb had been depressed over his inability to land a job at another newspaper and had sold his house the week before his death because he was unable to keep up with the mortgage.

The End of an Epidemic

Eventually, like all epidemics, the crack epidemic ended: users overdosed because crack was too pure to handle, many others were imprisoned, and the amount of horrific press crack got meant that the new generation who was starting to experiment with drugs stayed away. It burned out, just like a virus.

PLAGUES, PANDEMICS AND VIRUSES

CRACK IS WACK

The wild colors of artist Keith Haring's famous mural *Crack Is Wack* can be seen from Manhattan's major east-side artery, the FDR Dive, at East 128th Street and the Harlem River Drive. Painted in 1986 at the height of the crack epidemic, it features Haring's trademark animated figures as a skull, drowning addicts, a $0 bill, and a crack pipe that spews out the title of the mural.

At the time, Haring's studio assistant, Benny Soto, had become addicted to crack, inspiring Haring to paint the mural after many failed attempts to help Benny get clean. Haring, who often drove by an abandoned handball court in a park near Harlem River Drive, decided to use its wall to show his frustrations with the way the government was handling drug-related issues.

In the summer of 1986, without any legal permission to paint a mural, Haring climbed a ladder and finished the painting in one day. Surprisingly enough, he wasn't stopped or questioned by the police while he painted and even presumed that "when you have a van, ladders, and paint, policemen don't even consider asking whether you have any permission, they just assume you do."

Keith Haring died of AIDS on February 16, 1990, at the age of 31. Although the crack epidemic is long over, his mural still stands.

What of the victims left behind: the babies born to addicted mothers? Early studies reported that those who had been exposed to crack *in utero* would be severely emotionally, mentally, and physically crippled; this belief extended into the scientific and lay communities. Another prediction was that a generation of crack babies was going to put an enormous strain on social services and society as a whole once they were no longer babies because how could a baby exposed to crack—as a fetus, no less—not have severe physical and mental disabilities? Well, as it turns out, for the most part, they didn't.

Small samples and flawed testing had been the culprits as well as racism and classism. Scientists now realize that the discoveries published from early studies were highly exaggerated, and most, but not all, people who were exposed to crack *in utero* do not have disabilities or direct, long-term effects on language, growth, or development as measured by test scores. Prenatal cocaine exposure

PLAGUES, PANDEMICS AND VIRUSES

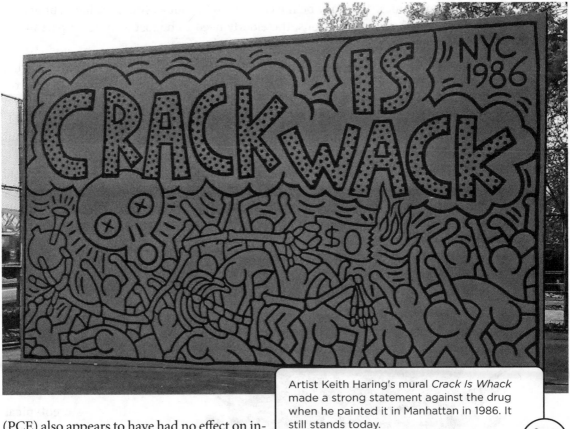

Artist Keith Haring's mural *Crack Is Whack* made a strong statement against the drug when he painted it in Manhattan in 1986. It still stands today.

(PCE) also appears to have had no effect on infant growth. What are directly tied to PCE, however, are premature birth and attention deficit hyperactivity disorder (ADHD). These results also happen to babies born to mothers who smoked while pregnant and are actually less severe than the effects on babies born to mothers who drank alcohol excessively while pregnant. No difference between crack and powder cocaine was evident when it came to fetal harm.

Studies suggest that the environment in which a child grows up makes a more important contribution in cognitive and behavioral outcomes than does cocaine exposure itself. How to tackle that is still a problem.

THE OPIOID EPIDEMIC

When it comes to drug and alcohol rehabilitation centers, the assumption exists that the patients are either young people who became addicted to hard drugs or moms and dads who way overdid it with the gin and tonics. That may be the case for some, but as you'll see later about sexually transmitted infections, the elderly need to be just as much a part of the equation.

The opioid epidemic began in the late 1990s. Americans were told that their aches and pains could be greatly reduced with the help of opioid pain relievers. They'd work better than the usual ibuprofen and were nonaddictive. Old and injured alike would be up and running in no time. Between 1991 and 2011, a near-tripling of opioid prescriptions was dispensed by U.S. pharmacies: from 76 to 219 million.

This was the same story that pharmaceutical companies had previously told health-care providers. Eventually, America became the world's leader in opioid prescriptions because doctors were more frequently prescribing opioids to new patients in addition to those who'd become addicted.

This is where the elderly contingent come in. It should be noted that the word "elderly" evokes images like Grandma sitting in a rocking chair with a shawl around her shoulders or Grandpa smoking a pipe on the front porch and reading the newspaper. These are, indeed, elderly people—but the 65-year-olds of today are much different from the 65-year-olds of even the 1990s; compare family photos for evidence.

When it comes to sex and drugs, the elderly are an invisible population, which is why it doesn't often occur to doctors to screen them for STIs....

This stereotypical image of the "Get off my lawn!" geriatric is what allows the younger set to believe that old people don't have sex, can't get or transmit STIs, and can't get addicted to drugs or alcohol. When it comes to sex and drugs, the elderly are an invisible population, which is why it doesn't often occur to doctors to screen them for STIs or imagine that they'll become drug addicts even though many of this generation grew up with rock 'n' roll, free love, and LSD.

In fact, the elderly are at risk for addictive behavior in part because they, too, believe that they're out of the woods since they've made it this far. However, excessive drinking to cope with the loss of a spouse can lead to alcoholism; widowers over the age of 75 have the highest rate of alcoholism in the United States. Unprotected sex at any age can lead to an STI, and opioid use can turn Grandma and Grandpa into drug addicts. They can't even believe it themselves. The number of elderly patients receiving opioid prescriptions increased ninefold between 1996 and 2010, according to *Psychiatric Times*, and more than one in three individuals over 50 reported that they had misused opiates in the previous month, causing the hospitalization rate for misuse to increase fivefold over the last two decades.

As we age, our metabolism slows down, which means that we also metabolize alcohol and drugs at a slower rate. An older person will feel these effects more intensely and for longer periods of time than younger people, and older patients, who are more likely to be prescribed multiple pain relievers, risk developing addictions within a shorter period of time. This can also affect their memories and cause them to take more than the prescribed dosage because they forgot they'd already taken it, so millions of older Americans are now filling prescriptions for many different opioid medications at the same time, while hundreds of thousands are winding up in the hospital with opioid-related complications.

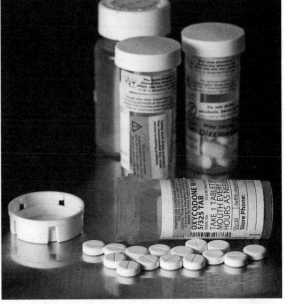

Prescription drug abuse of medications such as the opioid oxycodone has become a widespread problem in the United States.

Opioid abuse is notably more common among seniors who live in poor, rural, or or low-income areas and are insured through Medicare or another form of public insurance. Opioid use also went up dramatically depending on a person's perceived health status. For example, only 9 percent of seniors in "excellent" health filled out opioid prescriptions, compared to nearly 30 percent in "fair" health and 40 percent in "poor" health. Adults aged 65 and older make up 13 percent of the U.S. population, but they constitute 33 percent of outpatient spending on prescription drugs.

The challenge, said Dr. Arlene Bierman, director of the Agency for Healthcare Research and Quality, "is safe-prescribing for those who need opioids for pain, while avoiding overuse or misuse." An alternative is "using non-opioid pain medications and non-pharmacologic treatments before considering the use of opioids." She also suggested that if and when opioids are needed, "the lowest possible dose should be used."

In 2017, drug police expert Keith Humphries gave this assessment during the conference Stanford Medicine X:

> The biggest misconception is that the U.S. is normal in how it handles prescription opioids. So, let's compare ourselves to another country. Japan, for example. Older population than us; you would think more aches and pains. Universal access to health care, so more opportunities to prescribe.

> So consider the amount of standard daily doses of opioids consumed in Japan. And then double it. And then double it again. And then double it again. And then double it again. And then double it a fifth time. That would make Japan No. 2 in the world, behind the United States.

> Every other developed country does at least as good or as poor a job as we do when managing pain—while not using opioids at anywhere near the same level.

In 2015, nearly 35,000 drug overdoses occurred due to opioids like Percocet, OxyContin, heroin, and fentanyl. That's two-thirds of the overall drug-overdose deaths. This meant that more overdose deaths occurred that year than any other time in American history, including the meth epidemic or even the crack epidemic.

In 2016, 50 elderly people overdosed on opioids every day.

Big Pharma

It all started with Big Pharma. Its story of the efficacy of opioids sounded plausible to medical associations and the government. Doctors were pressured by medical associations and government agencies like the Veterans Health Administration to combat pain more quickly and effectively. They were also under the gun from insurance companies who wanted them to treat the doctor's office like a revolving door of opioid distribution. "Most doctors just want to keep you alive—they aren't helping you live your best life," Dr. Robin Berzin told Yahoo! Finance. "We're basically just trained to save lives—to prescribe pills and avoid catastrophic events that end life." In short: get patients in, prescribe meds, get them out, bill the insurance company.

Addiction specialist Anna Lembke agreed. The author of *Drug Dealer, MD*, she described the "tremendous pressure on doctors within these large integrated health care centers to practice medicine in a certain way and get patients out in a timely fashion to be able to bill insurers at the highest possible level and to make sure that their patients were satisfied customers."

Opioids answered both doctor and patient problems. Doctors could relieve the pressures put on them by the health-care industry, and the patient would be relieved of pain. This was the short-term answer to a long-term issue that still plagues us today, nearly 30 years later.

In some situations, doctors simply prescribed too much, giving weeks or even monthslong prescriptions for something like a wisdom tooth removal when only a few days' worth was needed—or when the pain could have also been treated with ibuprofen. In other cases, the doctors involved were outright malicious—setting up "pill mills," where they gave away opioids in order to get money in their pockets. In concert with this increase, a near-tripling of opioid-related deaths also occurred.

This is what happened in the case of Michael Jackson, who died on June 25, 2009, from a mixture of propofol and the antianxiety drugs lorazepam, midazolam, and diazepam. According to a July 22, 2009, search warrant, Jackson's personal physician, Conrad Murray, gave him propofol diluted with lidocaine shortly before Jackson's death. Propofol is normally administered in a hospital as general anesthesia during surgery and is only given by anesthesiologists, nurse anesthetists, or anesthesia assistants who have extensive training. Murray had no such training, as he was a cardiologist, not an anesthesiologist. He was sentenced to four years in prison for involuntary manslaughter but was paroled after two.

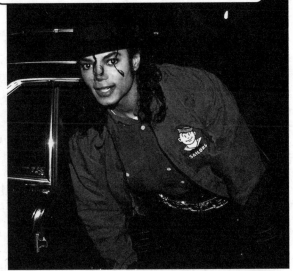

King of Pop entertainer Michael Jackson died from an overdose of propofol prescribed by his personal physician, Dr. Conrad Murray, who only served two years in prison for his crime.

What were some of the circumstances leading up to Murray giving Jackson propofol? At the time that he began working for Jackson, Murray had reportedly fathered seven children by six women; was behind on the mortgage for the Las Vegas home of his ex-wife and their children; owed child support to the mothers of the children he fathered outside of his marriage; and was paying the rent for Nicole Alvarez, whom he met at a gentleman's club and who gave birth to their son in March 2009. Murray was at risk of losing his California medical license due to unpaid child support and was a defendant in numerous civil lawsuits (though none for medical malpractice). By 2008, he had amassed more than $600,000 in court judgments against him for unpaid rent for his practices in Texas and Nevada. He also owed $71,000 in student loans at Meharry Medical College. Michael Jackson hired him as his personal physician in May 2009, and a month later, Jackson was dead.

Chasing the High

Over time, users began to use more potent kinds of opioids, like heroin and fentanyl. The reasons varied: they lost access to painkillers, had built up an opioid tolerance and needed something stronger, or had no idea what exactly they were taking. Fentanyl—which is so strong that it's used to treat agonizing pain in late-stage cancer patients—has become increasingly popular over the last several years. As a recreational drug, it's deadly—it's 50 to 100 times stronger than morphine. A fentanyl overdose killed Prince in 2016 at the age of 57. It is not known whether Prince obtained fentanyl by prescription or illegally, but an investigation revealed that he had been in significant pain for a number of years and had hundreds of painkillers of various types in his house. Apparently, Prince had also thought that he was taking the prescription drug Vicodin when, in fact, he was taking counterfeit Vicodin that was laced with fentanyl.

Nearly two years later, Tom Petty also died from an accidental drug overdose. A combination of opioids (fentanyl, oxycodone, acetylfentanyl, and despropionyl fentanyl), sedatives (temazepam and alprazolam), and citalopram (an antidepressant) were found in his system. Petty's wife and daughter said that he had multiple medical problems, "most significantly a fractured hip." He was prescribed pain medication for these problems and informed on the day of his death that his hip had severely deteriorated. A statement from the family read, "It is our feeling that the pain was simply unbearable and was the cause for his overuse of medication.... We feel confident that this was, as the coroner found, an unfortunate accident."

Not all painkiller users overdose and not all opioid users started with painkillers, but statistics suggest that many did: a 2014 study in *JAMA Psychiatry* found that 75 percent of heroin users in treatment started with painkillers, and CDC analysis from 2015 found that those addicted to painkillers are 40 times more likely to become addicted to heroin.

Increases in heroin and fentanyl availability and cutbacks in painkillers are both factors that have led to heroin and fentanyl booming across the United States. The result is that as the number of opioid painkiller deaths leveled off over during the 2010s, heroin and fentanyl deaths have rapidly increased because they are so terribly potent. Fentanyl—which you can now get on the street—is currently linked to more overdose deaths than any other drug in the United States.

Of the 64,000 drug-overdose deaths in 2016, opioids were responsible for 42,000 of these, which can involve both prescription and illegal opioids. The opioid overdose epidemic has also contributed to increased rates of nonfatal opioid overdoses, an increase in emergency department visits attributed to drug misuse, widespread outbreaks of infectious diseases linked to intravenous drug use, and heavy economic costs from death, lost productivity, and health-care spending.

Increases in heroin and fentanyl availability and cutbacks in painkillers are both factors that have led to heroin and fentanyl booming across the United States.

Between 1999 and 2014, rates of opioid misuse by pregnant women more than quadrupled to 6.5 per 1,000 births in the United States. In 2014, $563 million was spent on treatment of neonatal opioid withdrawal syndrome (NOWS); 82 percent of these charges were paid by state Medicaid programs, showing a greater tendency of mothers from lower-income communities to use opioids during pregnancy. About every 15 minutes in the United States, a baby is born suffering from opioid withdrawal.

If nothing is done, we can expect a lot of people to die: a forecast from the health media company STAT showed that as many as 650,000 people will die over the next decade from opioid overdoses. That's more people than the entire population of Baltimore, Maryland. The United States risks losing the equivalent of a whole American city in just one decade.

Also, the opioid epidemic was a major contributor to America's life expectancy dropping for two years in a row—in 2015 and 2016—the first time a two-year drop has occurred since the early 1960s. Getting high in the United States is a lot easier than getting help.

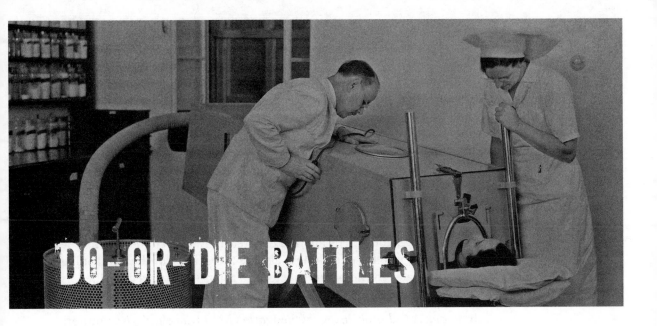

DO-OR-DIE BATTLES

Some diseases that afflict humanity can be viewed not as pandemics that flare up on occasion throughout history but, rather, as ongoing plagues that have been with us from the beginning of recorded history. Like other diseases discussed in this book, rabies, cholera, tuberculosis, and polio have left their mark on history, influencing everything from medical science to literature, movies, and cultures in general.

RABIES

"Alyssa" is an ultrafeminine name originating in Greece. It evokes images of a young girl playing in a field—a gentle, friendly type— and, in a way, the name says it all because when broken down into its two parts, it's *a*, which in Greek is a negative prefix, as in "not"; and *lyssa*, which is Greek for "rage" or "mania": literally, "not a maniac." It originates from the flower "alyssum," which was thought to cure the rage and mania that is rabies.

Euripides lived in Greece in the fifth century B.C.E. and was a famous tragedian—he specialized in tragic tales of gods and heroes. Lyssa was the spirit of rage and frenzy, driving humans insane and animals rabid. (Rabies was indeed written about in the time of the ancient Greeks.) Lyssa is said to have sprung from the blood that gushed after the god Uranus was castrated—just to bring home that point of where a furious woman can cause a man the most damage.

In his play *Herakles*, Lyssa is told by the goddess queen Hera that she must cause the title character to go insane, and though this is not something that brings her joy, like a good soldier, she sends Heracles into a lunatic rage that causes him to murder his wife and children.

In a tragic plot from an anonymous author, the hunter Actaeon accidentally sees the goddess Artemis bathing in a river. When she catches him staring at her nakedness, she's so enraged that she turns him into a deer and inflicts his hunting dogs with *lyssa*, in this case "wolf's madness," and they tear him apart. Lyssa is not a force to be trifled with.

The Iliad has the honor of appearing in two sections of this book: the chapter on the Plague of Athens and the chapter on rabies. Homer opens *The Iliad* with a plague: Apollo's punishment against the Greeks for the kidnapping of a Trojan girl. Later in the poem, Hector, a Trojan warrior, is described as being "possessed" in battle with a "strong fury" that has overcome him.

In *Rabid: A Cultural History of the World's Most Diabolical Virus* authors Bill Wasik and Monica Murphy ask:

> What is this peculiar fury that, in Odysseus's view, has possessed Hector, spurring him to unstoppable acts of martial courage but also to a mortal vulnerability? It is no ordinary anger. Homer's epics are awash in anger, with no fewer than nine terms employed to describe all the subtle flavors of fury. In *The Iliad* this litany begins with the poem's very first word, *menin*, which so famously frames the entire epic around the "rage" of Achilles. But here in Odysseus's presentation to Achilles, the term for what has provoked Hector to such frenzy—*lyssa*—is something rather more primal. It has not been invoked anywhere in the poem before this scene, and with one notable exception the term will not appear again during the tale. It is a term closely linked to the word *lykos*, or "wolf," and is used to connote an animal state beyond anger: an insensate madness, a wolfish rage.

It's no coincidence, then, that rabies belongs to the genus *Lyssavirus*. The bullet-shaped virus penetrates the body like a bullet, through a bite or scratch, and replicates by entering a cell with the correct receptors. However, what sets rabies apart is that it doesn't travel through the bloodstream; it travels through the nervous system. This causes it to move slower, as it's not propelled by your beating heart, but the bloodstream contains your immune system, and it would put up a hell of a fight. Because rabies is what's known as a neurotropic virus, meaning it infects the nerve cells, no blood test exists for it. If you're bitten by an animal like a raccoon and you can't catch it, the best course of action is to immediately get rabies shots as a precautionary measure. If that raccoon is rabid and you now have rabies, it will not eventually subside, like the flu—it will eventually cause agony, madness, and death, so it's best to make sure to get the vaccine right away. Once symptoms begin, death is next.

If no blood test exists, how can one determine whether or not an animal is rabid? Symptoms like aggression, difficulty walking, and foaming at the mouth indicate rabies, but the only way to make a positive diagnosis is to get a sample of brain tissue, and to do that, the animal must be dead—and that goes for humans as well. If the animal dies after biting, its head is removed and the brain tissue is tested for rabies. The same holds true if it's captured by animal control—except that it's put down first.

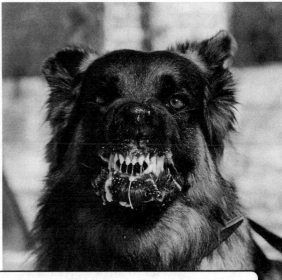

Aggressive behavior and foaming at the mouth are two clear indications that an animal could be rabid.

Let's break this down like we did with the name Alyssa.

A motor neuron is located in the spinal cord. When you decide to move a part of your body, your brain sends a command to the motor neuron inside your spinal cord.

This motor neuron fires an impulse, then travels through a long protrusion called an axon to the muscles.

When the tip of the axon comes into proximity with a muscle fiber, a connection, or synapse, forms with that fiber. This connection is called the neuromuscular junction.

Through a series of chemical reactions at the junction, the muscle contracts, and that part of your body moves.

When the rabies virus enters the body, it binds to receptors that surround a cell in the peripheral nervous system. The peripheral nervous system is located outside the brain and spinal cord—for instance, in the arms and legs—and is probably where you've been bitten. The virus is then drawn into the cell, where its RNA is released and replication begins. This continues as the virus begins its journey to the brain and spinal cord.

Since it doesn't have the benefit of the heart pumping it through the bloodstream, the rabies virus must find another means of transport: enter the axons. More than 99 percent of the volume and surface area of the neuron is in the axon and its branches. The axon is like a freeway on which the virus travels from the peripheral nervous system to the central nervous system.

(Compare the rabies virus to HIV and see how something as simple as a virus can behave so differently. HIV lives in the bloodstream and cannot live for long outside the body. The saline content in saliva also kills HIV. Rabies lives in the nervous system and thrives in the salivary glands. It uses saliva as a way to infect a new victim. HIV dies in saliva, and rabies would die in the bloodstream.)

This is a pretty slow freeway, however. The virus travels through the nervous system at a speed of about 1 to 2 centimeters per day, so it could take weeks or months for it to reach the central nervous system. This is called the incubation period. When the virus reaches the brain, it shuts off critical neuronal genes, which ultimately leads to the deterioration of brain function. This is when symptoms begin.

It starts with a fever and a sore throat, almost like the flu. Then, it progresses to anxiety, confusion, and hallucinations, both sight and sound. Muscle-churning spasmodic episodes, along with sleeplessness, excitability, fever, rapid pulse, and labored breathing, are all part of the illness, and at this point, the victim is literally losing their mind. Then, a bizarre, yet completely logical, symptom occurs—many believe it to be hydrophobia, or fear of water. This is because the victim may be tremendously thirsty, but they will not drink water or any liquid. They become hysterical just from looking at it.

It's not the liquid that strikes terror in a rabies victim, though—it's really the act of swallowing. The rabies virus affects the neurons responsible for swallowing, causing a condition known as dysphagia—from the Greek word *dys*, meaning "disordered," and *phag*, meaning "eat." The rhythmic and syncopated actions involved in swallowing that we're not normally conscious of are lost, and the act of swallowing becomes far too painful, no matter how thirsty the victim is.

From the virus's perspective, dysphagia makes perfect sense since saliva is the most common way rabies moves from one host to another. If the victim were able to drink, the viruses in the saliva would become diluted, the potency of the disease would be lessened, and all that work traveling through axon after axon would be for naught, as the virus would not be able to move to the next host. It's as though the *virus* fears water—as much as viruses can fear anything—but it uses the victim's nervous system as a shield to protect itself so that the *victim* then fears water.

Once the virus starts replicating in the brain, it spreads outward to the salivary glands, causing them to work overtime. Since the victim is still not drinking, the resulting foaming at the mouth is producing more and more lyssa-filled saliva that will enter a wound at first bite. Rabies also attacks the central pattern generators (CPGs),which is a neural network that allows us to do things like swallow without thinking about it. The CPGs that handle actions like breathing and chewing are all affected as rabies attacks the medulla oblongata, the part of the brain that's responsible for involuntary actions.

Eventually, the mania and aggression leave the victim exhausted, after which they have seizures, fall into a coma, and die.

Eventually, the mania and aggression leave the victim exhausted, after which they have seizures, fall into a coma, and die.

Rabies may have a longer incubation period than other diseases, but it ends somewhat quickly, though not fast enough. The victim still suffers terribly until death results from cardiac arrest or organ failure, which takes between three and ten days.

Having said this, a bite from a rabid animal (or person) does not mean certain death. The incubation period varies depending on where the victim is bitten. The closer to the brain, the shorter the incubation period since the virus has a shorter distance to travel, but if, for instance, a person were bitten on the toe, it would take much longer for the virus to travel all the way to the central nervous system. A person bitten on the face might only have weeks before symptoms begin; a person bitten on the foot might have months. In that time, it's critical that they get postexposure prophylaxis (PEP), which is the rabies vaccine, along with rabies immune globin (RIG).

Humans are actually a terrible host for rabies, as we tend not to bite when infected, unlike a dog, raccoon, bat, or otter. Also, compared to these animals, we have lousy teeth. However, writer Zora Neale Hurston in her 1937 novel *Their Eyes Were Watching God* frighteningly yet enthrallingly describes the scene between the main character, Janie, and her lover, Tea Cake. Having been bitten by a rabid dog, Tea Cake has turned rabid himself:

He steadied himself against the jamb of the door and Janie thought to run into him and grab his arm, but she saw the quick motion of taking aim and heard the click. Saw the ferocious look in his eyes and went mad with fear as she had done in the water that time. She threw up the barrel of the rifle in frenzied hope and fear. Hope that he'd see it and run, desperate fear for her life. But if Tea Cake could have counted costs he would not have been there with the pistol in his hands. No knowledge of fear nor rifles nor anything else was there. He paid no more attention to the pointing gun than if it were Janie's dog finger. She saw him stiffen himself all over as he leveled and took aim. The fiend in him must kill and Janie was the only thing living he saw. The pistol and the rifle rang out almost together. The pistol just enough after the rifle to seem its echo. Tea Cake crumpled as his bullet buried itself in the joist over Janie's head. Janie saw the look on his face and leaped forward as he crashed forward in her arms. She was trying to hover him as he closed his teeth in the flesh of her forearm. They came down heavily like that. Janie struggled to a sitting position and pried the dead Tea Cake's teeth from her arm.

The Rabies Vaccine

Louis Pasteur had already established himself as a leader in the study of infectious diseases and in 1877 was studying chicken cholera, a disease that, as it similarly does with humans, caused diarrhea and death. Pasteur was influenced by Edward Jenner, who'd developed the smallpox vaccine in 1796. Pasteur believed that if a vaccine could be found for smallpox, it could be found for any other disease, and, indeed, in 1879, he developed a chicken cholera vaccine and in 1881 an anthrax vaccine for sheep, goats, and cows.

Rabies, though, was a whole other ball game. For starters, chicken cholera and anthrax are bacterial diseases; rabies is viral. Even though Pasteur's team discovered that the pathogen was located in the central nervous system and the salivary glands, they failed to isolate and grow a new pathogen from either location.

The path to a vaccine was extremely treacherous.

In order to start developing the rabies vaccine, Pasteur and his assistants acquired sick dogs from kennels at the national veterinary school at Maisons-Alfort, France, and from veterinary offices around the city. Because rabies could not be grown like bacteria, this meant that it had to be collected from the cells

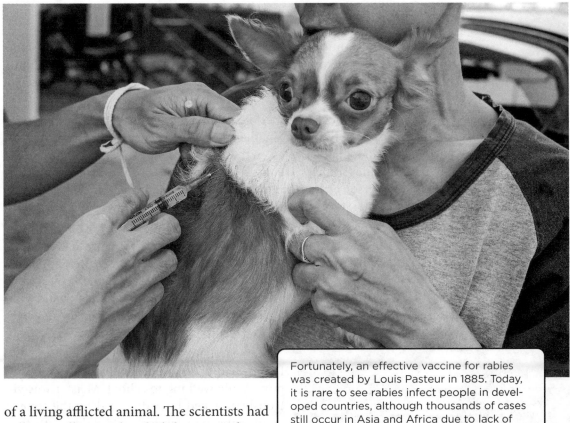

Fortunately, an effective vaccine for rabies was created by Louis Pasteur in 1885. Today, it is rare to see rabies infect people in developed countries, although thousands of cases still occur in Asia and Africa due to lack of medical treatment.

of a living afflicted animal. The scientists had to repeatedly wrestle rabid dogs in order to collect their saliva.

"At the beginning of each session a loaded revolver was placed within their reach," said Mary Cressac, the niece of Pasteur's collaborator, Emile Roux. "If a terrible accident were to happen to one of them, the more courageous of the two others would put a bullet in his head."

According to Pasteur's son-in-law, René Vallery-Radot:

"We absolutely have to inoculate the rabbits with this slaver," said M. Pasteur. Two helpers took a cord with a slip knot and threw it at the dog as one throws a lasso. The dog was caught and pulled to the edge of the cage. They seized it and tied its jaws together. The dog, choking with rage, its eyes bloodshot, and its body racked by furious spasms, was stretched out on a table while M. Pasteur, bending a finger's length away over this foaming head, aspirated a few drops of slaver through a thin tube. It was … at the sight of this awesome tête-à-tête that I saw M. Pasteur at his greatest.

In order to continue their work without endangering his life and the life of his team, a different tack was taken: healthy dogs had the virus injected into their brains. This also shortened the incubation period, as dogs became rabid within about two weeks.

A shortened incubation period also meant increased virulence, or severity: the more severe the infection, the quicker it will engulf the victim. Pasteur knew that he had to markedly lessen the virus's potency in order for it to be effective as a vaccine (similar to Jenner's less dangerous cowpox virus being used to vaccinate a person against the much deadlier smallpox vaccine).

In March 1885, Pasteur wrote to his friend, "I have not yet dared to treat human beings after bites from rabid dogs; but the time is not far off, and I am much inclined to begin with myself." However, Pasteur never did test the vaccine on himself since enough people with mad dog bites were always available whose families would volunteer them for experimentation.

Nine-year-old Joseph Meister would become to Louis Pasteur and rabies what James Phipps had been to Edward Jenner and smallpox. While walking to school, Meister was viciously attacked by a dog, and by the time a good Samaritan fended off the dog with two iron bars, Meister had suffered fourteen bites to his thighs, legs, and hand. Later that day, after cauterizing the bite wounds with carbolic acid, Meister's physician sent the boy and his mother from their village in Alsace about 300 miles to Paris to see Louis Pasteur.

Interestingly, Louis Pasteur had never been trained as a doctor and did not have a medical license, so he therefore could not hold the syringe for the first modern laboratory vaccine for humans. "On 6 July, at eight o'clock in the evening, 60 hours after the bites of 4 July, and in the presence of Drs. Vulpian and Grancher, we inoculated into a fold of skin over young Meister's right hypochondrium half a

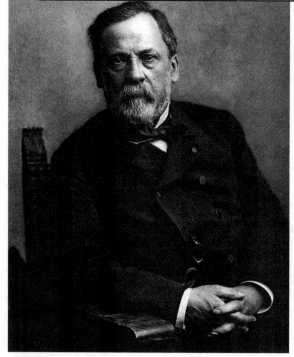

French biologist and chemist Louis Pasteur was a key figure in developing vaccinations for diseases and, of course, developing what we now call pasteurization to remove harmful bacteria from dairy foods and wine.

PHYSICAL EVIDENCE OF VIRUSES

Although both Louis Pasteur (in 1885) and Edward Jenner (in 1796) developed the first vaccines to protect against viral infections, they never saw a virus. The first evidence of the existence of viruses came from experiments with filters that had pores tiny enough to retain bacteria. In 1892, Dmitri Ivanovsky used one of these filters to show that filtered sap from a diseased tobacco plant could still infect healthy tobacco plants. Martinus Beijerinck called the filtered, infectious substance a "virus" (from the Latin *virus*, meaning "poisonous secretion" or "venom"), and this discovery is considered to be the beginning of virology.

Pravaz syringe of the spinal cord from a rabbit dead of rabies on 21 June; the cord had since then—that is, for fifteen days—been kept in a flask of dry air," Pasteur wrote in his notebook. The treatment lasted for ten days and consisted of thirteen inoculations, which included the spinal tissue from a deceased rabbit that had rabies.

On July 16, 1885, Meister received his final inoculation. Each successive inoculation had been increasingly virulent, preparing the little boy's immune system for the most potent of them all. Such a dangerous inoculation would provide a convincing test of Meister's immunity: if they'd started with this dosage, Meister would have contracted rabies within days. Pasteur's son-in-law said:

> Cured from his wounds, delighted with all he saw, gaily running about as if he had been in his own Alsatian farm, little Meister, whose blue eyes now showed neither fear nor shyness, merrily received the last inoculation; in the evening, after claiming a kiss from "dear Monsieur Pasteur," as he called him, he went to bed and slept peacefully. Pasteur spent a terrible night of insomnia; in those slow dark hours of night when all vision is distorted, Pasteur, losing sight of the accumulation of experiments which guaranteed his success, imagined that the little boy would die.

Instead, Louis Pasteur's work in virology led to vaccines—comprising a weakened version of a virus—for a number of diseases, including diphtheria (1888), plague (1897), tuberculosis (1927), yellow fever (1936), measles (1963), mumps (1967), rubella (1969), and chicken pox (1995)—after a much-needed rest from having tested a rabies vaccine on a nine-year-old boy.

CAUTERIZATION DISPROVED AS A RABIES TREATMENT

When Louis Pasteur was about the same age as Joseph Meister, the eastern French village he lived in, Arbois, was terrorized by a rabid wolf. Pasteur and his friends saw one victim brought to the blacksmith's shop to have his wound cauterized for treatment. It left an impression— and the eventual realization that this form of torturous treatment did nothing to help the victim.

Myths and Rabies

A disease this terrifying has also been inspiring writers from the time of Euripides to today. The myths of the werewolf, the vampire, and the zombie can draw their roots back to rabies. The late-stage aggression and dementia could have caused people to think that the infected person was becoming bestial or living in some world that lay between the dead and the living.

Also, the growing emphasis on the bestial/sexual nature that went along with rabies brought lurid details of how animalistic a human could become. In the nineteenth century, nymphomania began to appear in lists of hydrophobia symptoms. Often, these reports were accompanied by an anecdote about a man taken over by extreme sexual madness, ravishing a woman.

On August 8, 1855, the *Brooklyn Daily Eagle* reported on the gruesome murder of a bride by her husband, Peyron, on their wedding night. The story came from Lyons, France, where the woman's parents had initially prevented the couple's engagement "on account of the strangeness of conduct sometimes observed in the young man."

Peyron's mother convinced them to reconsider, after much begging, because "his passion for the girl became at length so violent that he declared he could not exist without her." Although the wedding took place "with all the rustic pomp and ceremony common in that part of the provinces," something happened on their wedding night. "Cries were heard from the nuptial chamber." "Fearful shrieks" came from their quarters. People quickly arrived to find "the poor girl … in the agonies of death—her bosom torn open and lacerated in a most horrible manner, and the wretched husband in a fit of raving madness and covered with blood, having actually devoured a portion of the unfortunate girl's breast." Shortly afterward, the bride died, as did Peyron, after "a most violent resistance."

According to witnesses, Peyron had previously "been bitten by a strange dog." The *Eagle* determined that the deaths were caused by "a sad and distressing case of hydrophobia," aka rabies. This article had it all: the terror of a werewolf and vampire tale, and the bite of a rabid dog, transforming a man into a beast whose sexual desire exploded into violence.

Variations on the tale of Peyron and his doomed bride were written about in newspapers as late as the 1890s. The *Eagle* was just one of many tabloids that turned a folktale about mad dogs into news. Other diseases like cholera, typhoid, and diphtheria killed far more people in the nineteenth century, but rabies caused a singular kind of panic because it was a disease transmitted by snarling, violent animals that stole away a person's humanity. Without knowing about viruses, the supernatural and the belief that evil forces turned people into monsters seemed as logical an explanation as any for the victim's transfor-

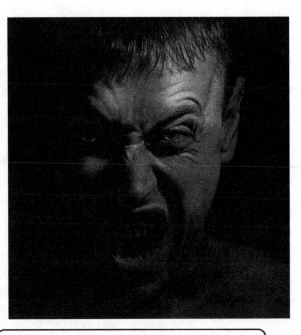

Zombie and werewolf myths can trace their origins back to people's very real fears of rabies and the madness it can cause.

mation. It could go as far as to be like demonic possession. Even knowing about viruses today doesn't make rabies any less terrifying; perhaps it's less malevolent now in the spiritual sense—viruses are only in it for the replication, not for infamy—but it's still terrifying knowing the sheer power that pathogens have over us.

Nineteenth-century American reports never claimed outright that a supernatural force was at work, but the Gothic descriptions of cases allowed people to read between the lines where the disease left the soul of a wild animal and entered into that of a suffering human. Hallucinations, respiratory spasms, and out-of-control convulsions produced fearful impressions of an evil spirit within the human body—and the descriptions of those who had rabies were often paired with the animal that bit them, so those who caught rabies from dog bites were barking mad, while those who caught rabies from a rabid cat would scratch and spit. Folk remedies included killing the rabid dog that bit someone not just to stop the spread of rabies but as a way to cure the victim (like killing the head vampire). Don't forget: even today, you're still likely to die of rabies once symptoms begin.

PLAGUES, PANDEMICS AND VIRUSES

CHOLERA: THE BLUE DEATH

Back in the 1800s, physicians drew the same conclusions about cholera that their predecessors did about the plague—they thought it was caused by that bad air, or miasma, rising up from places like sewers and open graves. New York City banned burials in Manhattan because of this, which is why most cemeteries in the city are located in an area known as the outer boroughs—like the border of Brooklyn and Queens, also called the Cemetery Belt, which back then was mostly farmland.

A British physician named John Snow believed that something else was at hand because unlike diseases such as plague or influenza, the lungs were not attacked, so the cause couldn't be inhaled. It was the digestive tract that was stricken, so the cause was probably something people ingested.

Snow was familiar with unsanitary conditions because he grew up around them in a town called Mickelgate, which was within the northern English city of York. At the time, York was still a walled city like London was, a remnant from when it, too, was occupied by the Romans. York was also the northern English capital because it lay at the junction of two rivers, the Ouse and the Swale. Again, this is great for commerce but bad for living. During Snow's childhood, most of the streets in Micklegate were unsanitary because of a cultural lack of hygiene that led to the rivers being contaminated. The locals drew water directly from them even though they were polluted from raw sewage. Intermittent flooding also occurred, which brought all that filth back into town.

It is no wonder that people blamed illness on smells. Can you imagine what a town flooded with sewage smells like or a city like London, with no organized measures of sanitation, with trash and waste smeared about?

Luckily for Snow, his talent for math and science gained him a one-way ticket out of Mickelgate and an apprenticeship as a surgeon-apothecary ("apothecary" meaning "pharmacist") when he was only fourteen years old in the industrial city of Newcastle-upon-Tyne. In 1832 at the age of nineteen, Snow encountered a cholera epidemic for the first time in a nearby coal-mining village. Snow treated many victims of the disease and studied its symptoms. By the time the epidemic lessened later that year, several Newcastle physicians and surgeons had founded a medical school. Snow was one of first eight students who enrolled.

Before he became the hero of London's cholera epidemic, John Snow helped the sick in the morgue, of all places. At the time, arsenic was one of the ingredients used to embalm medical school cadavers before they were dissected, and students studying the cadavers were becoming ill. Snow designed a series

PLAGUES, PANDEMICS AND VIRUSES

of experiments which revealed that the illnesses were caused by inhaling arsenic vapor. The result was an end to the use of arsenic to preserve bodies. This discovery also led to the discontinuation of candles laced with arsenic. These particular candles burned brighter than regular ones, but they, too, emitted a toxic arsenic vapor.

It's intriguing to note that one of Snow's earliest medical victories had to do with inhaling bad air, while his greatest achievement—which most thought had to do with inhaling bad air—had nothing to do with inhaling anything.

John Snow became a doctor in what was then the new field of obstetrics but specialized in respiration. He studied its effects on circulation along with the chemistry and physics of inhaled gases with a unique interest in anesthetic gases and how they applied to childbirth. At the time, using anesthetics to ease the pain of delivery was considered unethical by everyone from the medical community to the Church. This was nothing new. In 1591, a Scottish woman, Euphanie Macalyane, unable to bear the pain of childbirth, asked her midwife to give her something to relieve the pain. When King James VI— after whom the King James Bible is named —heard about this, he had her burned alive on Castle Hill, Edinburgh, as a warning to those who dared evade the curse of Eve. As per Genesis 3:16: "The Lord God said to [Eve] … 'I shall greatly increase your pangs in childbearing; in pain you shall bring forth children.'"

Three hundred years later, in the nineteenth century, priests from the Church of England—who never experienced childbirth themselves—still preached against any kind of childbirth anesthetic, still citing Genesis 3:16. However, on April 7, 1853, Queen Victoria, who was about to give birth to her eighth child, asked John Snow to give her chloroform analgesia during the delivery. The amount of pressure on John Snow in this endeavor must have been astronomical, yet the birth was such a success (she even gave birth to a boy!) that it was repeated

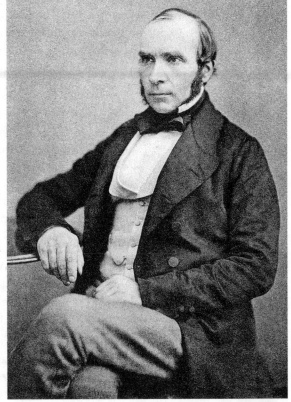

English epidemiologist John Snow, a pioneer in the area of medical hygiene as well as anesthesia and obstetrics, was famous for his work in figuring out how water pollution resulted in a cholera outbreak in Soho, England.

three years later. Obstetrical anesthesia now had the royal blessing, and medical and religious communities had no choice but to follow.

You Know Nothing, John Snow

A cholera epidemic hit London in the fall of 1848 and was the worst cholera outbreak in the city's history, claiming 14,137 lives. Locals, still believing in the theory of miasma, blamed it on those who worked in places like slaughterhouses, rendering plants, or cemeteries. John Snow wasn't so sure. If inhaling miasma was causing the disease, why weren't the slaughterhouse or rendering plant workers not immediately dropping dead from it? Snow believed that cholera was instead transmitted by ingesting—not inhaling—"morbid matter" that contained the disease. Specifically, he believed it was something in the water.

Snow conducted the world's first study on cholera's mortality rates within 32 London subdistricts. He reported that houses whose water supply came from the part of the River Thames that ran above London had far cleaner water and fewer instances of cholera compared to houses whose water supply came from the lower parts of the Thames, which contained human fecal matter. According to Snow, this meant, among other debris, that those who were drinking water from the lower Thames were also drinking bits of other people's fecal matter.

The theory was decidedly unpopular. Snow nevertheless first published his theory in an 1849 essay, "On the Mode of Communication of Cholera":

> Having rejected [miasma] and the poisoning of the blood ... and being led to the conclusion that the disease is communicated by something that acts directly on the alimentary canal, the excretions of the sick at once suggest themselves as containing some material which, being accidentally swallowed, might attach itself to the mucous membrane of the small intestines, and there multiply itself by the appropriation of surrounding matter.

The epidemic lasted for two years.

By the time of the 1854 outbreak, the gloves were off, and John Snow undertook another extensive study to connect cholera deaths with the actual source of water. He wanted to pinpoint the place of infection rather than devising a more general theory that it's from part of the River Thames.

Soho, a suburb of London, was hit particularly hard. This also happened to be where Snow lived. He mapped the reported cases of cholera and learned that the outbreak was radiating from one spot. This spot was like the epicenter of an earthquake. It was the Broad Street water pump. The highest number of cholera cases surrounded it, which led Snow to believe that Broad Street-contaminated water was the culprit. "Within 250 yards of the spot where Cambridge Street joins Broad Street there were upwards of 500 fatal attacks of cholera in 10 days," Snow wrote. "As soon as I became acquainted with the situation and extent of this irruption of cholera, I suspected some contamination of the water of the much-frequented street-pump in Broad Street."

Tirelessly, Snow worked to gather information from hospitals and public records, to schools, restaurants, and pubs. Snow suspected that those who lived or worked near the pump were the most likely to use the pump and therefore contract cholera. He also used the data within the Registrar-General's *Weekly Returns of Deaths in London* to argue that workers in "nuisance trades" suffered no more ill health than those in other occupations.

Snow also investigated those who lived or worked near the water pump but did not get cholera. What was the difference? Where were they getting their water? Snow found several critical examples, including a prison near Soho that had 535 inmates and almost no cases of cholera: the prison had its own well.

Also, men who worked in a Broad Street brewery escaped cholera. The owner told Snow that the men drank the liquor they made or water from the brewery's own well and not water from the Broad Street pump. None of the men had cholera.

In an 1854 letter to the editor of *The Medical Times and Gazette*, John Snow wrote:

JOHN SNOW'S CHOLERA MAP

Snow's type of mapping began around the time the Bills of Mortality had stopped. According to Dr. Richelle Munkhoff, "John Snow's way of mapping had a sense of continuity but also change. The [plague] that they designed the Bills to keep track of over long periods of time wouldn't necessarily work with cholera. Snow's map is different because cholera's so fast, and his map is showing you the street [where the outbreak is coming from]. The Bills of Mortality broke plague down by parish and they were writing the location but weren't *showing* the location. So you had to have a map of London in your head to know where not to go."

Dr. Munkhoff also draws parallels between both these maps and the ones being used today to show the spread of COVID-19. "Our maps with this pandemic use both kinds. We want to see the daily tally but we also want to see a geographic map."

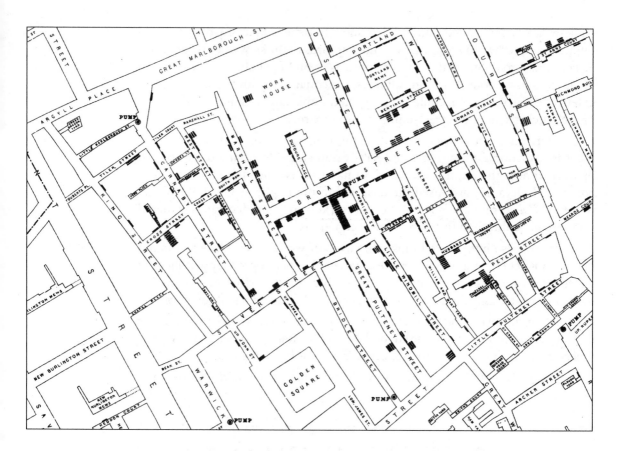

A close-up of Dr. Snow's cholera map shows how he kept track of cases (the short, black lines each indicate a patient) and found that they centered around a pump located on Broad Street.

On proceeding to the spot, I found that nearly all the deaths had taken place within a short distance of the [Broad Street] pump. There were only ten deaths in houses situated decidedly nearer to another street-pump. In five of these cases the families of the deceased persons informed me that they always sent to the pump in Broad Street, as they preferred the water to that of the pumps which were nearer. In three other cases, the deceased were children who went to school near the pump in Broad Street....

With regard to the deaths occurring in the locality belonging to the pump, there were 61 instances in which I was informed that the deceased persons used to drink the pump water from Broad Street, either constantly or occasionally....

PLAGUES, PANDEMICS AND VIRUSES

The result of the inquiry, then, is, that there has been no particular outbreak or prevalence of cholera in this part of London except among the persons who were in the habit of drinking the water of the above-mentioned pump well.

I had an interview with the Board of Guardians of St James's parish, on the evening of [7 September], and represented the above circumstances to them. In consequence of what I said, the handle of the pump was removed on the following day.

On September 7, 1854, Snow took his research to the town officials and convinced them to dismantle the pump, making it impossible to draw water. The officials, though reluctant to believe him, took the pump handle off with the idea that "we'll try anything once." Reports of new cholera cases almost immediately ceased.

Before you think that John Snow was then carried around Broad Street on the shoulders of its grateful citizens, though, think again.

Although they were living amid terrible hygienic conditions, people still didn't want to believe they were drinking water contaminated with feces—that was a bridge too far away to be crossed just yet.

Also, the theory of miasma was believed to be a perfectly good theory, held by smart men for so long, that it was nearly impossible to get people—including those in the medical community—to dismiss it. Dr. William Farr, member of the Scientific Committee for Scientific Enquiries in Relation to the Cholera Epidemic of 1854, believed that the source was miasma, which rose from the soil surrounding the River Thames and contained decaying organic matter, including miasmatic particles that were released into the London air. Farr and his committee wrote:

> In explanation of the remarkable intensity of this outbreak within very definite limits, it has been suggested by Dr. Snow, that the real cause of whatever was peculiar in the case lay in the use of one particular well, situated at Broad Street in the middle of the district, and having (it was imagined) its waters contaminated with the rice-water evacuations of cholera patients. After careful inquiry, we see no reason to adopt this belief. We do not feel it established that the water was contaminated in the manner alleged; nor is there before us any sufficient evidence to show whether inhabitants of that district, drinking from that well, suffered in proportion more than other inhabitants of the district who drank from other sources.

Even the storied medical journal *The Lancet* published a harsh criticism of John Snow by its founder, Thomas Wakley, who exclaimed, "In riding his hobby very hard, he has fallen down through a gully hole and has never since been able to get out again" and, "Has he any facts to show in proof? No!".

Although Snow believed that it was the Broad Street pump that was the site of the problem, he couldn't determine what contaminated it. Officials contended that it was impossible for sewage from town pipes to have leaked into the pump, and even Snow himself said that he couldn't figure out whether the sewage came from open sewers, drains underneath houses or businesses, public pipes, or cesspools. In the meantime, the pump handle that Snow had managed to have taken off was promptly replaced.

Researchers later discovered that the pump had been dug only three feet from an old cesspit, which had begun to leak fecal bacteria. It began when a woman, whose child had contracted cholera from another source, washed the baby's soiled diapers in water—water that she then dumped into the cesspool, which traveled into the Broad Street pump, where the bacteria proliferated.

On June 10, 1858, John Snow suffered a stroke while working in his London office. He was 45 years old at the time. He died six days later.

By 1866, eight years after the death of John Snow, medical opinion had changed to support the germ theory of cholera and its waterborne transmission. Former critic William Farr wrote a detailed report that year where he publicly acknowledged that water was the most important means of transmission, not miasma. The revelation came while he was investigating another outbreak of cholera in East London and gave immediate orders that water must be boiled before drinking.

Each September, the John Snow Society Pumphandle Lecture takes place in London to celebrate the memory of John Snow. The ceremony includes the removal and replacement of the Broad Street pump handle as a reminder of the continuing challenges facing public health. A plaque affixed to a pub near the pump reads: "The Red Granite kerbstone mark is the site of the historic Broad Street pump associated with Dr John Snow's discovery in 1854 that cholera is conveyed by water."

In 2013, *The Lancet* printed a correction of its all-too-brief obituary of Snow, originally published in 1858. The obituary originally read:

Dr John Snow: This well-known physician died at noon, on the 16th instant, at his house in Sackville Street, from an attack of apoplexy. His researches on chloroform and other anaesthetics were appreciated by the profession.

In 2013, Sandra Hempbel, on behalf of *The Lancet*, wrote:

The journal accepts that some readers may wrongly have inferred that *The Lancet* failed to recognise Dr Snow's remarkable achievements in the field of epidemiology and, in particular, his visionary work in deducing the mode of transmission of epidemic cholera. The Editor would also like to add that comments such as "In riding his hobby very hard, he has fallen down through a gully hole and has never since been able to get out again" and "Has he any facts to show in proof? No!", published in an Editorial on Dr Snow's theories in 1855, were perhaps somewhat overly negative in tone.

Others were more generous about Snow than Wakley had been. After the obituary, *The Lancet* published letters from former colleagues in support of Snow's contribution. Dr Hooper Attree, a former house surgeon at the Middlesex Hospital where some of the Broad Street cases were taken, wrote: "I trust that the profession will evince some public testimony towards the late Dr John Snow. Who does not remember his frankness, his cordiality, his honesty, the absence of all disguise or affectation under an apparent off-hand manner? Her Majesty the Queen has been deprived of the future valuable services of a trustworthy, well-deserving, much-esteemed subject, by his sudden death. The poor have lost in him a real friend in the hour of need." And the medical officer of the Poland Street workhouse, John French, remarked that "although ephemeral criticism has been uniformly against him, yet I venture confidently to predict, that the facts which have been brought to light by his indefatigable industry will prove to posterity that he was by far the most important investigator of the subject of cholera who has yet appeared". Here the workhouse medical officer was to prove more visionary than [*The Lancet* founder] Thomas Wakley.

Cholera Today

Cholera is a contagious infection caused by the bacterium *Vibrio cholerae*. This can cause severe gastroenteritis and excessive, watery diarrhea for several days. Rapid dehydration and electrolyte imbalances can be fatal, as was suspected in the death of James Polk, the eleventh president of the United States, and Charles X, the king of France. (Electrolytes are electrically charged minerals that help balance your body's acid/base, or pH, level.)

Under a microscope, *V. cholerae* bacteria look like tiny commas: they're curved and rod-shaped. They're prokaryotic cells, meaning that they lack a membrane around the nucleus. Their components, like DNA and proteins, float freely within the cytoplasm, all encased within a cell membrane. *V. cholerae* also have a flagellum, which is a tail that propels it through the gastrointestinal tract, and a slime capsule, which is a kind of goo they release that allows them to slide around their environment. The slime also protects them from stomach acid so that they can get to the small intestine.

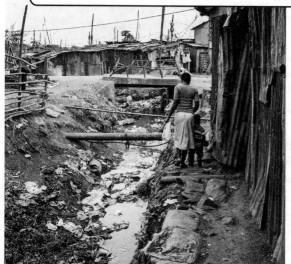

Poverty-stricken shanty towns, where clean water is a rarity, remain hot spots around the world for cholera.

Transmission usually occurs on a fecal-to-oral route. Does this mean that someone who has cholera ate poop? The answer is: not intentionally. The fecal matter may be in food that someone unknowingly eats, though people mainly get cholera through contaminated water. Other ways to get cholera include drinking untreated sewage water or anything that comes into contact with it like raw or uncooked fish, or improper hygiene, such as a lack of hand washing after a bowel movement. Cholera bacteria in the water can even contaminate the soil and get transmitted to the surface of food by flies or by touching it with your hand.

Our stomachs contain a fluid called "chyme" that breaks down food using its highly

PLAGUES, PANDEMICS AND VIRUSES

acidic properties. (A word about pH: pH is a chemical ruler that specifies how acidic or basic a liquid is. The scale runs from 0 [most acidic] to 14 [most basic]. An example of a liquid with a pH level of 0 is battery acid. One with a pH value of 14 is drain cleaner. Blood typically has a pH level of 7, which means it's equally balanced.)

Some parts of our bodies need to be acidic. Our stomach lining has a very acidic pH level of 2 (the same as vinegar), which aids in digestion and also kills cholera bacteria. The majority of the bacteria will quickly die off, but some can survive, and when they pass into the small intestine, they encounter a pH of around 8.5.

This basic level is the perfect pH for cholera bacteria to grow, thrive, and ultimately infect the epithelial cells found in the small intestine. When a *V. cholerae* bacterium enters the stomach, it halts its own protein production to conserve energy and successfully survive the acidic environment, but once in the intestines, it uses its flagellum to swim to the intestinal walls, where it releases toxins that attach to an epithelial cell on the small intestine. A chemical reaction takes place, and the toxin is engulfed through the membrane into the epithelial cell, just like a virus would be engulfed into a cell.

The type of toxin depends on the strain of *V. cholerae*. Some strains release toxins that will cause mild to no symptoms. If you were to take ten people infected with *V. cholerae*, about one person would fit into this category. The other nine could be healthy, then die within hours. These are the ones infected with toxins called choleragen, which is most often the cause of significant clinical symptoms. When choleragen enter the epithelial cells, they disrupt that critical pH balance between the intestines and surrounding tissue, so water, bicarbonate, and potassium rush into the intestine to try to bring the pH levels back to normal. This causes vomiting and voluminous amounts of watery diarrhea, which is filled with high levels of *V. cholerae*, ready to infect another individual.

Typically, no fever, pain, or cramping occurs. While the incubation time for *V. cholerae* can take anywhere from a few hours to two to three days, severe dehydration and depletion of electrolytes can happen within 4 to 12 hours after the first bout of diarrhea or vomiting. These chemical imbalances can then cause disorientation, dry mouth, swollen tongue, clammy skin, or shriveled and dried hands and feet.

Even more severe and fatal complications begin to arise from depleted electrolytes and water in the blood. This causes hypovolemic shock, or an extreme loss of the body's fluid, making the blood thicken, which causes problems with circulation and allowing the blood to reach internal organs.

PLAGUES, PANDEMICS AND VIRUSES

When people lose so much water, they start to look different. Their eyes sink and their teeth protrude, like a skeleton. The skin turns blue due to massive dehydration. This is how cholera got the nickname "The Blue Death."

Cholera is alive and well and is the most common cause of bacterial gastroenteritis (an infection of the gut) in parts of the world such as Africa, India, and Haiti, where many sites are overcrowded and lack sanitation. When someone is infected with *V. cholerae*, it's like an explosion has gone off inside them, forcing them to spew wave upon wave of vomit and diarrhea—in some cases up to five gallons of diarrhea a day—until death from dehydration comes as a miserable relief. However, the victim has then left behind a deadly corpse, for to touch a person who has died of cholera is to expose yourself to the bacteria. Touching the body, then touching your eyes or mouth, means that you may be the next victim.

If any chance of survival is possible, the patient must be quickly rehydrated. Depending on the severity of the case, this would be done intravenously or by drinking oral rehydration salts (ORS). The ORS recipe is:

- 5 cups of clean water
- 6 teaspoons of sugar
- 12 teaspoons of salt

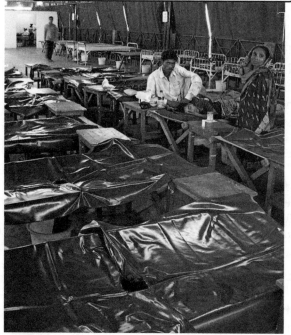

These "cholera beds" in Dhaka, Bangladesh, are low-tech beds covered in plastic with a hole for elimination that permits minimally trained health workers to measure fluid output.

That's it. Salt might be a surprising ingredient, but it's because our bodies need sodium for critical tasks like sending nerve impulses, contracting and relaxing muscle fibers (including those in the heart and blood vessels), and maintaining a proper fluid balance. The ORS dosage level can vary depending on the size of the victim, as cholera can strike babies or adults.

According to the WHO, cholera infects three to five million people every year and causes between 100,000–220,000 deaths worldwide.

If you're diagnosed with cholera and treated immediately, your chance of survival is higher than 99 percent. If you're not treated, your chance of survival is 50 percent. Although cholera treatment is about as simple as treatments can get, it's still not available in many parts of the developing world, largely for lack of clean

PLAGUES, PANDEMICS AND VIRUSES

water. To make matters worse, certain African countries, such as Guinea-Bissau, have funerary rites that perpetuate the disease: Those who have died of cholera are often washed by family members, who then go on to prepare funeral feasts held very soon after the victim's death. *V. cholerae* spreads from such funeral feasts because the corpse handlers cannot properly clean themselves before preparing the meal. The bacteria are transferred from the corpse to the handler to the food and water used with the meal to the visitor at the feast. Then, the bacteria begin to replicate in a new host and cause disease again.

TUBERCULOSIS

It was July 1939 in Staten Island, New York, and a man stood smiling at his living room window, knocking gently on it and waving. Looking onto the front porch, he saw his first grandchild, Rita, smiling in a baby carriage. This would be the first and only time he'd see her. Five months later, Fred Siller would be dead from tuberculosis, which was also the reason he was separated from his granddaughter by a window, unable to hold her; able only to wave "hello." He would never get to hold 20 subsequent grandchildren, either.

Roughly 100 years earlier, in the absence of germ theory, the symptoms of tuberculosis (also known as "the consumption" or TB) were thought to have been caused by a mystical state rather than disease—a consequence of being one of the beautiful, the artistic, the damned. A nobility was contained within its fatality, ranking up there with the greatest of tragedies, the melancholy of the soul. It led to women wearing bright red lipstick to offset their complexion, to excessively powder a face that wasn't pale enough, and to don nightgownlike dresses that made them appear ghostly. It was the nineteenth-century version of 1990's "heroin chic."

"Consumption, I am aware, is a flattering malady," wrote Charlotte Brontë in 1849. (She also wrote *Jane Eyre*.) Charlotte was referring to the phantomlike pallor of the skin, set off by blood-red lips and pulsing veins that characterized the ideal TB victim. (This is similar to one of Dracula's victims—the novel by Bram Stoker would be published 48 years later.) Of the six Brontë children—five girls and one boy—all were wildly talented, and all but Charlotte died of the consumption (though many believe that TB took Charlotte as well). Charlotte's talk of the "flattering malady" was in regard to her sister, Anne, the youngest Brontë and author of *The Tenant of Wildfell Hall*. Anne would die of TB later that year at 29 years of age. Her sister, Emily Brontë, best known for the Gothic novel, *Wuthering Heights*, died of TB in December 1848 at the age of 30. Their brother, artist Branwell Brontë, died of a combination of TB and se-

Charlotte was referring to the phantomlike pallor of the skin, set off by blood-red lips and pulsing veins that characterized the ideal TB victim.

vere alcoholism in 1848 at the age of 31. (The oldest sibling, Maria, had died several years earlier of TB at the age of eleven.) The Brontës' father, Patrick Brontë, would survive them all.

Fred Siller was a one-eyed alcoholic from Brooklyn, New York. He brought to those around him hilarity and spurred imaginations with tales of his days as a vaudevillian. He also caused disappointment and heartbreak when he'd be seen by his daughter stumbling drunk in the early afternoon while she was in fifth grade at recess or when she'd hear him stumbling up the stairs at night. Siller had lost his eye from an injury on the job and was awarded the equivalent of more than $500,000 today, but he lost it trying to run a fish market. It's unknown where Siller got TB from, but between his alcoholism and heavy smoking, it came as no surprise when he tested positive; it was just tragic.

So, why was such a horrible fate ever considered flattering?

When Death Was Cool

As people are so fond of saying, "Blame the media." In the nineteenth century, the arts made up much of the media. Thomas Gainsborough's 1770s painting of the pallid "Honourable Mrs. Graham" was completed right before her death from TB. Although she died by drowning, who embodied the vision of the consumptive body better than the noblewoman Ophelia, the doomed character from William Shakespeare's *Hamlet*? A mid-1800s painting of Ophelia by British artist John Everett Millais shows her just before she sinks below the water's surface, looking as delicate as the flowers still in her grasp, with flowing, red locks complemented by poppies (signifying death) amid a lush world of field and stream. This isn't death as much as a death wish, the epitome of pre-Raphaelite art that was so popular back then.

The pallor of the victim gave TB the moniker "The White Plague" in Victorian England. It was "an excess of passion, burning away inside the body, [purifying] the creative soul with suffering." Since people at that time didn't know that TB was spread by bacteria, they believed that it was perhaps spread by the gentle touch of the muses. When looking into a mirror, the poet Lord Byron said to a friend, "I should like, I think, to die of consumption." When his friend asked why, Byron said, "Because then all the women would say 'See that poor Byron, how *interesting* he looks in dying.'" (Victor Hugo, author of *Les Misérables,* was told that he'd be a better writer if he were more consumptive.)

TB was romanticized by poets like Percy Bysshe Shelley and writers such as Edgar Allan Poe, Robert Louis Stevenson, and Emily Brontë—many of whom would themselves die from it. In Katherine Byrne's book *Tuberculosis and the Victorian Literary Imagination*, she refers to the romantic poetry of Keats and Shelley, which "sought to find beauty in the horror and melancholy of consumption." Such works of the time were sometimes called "graveyard poetry." Poets including John Keats, Elizabeth Barrett Browning, and Henry David Thoreau did die of TB but not because they were talented writers. John Keats wrote in 1819, "Youth grows pale, and spectre thin, and dies." Keats died of TB in 1821 when he was 26 years old. On a winter evening in 1818, when Keats was returning to his home in Hampstead Heath from London, he felt ill and immediately went to bed. He suddenly coughed blood onto his pillow and said to his friend, John Arbuthnot Brown, "I know the color of that blood. It is arterial blood, I cannot be deceived by its color. It is my death warrant. I must die."

Edgar Allan Poe described his wife, Virginia, who suffered from TB, as being "delicately, morbidly angelic." In 1842, while they were having dinner, Virginia had a sudden coughing fit, and Poe remarked, "Suddenly she stopped, clutched her throat and a wave of crimson blood ran down her breast.… It rendered her even more ethereal." Emily Brontë described the tuberculous character in *Wuthering Heights* as

TB was sometimes romanticized in the arts, such as in the Puccini opera *La Bohème*, which was also adapted as the Broadway musical *Rent* and into the movie musical *Moulin Rouge.*

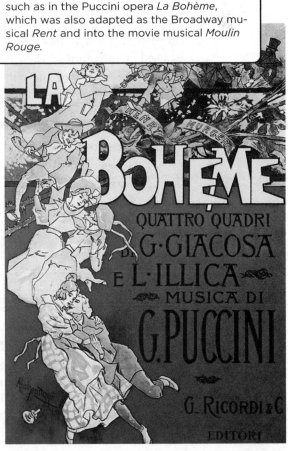

"rather thin, but young and fresh complexioned and her eyes sparkled like diamonds." (Recall that Emily, three of her four sisters, and her brother Branwell all died in young adulthood of TB. It was an obsession that bore fruit.)

TB inspired Alexandre Dumas's novel *Camille* (1852), which inspired Guiseppi Verdi's *La Traviata* (1853). Giacomo Puccini's opera *La Bohème* (1896) and a lesser-known opera of the same name by Rugerro Leoncalvo in 1897 were both based on Henri Muger's series of stories from 1848 called *Scenes of a Bohemian Life*. All have female protagonists who die of TB. (In turning the notion of a "good death" on its head, Jonathan Larson's wildly popular 1994 musical, *Rent*, was inspired by *La Bohème*, but these "bohemians" were outcasts who died of HIV/AIDS.)

Susan Sontag wrote in *Illness as Metaphor* that "all the evidence indicates that the cult of TB was not simply an invention of romantic poets and opera librettists but a widespread attitude, and that the person dying (young) of TB really was perceived as a romantic personality…. Sickness was a way of making people 'interesting'—which is how 'romantic' was originally defined." Perhaps Lord Byron wasn't too far off. (He would die from a fever that was possibly caused by infection in 1824 at the age of 36.)

The vision of the consumptive was exploited by nineteenth-century writers, who began the literary tradition of vampirism, especially in consumptive areas of the world where such folklore abounded, such as New England and Yorkshire, where it was whispered that people who were suffering from what were actually symptoms of TB—wasting and extreme pallor—were actually vampires.

However, all fads must come to an end, as did "consumptive chic" once it was discovered to have come from bacteria, not muses, and was then down-

---

FUNNY GIRL TB

In the 1964 musical *Funny Girl*, which is about the actor/singer/comedian Fanny Brice, the song "I'm the Greatest Star," written by Jule Styne and Bob Merrill, includes the lines:

> Now, can't you see to look at me
> That I'm a natural Camille?
> As Camille I just feel
> I've so much to offer
> Kid, I know I'd be divine
> Because I'm a natural cougher

PLAGUES, PANDEMICS AND VIRUSES

graded to the lower classes. By the time Fred Siller contracted TB, it was long past its glamorous phase.

Ancient Lungs

TB is an ancient disease. In the third millennium B.C.E., a "wasting disease" was described in one of the earliest medical works, the Chinese *Huang Ti Nei-Ching*, or *Yellow Emperor's Inner Canon*. A much later Chinese medical text, *Huangdi Neijing* (c. 400 B.C.E.–260 C.E.), describes a disease that has all the characteristics of TB, called *xulao bing*, or "weak consumptive disease." Its symptoms are severe coughing, fever, unhealthy pallor, and shortness of breath. More symptoms were described dramatically as *lao ji* ("exhausted sacrifice"), *shi zhu* ("corpse infection"), *gui zhu* ("ghost infection"), *huaifu* ("bad palace"), and *wugu* ("innocence").

However, all fads must come to an end, as did "consumptive chic" once it was discovered to have come from bacteria, not muses....

The *Huangdi Neijing* describes TB as such: "As for a string which is cut, its sound is hoarse. As for wood which has become old, its leaves are shed. As for a disease which is in the depth [of the body], the sound it [generates] is hiccup. When a man has these three [states], this is called 'destroyed palace.' Toxic drugs do not bring a cure; short needles cannot seize [the disease]."

In the second millennium B.C.E., King Hammurabi of Babylonia wrote of a chronic lung disease that may have been TB, and Homer's famous *Odyssey* from the eighth century B.C.E. refers to "grievous consumption which took the soul from the body," which caused a person to "lie in sickness ... a long time wasting away."

TB has also left behind traces of itself in Egyptian mummies dated between 3000 and 2400 B.C.E. The most convincing case was found in the mummy of the priest Nesperehen, discovered in 1881, which had evidence of spinal tuberculosis. Similar TB features were found on other mummies throughout the

PLAGUES, PANDEMICS AND VIRUSES

cemeteries of Thebes, a former city along the Nile River. It also seems likely that Egyptian pharaoh Akhenaten and his wife Nefertiti died of TB, and evidence has even been found that TB hospitals existed in Egypt back as far as 1500 B.C.E.

The Ebers papyrus, an important Egyptian medical discourse from around 1550 B.C.E., describes a pulmonary disease associated with swollen neck lymph nodes. The recommended treatment was the application of a mixture of acacia leaves, peas, fruits, animal blood, insect blood, honey, and salt upon the neck.

In Book 1 of *Of the Epidemics* (410–400 B.C.E.), Hippocrates describes a disease of "weakness of the lung" with fever and cough, which he refers to as *phthisis* (from the Greek word *phthiein*, meaning "to waste away"):

> Early in the beginning of spring, and through the summer, and towards winter, many of those who had been long gradually declining, took to bed with symptoms of phthisis; … Many, and, in fact, most of them died, and of those confined to bed, I do not know of a single individual survived for any considerable time, …

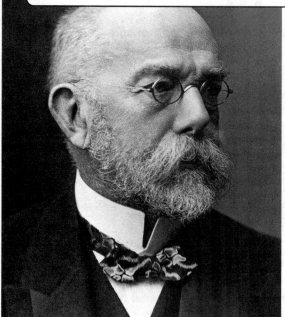

Dr. Robert Koch, a Nobel Prize-winning German microbiologist and physician who was one of the founders of bacteriology, discovered the bacteria that causes TB. He also found the causes of anthrax and cholera.

> Consumption was the most considerable of the diseases which then prevailed, and the only one which proved fatal to many persons. Most of them were affected by these diseases in the following manner; fevers accompanied with rigors, … constant sweats, … extremities very cold, and warmed with difficulty; bowels disordered, with bilious, scanty, unmixed, thin, pungent, and frequent dejections. The urine was thin, colorless, unconcocted, or thick, with a deficient sediment. Sputa small, dense, concocted, but brought up rarely and with difficulty; and in those who encountered the most violent symptoms there was no concoction at all, but they continued throughout spitting crude matters.

Hippocrates recognized the predilection of the disease for young adults: "Phthisis makes its attacks chiefly between the age of 18 and 35."

The Greeks called it *phthisis*. The Incas called it *chaky oncay*. The English would eventually call it tuberculosis. *Mycobacterium tuber-*

culosis, or *M. tuberculosis*, is the bacteria that causes TB, which was discovered in 1882 by German physician Robert Koch. A person may develop TB after inhaling *M. tuberculosis*.

A person can have TB bacteria in their body and never develop symptoms. In most people, the immune system can contain the bacteria so that it does not replicate and cause disease. In this case, a person will have the TB infection but not the active disease—this is called a latent phase. Others may develop TB long after infection, when the immune system is weakened due to illness or the use of certain medications. This is called its active phase. When this happens, the bacteria can replicate and cause the characteristic symptoms of TB. Without medical intervention, TB becomes active in 5–10 percent of infected people. Although people with latent TB cannot spread the infection, people with active TB can.

M. tuberculosis typically travels through the air and into our nasal passageways. It eventually reaches the lungs and is engulfed by macrophages that are part of our immune system. This is usually enough to wipe out the bacteria. For those with other medical conditions, though, the immune response may not be enough to destroy the intruder. If this is the case, *M. tuberculosis* will multiply and form what are known as "colonies" within the lungs. Symptoms include coughing for more than three weeks, coughing up blood, loss of appetite and weight, tiredness, fever, night sweats, and chest pain. As they infect more cells, the bacteria use enzymes that destroy the infected lung tissue, which causes chest pain and blood in the spittle. Because TB is an airborne disease, an infected person who coughs or sneezes risks infecting someone else since the bacteria can stay airborne for several hours.

Though Koch's research had proven that TB was caused by bacteria, the general public was slow to understand this critical fact....

The bacteria can also travel to the skeletal system, causing back pains and difficulty

PLAGUES, PANDEMICS AND VIRUSES

TB AND ARCHITECTURE

Medical professionals believed a TB patient's best chance of recovery was to live where they could get plenty of fresh air, sunlight, rest, and food. As form follows function, the design of TB sanitoriums reflected this. TB sanatoriums began in Europe in the mid-1800s in Poland, Germany, and Switzerland. Although they began as collections of cottages in mountainous locales, they evolved into modernist buildings that would allow for fresh air and sunlight. The first TB sanatorium in the United States was founded in 1885 by Dr. Edward Livingston Trudeau in Saranac Lake, New York. Dr. Trudeau—who had TB himself—made sure the buildings had a glass-enclosed deck, known as a "cure porch." Patients would spend much of their time resting on recliners on these porches, especially in the dry, winter air, under blankets.

Sanatoriums coincided with Modernism and brought forth architectural elements like terraces and balconies and white- or light-painted rooms. Like the sanatorium, this new architectural style was intended to cure the anxiety caused by living in crowded cities. In 1925, Swiss architect Le Corbusier described his vision of a city where "there are no more dirty, dark corners. Everything is shown as it is. Then comes inner cleanliness.…"

This belies the idea that Modernism was meant to be sterile and cold. On the contrary, Modernists like Charles and Ray Eames paid close attention to the dimensions and comfort of the human body. "One of the very common criticisms of modern architecture," said Peter MacKeith, dean of architecture at the University of Arkansas, "is that it's usually presented and understood as being derived from a very mechanistic approach. As opposed to an architecture that's much more derived [from human] anatomy itself and all of the interrelated systems that we have."

moving. It can infect the kidneys and intestines, causing terrible abdominal pain. It can also travel to the brain, leading to headaches and the repeated fainting spells that made healthy Victorians swoon. Finally, the infected reached that classic consumptive look of weight loss and pale skin.

At the end of the nineteenth century, one in seven people around the world had died of TB, and it was the third-leading cause of death in the United States. Though Koch's research had proven that TB was caused by bacteria, the general public was slow to understand this critical fact, and most paid little attention to how the disease was spread. They didn't understand that the things they did could make them sick. S. Adolphus Knopf, an early TB specialist, wrote in his book *Pulmonary Tuberculosis: Its Modern Prophylaxis and the Treatment in Special Institutions and at Home* that he had once observed several of his patients in New York City sipping from the same glass as other passengers on a train, even as "they coughed and expectorated a good deal." Back then, it was all too common to share a drinking cup with family members or even strangers.

With Knopf's guidance, in the 1890s, the New York City Health Department launched a massive campaign to reduce transmission. Educating the public around the world about its own health became a vital tool in controlling TB and led to curbing habits like spitting on the ground. "War on Tuberculosis" posters showed such scenes as a father closing the door on a deathly figure trying to enter his home, or French mothers with a line of numerous children—one of whom has a flag tied to his shirt that says, "*Allons-tous à la consultation*," or "Let's go see the doctor." Public-health campaigns discouraged cup sharing and prompted states to ban spitting inside public buildings and on public transit, sidewalks, and other outdoor spaces—instead encouraging the use of special spittoons to be carefully cleaned on a regular basis. (In the Soviet Union, one poster shows an organ grinder named Dirty Vlas showing that people who spit spread TB and are therefore enemies of the people's health.) Before long, spitting in public spaces came to be considered filthy. Changes in public behavior helped to successfully reduce the prevalence of TB.

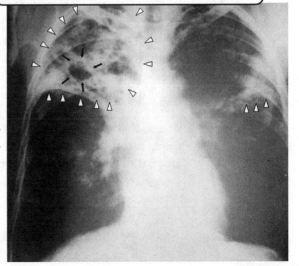

A chest X-ray indicates advanced tuberculosis in a patient, including bilateral pulmonary infiltrate (white arrows) and a caving formation (black arrows) that are signs of severe organ damage.

In 1895, Wilhelm Röntgen invented the X-ray (an achievement that earned him the very first Nobel Prize for Physics in 1901). This allowed physicians to diagnose and track the disease's progression throughout the lungs and body.

In 2014, scientists from the University of Tübingen were able to recreate the genome of bacteria from remains of skeletons in Peru. Although the skeletons were a thousand years old, the DNA of *M. tuberculosis* found in these skeletons was around five thousand years old. The team members also believe that humans acquired the disease in Africa about five thousand years ago from domesticated animals. Seals acquired it when coming up on African beaches for breeding and carried it across the Atlantic, which is why it showed up in Peruvian skeletons. In addition, TB was spread via the trade routes within the Old World.

TB Treatment

Unlike other bacteria, *M. tuberculosis* doesn't exchange immunity through horizontal gene transfer. Between that and its low rate of multiplication and evolution, resistance to antibiotics has been relatively slow compared to, say, gonorrhea, a venereal disease that is now immune to almost all antibiotics.

Traditional treatments will take six to twelve months, requiring a high number of drugs and numerous side effects that are similar to TB symptoms, which also may include jaundice and rashes. This discourages people from finishing the full course of these drugs, and partial treatment only helps bacteria to develop resistance and TB to recur. A recurrence of TB is harder to treat because the medicines are now less effective, so the medications have to be taken for a longer period of time and may lead to more powerfully unpleasant side effects, and the chances of a cure are sharply reduced. However, more than 95 percent of patients are cured if they take the full course of their medications the first time around.

Although TB is a bacterial infection, a vaccine does exist for it. Bacilli Calmette-Guérin (BCG) is a weakened version of *Mycobacterium bovis*, a bacterium that causes TB in cattle and is related to *M. tuberculosis*. It was first used on humans in 1921. Today, it's primarily given to infants and small children in countries where TB is common such as India, China, Indonesia, the Philippines, Pakistan, Nigeria, Bangladesh, and South Africa; its effectiveness in adults varies widely.

TB remains one of the most infectious diseases on Earth, causing more deaths than malaria or AIDS, and is prevalent in more than 30 countries, mostly ones that suffer from other health crises that exacerbate TB. TB develops in about 8.5 million people worldwide every year, and about 15 percent of them die. Also, accessing treatment is difficult in many of these countries, and the stigma that goes along with TB can prevent people from getting the help they need. Faster-acting antibiotics and better health care in developing countries are part of what's needed to wipe TB off Earth forever.

POLIO

Polio is short for poliomyelitis, which is a disease caused by poliovirus. Like cholera, it has a fecal-to-oral route, but unlike cholera, it's viral, not bacterial. It belongs to the family *Picornaviridae—picorna* meaning "small RNA viruses." The viruses in this family can cause paralysis, meningitis, hepatitis, and polio. The genus that descends from this family, *Enterovirus*, is transmitted through the intestine, hence the fecal-to-oral route that holds true for the species, poliovirus. Poliovirus is strictly a human pathogen and does not naturally infect any other animals. The result, poliomyelitis, stands for *polio*, the virus; *myel* refers to the spinal cord, which is affected; and *itis* means inflammation. Today, it mainly infects children under the age of five.

As with cholera, the disease is bad enough, but the idea of a contracting it as a result of ingesting fecal matter is not something one would want to dwell on—and how does that happen, anyway?

Some examples of fecal-to-oral transmission routes include:

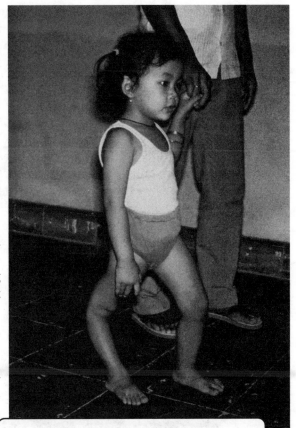

This young girl has suffered a severe leg deformity as a result of the polio virus.

- Shaking someone's hand that has been contaminated by stool
- Changing diapers
- Dealing with livestock or house pets
- Food that has been prepared in the presence of fecal matter
- Vectors like houseflies spreading contamination
- Not washing hands after using the bathroom
- Lack of cleaning anything that has been in contact with feces
- Sexual practices that may involve oral contact with feces
- Eating feces, whether it be children or adults with a mental disorder called corprophagia

It can also (rarely) be transmitted when an infected person sneezes or coughs, which spreads millions of viral particles through the air within the droplets. Once inside the body, the poliovirus binds to epithelial cells in the small intestine, enters the cells, uses the cells to make multiple copies of itself, then buds out from the cells and moves to the lymph nodes and bloodstream. The poliovirus prefers to bind to motor nerves, so it will leave the bloodstream and get into the muscle tissue. From there, the virus enters the motor neuron and travels retrograde—just like the rabies virus—meaning backward up through the axon to the spinal cord.

This causes an immune response that inflames and damages the spinal cord. As the muscles from the infected neurons die, the limbs stop getting signals from the brain, which causes them to shrivel and weaken. Depending on their age and the severity of the infection, an infected person may be paralyzed for life, need crutches, have weakened muscles, or have no symptoms at all. In fact, only 1 percent of polio victims progress to where it's a paralytic disease. It begins with a high fever, muscle spasms, and loss of muscle reflexes, eventually moving to paralysis. Diagnosis comes from the presence of poliovirus in a stool sample or throat swab or in the cerebrospinal fluid from a spinal tap.

In rarer cases, the poliovirus can infect nerves involved in speaking and swallowing and the motor nerves of the diaphragm. This type of polio, called bulbar polio, can make it impossible for the victim to breathe on their own, in which case they would need an iron lung. An iron lung is typically a large cylinder in which a person is laid with their head coming out of one end resting on a pillow. Their nose and mouth have access to the air around them, while the rest of their body is sealed inside the cylinder, where air pressure is continuously cycled up and down.

> In rarer cases, the poliovirus can infect nerves involved in speaking and swallowing and the motor nerves of the diaphragm.

To make a person inhale, air is pumped out of the cylinder, causing a slight vacuum, which causes their chest and abdomen to expand and the person to inhale. Then, the air inside the cylinder is compressed slightly, pushing on the chest and abdomen and forcing air out of the lungs as the patient exhales. (Due to the eradication of polio throughout most of the world, iron lungs are generally consid-

PLAGUES, PANDEMICS AND VIRUSES

DIANNE ODELL

Dianne Odell was a Tennessee woman who contracted bulbar polio in 1950 at the age of three and spent most of her life in an iron lung. Caregivers could still slide Odell's bedding out of her iron lung for basic nursing care but only briefly. Odell was confined to it for nearly 60 years, becoming one of the longest users ever of an iron lung; Odell's was 7 feet long and weighed 750 pounds.

Although Odell could not attend high school, she completed her work by having her classmates or teachers bring assignments home, where she would read the answers into a Dictaphone or have friends or family transcribe them. She also learned to write with her toes. Odell graduated from high school in 1965 and subsequently took long-distance classes from Freed-Hardeman University, where she received an honorary degree in 1987. She received the Paul Harris Fellow Award from the Jackson Rotary Club, one of the club's highest honors. In 1992, Odell was profiled in *Woman's World* magazine. After she was asked if she thought people were hopelessly shallow, Odell replied, "Not hopelessly."

Friends and family have said that despite her condition, Odell accepted what life handed her with grace. For one Halloween party, they decorated her iron lung as a pack of Life Savers and for another as a yellow submarine. In a 1994 interview with the Associated Press, Odell said, "I've had a very good life, filled with love and family and faith. You can make life good or you can make it bad."

Odell's life was threatened when power outages in 1957 and 1974 disabled her respirator. However, she survived with the help of her family, who hand-pumped the respirator until power was restored. In 1995, the Odell family received a generator large enough to power the house and the iron lung in case of future power outages. However, on May 28, 2008, the power failed both at home and in the backup generator. Family members tried to use the emergency hand pump, which they had done before, to keep her breathing, but their efforts were unsuccessful. Dianne Odell died at the age of 61.

ered obsolete, though the COVID-19 pandemic has brought iron lungs back to the fore as possible substitutes for hospitals that lack ventilators.)

PLAGUES, PANDEMICS AND VIRUSES

Polio Vaccine

Polio is a virus that's been doing damage at least since ancient times. Egyptian art shows adults with withered limbs and children with canes. English physician Michael Underwood gave the first clinical description in 1789, when he called it "a debility of the lower extremities." The disease was later called "infantile paralysis" due to children being more susceptible than adults.

Before the twentieth century, most cases of polio were diagnosed in children aged six months to four years. Poorer sanitation led to a constant exposure to the virus, which, in an oddly positive sense, enhanced people's immunity to it. But improvements in sanitation and clean water in developed countries ironically had a terrible drawback: they drastically reduced the exposure of populations to the poliovirus, thereby increasing the proportion of children and adults at risk of paralytic polio infection.

Epidemics began to appear in Europe and the United States around 1900, and outbreaks hit Europe, North America, Australia, and New Zealand for the next 50 years. By 1950, the peak age incidence of paralytic poliomyelitis in the United States had changed to children aged five to nine years; about one-third of the cases were reported in people over 15 years of age. The rate of paralysis and death due to polio also increased. The 1952 epidemic became the worst polio outbreak in the nation's history. Of the nearly 58,000 cases reported that year, 3,145 died and 21,269 were left with mild to disabling paralysis. Most hospitals at the time had limited access to iron lungs for victims who could no longer breathe on their own; respiratory centers designed to assist the most severe polio patients became the precursors of modern intensive care units.

The development of the polio vaccine became "the most elaborate program of its kind in history, involving 20,000 physicians and public health officers, 64,000 school personnel, and 220,000 volunteers," with over 1.8 million schoolchildren participating in the trial. A 1954 Gallup Poll revealed that more Americans knew about the polio field trials than could give the entire name of then president Dwight David Eisenhower.

Jonas Salk

Jonas Salk was one of those people in medicine, like Louis Pasteur, who was destined for greatness. His parents didn't receive a formal education, but Salk studied like mad in order to make it into the City College of New York (CCNY), which was at the time one of the most prestigious—and also free—schools in the country. At 15, Salk became a freshman at CCNY.

PLAGUES, PANDEMICS AND VIRUSES

After graduating in 1934, Salk enrolled in New York University to study medicine. In his last year of medical school, Salk said that he "had an opportunity to spend time in elective periods in my last year in medical school, in a laboratory that was involved in studies on influenza. The influenza virus had just been discovered about a few years before that. And, I saw the opportunity at that time to test the question as to whether we could destroy the virus infectivity and still immunize. And so, by carefully designed experiments, we found it was possible to do so."

In 1942, Salk worked at the University of Michigan School of Public Health on an Army-commissioned project to develop an influenza vaccine. He and virologist/mentor Thomas Francis Jr. eventually developed a vaccine that would become widely used at Army bases; annual variations on the vaccine are used today.

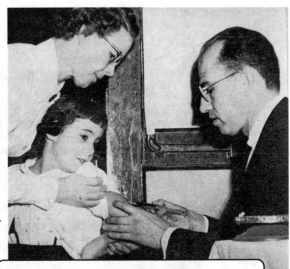

Dr. Jonas Salk is shown here injecting his polio vaccine into a young patient. He developed the vaccine in 1955, three years after a horrific outbreak of the disease.

In 1947, Salk was appointed director of the Virus Research Laboratory at the University of Pittsburgh School of Medicine. The following year, Harry Weaver, the director of research at the National Foundation for Infantile Paralysis, offered Salk space, equipment, and researchers to develop a polio vaccine. During the first year, Salk gathered supplies and a team, including Julius Youngner, Byron Bennett, L. James Lewis, and Lorraine Friedman. As time went on, Salk began securing grants from the Mellon family—of Pittsburgh's Carnegie-Mellon University—and was able to create his own virology laboratory.

Salk and his team devoted themselves to research for the next several years. The prevailing idea at the time was that a vaccine had to be made of a weakened version of a virus, as was the case with smallpox. Salk decided instead to test a safer "killed" virus, which could immunize a person with little to no chance of infecting them.

Salk and his team hypothesized that these viruses, though dead, would still be recognized by the body as "other," and therefore, the immune system would develop the ability to quickly respond to any subsequent encounters. By exposing a person to what's called an immunogen—like a killed poliovirus—in a controlled way, their body could learn to protect itself in what's called "active immunization." If the poliovirus appeared again, it would be covered by antibodies, and the virus would then be devoured by phagocytes, keeping motor neurons safe from infection.

> By exposing a person to what's called an immunogen—like a killed poliovirus—in a controlled way, their body could learn to protect itself....

In 1952, after successfully inoculating thousands of monkeys, Salk began the next step—trying to inoculate humans. In the first trial, Salk injected himself, his wife, and his three sons in their Pittsburgh kitchen after boiling the syringes on the stove. "He felt that he couldn't ask other parents to let him give this vaccine to their children if he wasn't willing to first try it on his own," said Dr. Darrell Salk, one of Jonas's sons—all of whom became doctors. This was regarded as a normal first stage, though today, it sounds horrifying.

How did Salk know whether or not he and his family were successfully inoculated? By repeatedly checking the antibody levels in his family's blood to see if enough of an immune response was produced. "I once hid under the bed," said Dr. Darrell Salk, who was then five years old. It wasn't the experimental vaccine that sent him hiding, it was all the blood tests. This first trial was a success.

On July 2, 1952, assisted by the staff at the D. T. Watson Home for Crippled Children, Salk injected 43 children with his killed-virus vaccine. (It was literally a do-or-die moment reminiscent of John Snow administering the then new chloroform analgesic to Queen Victoria while she was in labor.) A few weeks later, Salk injected children at the Polk State School for the Retarded and Feeble-Minded. In 1954, he tested the vaccine on close to one million children, known as "polio pioneers." The vaccine was announced as safe on April 12, 1955. In the two years before the vaccine was widely available, the average number of polio cases in the United States was more than 45,000. By 1962, it was down to 910.

Salk's monumental achievement brought him international fame; Edward R. Murrow told him, "Young man, a great tragedy has befallen you." Indeed, Salk loathed the spotlight. It was as though he'd become the movie star he

PLAGUES, PANDEMICS AND VIRUSES

never wanted to be. During a 1980 interview with *The New York Times*, Salk said, "It's as if I've been a public property ever since.… It's brought me enormous gratification, opened many opportunities, but at the same time placed many burdens on me. It altered my career, my relationships with colleagues; I am a public figure, no longer one of them."

Charlotte DeCroes Jacobs, author of *Jonas Salk: A Life*, said in an interview with the Oxford University Press:

> This wasn't done by a pharmaceutical firm or research institute, but by a single man [with] his research associates.… Heads of states around the world rushed to honor him [but] the scientific community remained ominously quiet. Basil O'Connor, the powerful director for the National Foundation for Infantile Paralysis, said that the scientists acted as if "Salk had halitosis or had committed a felony."

> It started out that Salk was quite junior and wasn't a member of the "scientific brotherhood" and he had made this vaccine and tested it really in secret, almost behind their back—at the same time challenging what was a closely held principle at the time that only a vaccine made with a live virus could prevent a disease for a lifetime, as smallpox had. And Jonas Salk made his from a killed [virus].

> [Also,] Jonas Salk reached out to the public as few scientists, maybe with the exception of Pasteur, ever had. And in that he had kind of crossed that imaginary line of proper academic behavior.… Although nominated many times, he never received the Nobel Prize; maybe even more egregious he was blackballed from the National Academy of Sciences, and some said that he really never made an important scientific discovery.

Salk agreed with how he was viewed by the medical community: "I couldn't possibly have become a member of the [Salk Institute for Biological Studies] if I hadn't founded it myself."

Nevertheless, Salk received rave reviews from his friends. A Washington newspaper reporter said, "He could sell me the Brooklyn Bridge, and I never bought anything before."

Most importantly, it was a time when the United States and much of the world felt like they were all in it together, that health and insurance companies didn't have a hand in someone's pocket, and that we no longer had to worry about something as terrifying as polio.

PLAGUES, PANDEMICS AND VIRUSES

On the CBS news show *See It Now*, which aired on April 12, 1955—the same day the vaccine was made available to the world—Edward R. Murrow asked Salk who owned the patent. "Well, the people, I would say," Salk answered. "There is no patent. Could you patent the sun?"

Salk continued his medical research through the Salk Institute for Biological Studies, which he founded 1963 with the help of a $20 million grant from the National Science Foundation and support from what had been the National Foundation for Infantile Paralysis, now known as the March of Dimes. Salk's final years were spent working on an HIV vaccine. He died in 1995 at the age of 80 in La Jolla, California.

Post-polio Syndrome

Post-polio syndrome (PPS) is a viral infection that occurs between 15 and 30 years after an initial polio attack. Symptoms include a decrease in muscular function, overall weakness, and memory loss. Most people who had polio become aware that they might have PPS due to extreme fatigue, where even throwing out the trash can cause punishing exhaustion. Increased activity during the time between the original infection and the onset of PPS can increase the symptoms, meaning that those who caught polio at a young age are more likely to have debilitating PPS symptoms than an adult who caught polio.

Even though a vaccine was developed for polio, scientists are still stymied as to the causes of PPS and why this condition flares up in the first place. It could be aging: as the neurons that had replaced the damaged neurons age, they begin to die, leaving the person with fewer muscle neurons. The most recent data from 2004 showed that up to 85 percent of polio survivors had symptoms of PPS.

The Who's Who of Polio

In 1977, 254,000 people living in the United States had been paralyzed by polio. According to doctors and local polio support groups, some 40,000 polio survivors with varying degrees of paralysis live in Germany, 30,000 in Japan, 24,000 in France, 16,000 in Australia, 12,000 in Canada, and 12,000 in the United Kingdom. Many notable individuals have survived polio and often credit the prolonged immobility and residual paralysis associated with polio as a driving force in their lives and careers. Polio survivors include violinist Itzhak Perlman; actors Alan Alda and Donald Sutherland; directors Ida Lupino and Francis Ford Coppola; folk and rock musicians Joni Mitchell, Judy Collins, Neil Young, and Donovan; dancer Gwen Verdon; and writer Arthur C. Clarke.

FDR: A FAMOUS VICTIM OF POLIO

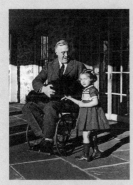

A rare photo of President Franklin D. Roosevelt shows him in a wheelchair.

President Franklin D. Roosevelt is perhaps the most famous polio victim ever. In 1921 at the age of 39, the disease crippled him from the waist down for life, though few knew the extent of the damage, as FDR was able to—with tremendous upper-body strength and stamina—stand and walk a couple of steps in front of enormous crowds, especially while campaigning for president. He would eventually be elected president four times and, as one of the leaders of the Allied Forces, see us through World War II. In 1938, in recognition of his illness, FDR founded what was then called the National Foundation for Infantile Paralysis but which is now known as the March of Dimes; it led to the development of polio vaccines.

Interestingly, a 2003 peer-reviewed study of FDR's illness leans toward Guillain-Barré syndrome (GBS), an autoimmune disease where the immune system mistakenly thinks the nerves in the peripheral nervous system (the part of the nervous system that extends from the brain and spinal cord into the skin, muscles, and organs) are pathogens and destroys them. Polio was at one of its lowest ebbs in the northeastern United States in 1921, so the probability of polio in FDR's age group in the United States in 1921 was much lower than at other times. It is possible that FDR was exposed to an infectious agent at a Boy Scout jamboree in late July 1921. The two-week interval before the onset of his illness was in keeping with both the incubation period of polio and with exposure to an infectious agent leading to GBS. No reports indicate that any scouts or adults at the camp were ill around the time of Roosevelt's visit. However, in 1912 and 1915, FDR had illnesses compatible with *Campylobacter jejuni*, a bacterium that is one of the most common causes of food poisoning. Those with recent *C. jejuni* infections are 100 times more likely to develop GDS than the general population.

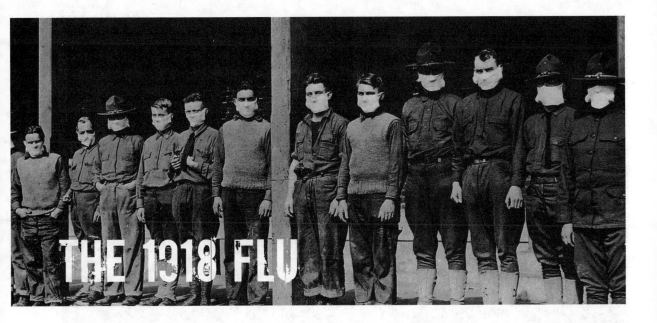

THE 1918 FLU

Ask someone what caused World War I, and you might be met with a blank stare. Ask that same person what caused the 1918 Spanish flu, and the look will probably be the same. These earth-shattering events had ranked rather low in the hierarchy of "popular" wars and diseases until COVID-19 launched them both back into the public consciousness. World War II had Adolf Hitler. World War I had leaders who were playing a real-life game of Risk—the kind that never seems to end. (Indeed, when describing what caused World War I, it's difficult to cite the players who were calling the shots. It's usually taught like this: "Britain fighting Germany fighting Russia fighting Austria-Hungary.")

World War I essentially began when Austria-Hungary's Archduke Franz Ferdinand's motorcade went the wrong way, so Serbian rebel Gavrilo Princip saw his once-in-a-lifetime chance and assassinated the archduke and his wife, though the seeds had already been planted for war.

World War I was a time of trenches and mustard gas, with new ways of killing each other yet with leaders still using old tactics. (If you want to think of a pandemic like a war, consider the Black Plague, where fourteenth-century doctors were working from medical texts written 1,000 years earlier. The results were similar.)

The 1918 flu pandemic erupted just as World War I was ending, though they are linked like a double helix of war and disease. Like a soldier charging into no-man's land, the flu spread rapidly worldwide, as opposed to the war itself, which had dragged on, ponderously, for years. (Although referred to as the "Spanish flu," the pandemic had nothing to do with Spain, though it did make

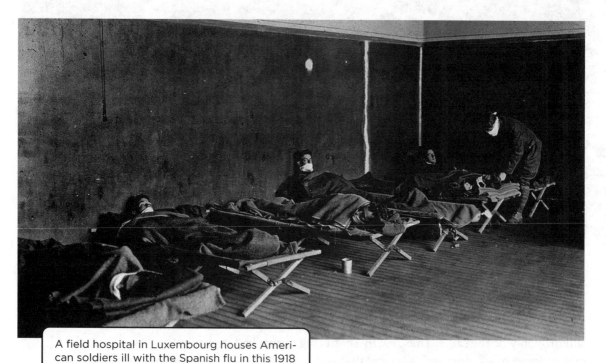

A field hospital in Luxembourg houses American soldiers ill with the Spanish flu in this 1918 photograph.

the Spanish king, Alfonso XIII, very sick.) The pandemic was completely unexpected; targeted healthy, young adults; infected more than a billion people worldwide; and killed between 50 and 100 million of them from remote tropical islands all the way to the Arctic. Adjusted for population, that would equal between 220 and 430 million people today.

Then, it vanished.

The 1918 flu is one of the worst natural disasters in recorded history, yet before COVID-19, few had heard about it. Why was it so deadly, and how could that make for such listless PR?

Because the 1918 flu began during World War I, reports of illness and mortality were embargoed in countries such as the United States, Great Britain, Germany, and France, as it was believed that news of illness and death *not* part of the war would be detrimental to the war effort. (Neutral Spain didn't partake in such censorship and was rewarded by having a pandemic bear its name.) This allowed the flu to spread rapidly since few knew to take precautions in order to stop it. By the time it finally made headlines, the disease was on a rampage.

Those who caught the 1918 flu experienced what most go through when they have the flu—fever, cough, runny nose, exhaustion, and achiness—but the

1918 flu didn't end there. Victims then developed pneumonia—a lung infection—which began as viral pneumonia and then often progressed to an additional bacterial pneumonia. At the time, no treatment was available for either disease—antibiotics had not yet been invented to kill bacterial infections, and no one knew that a virus was causing the viral flu. Struck with blistering fevers, nasal hemorrhaging, and pneumonia, patients would drown in their own fluid-filled lungs, a miserable process that took about 10–12 days. Not only was it shocking that healthy, young men and women were dying by the millions worldwide, but it was also shocking *how* they were dying.

Eldonna "Toni" Heath was living in Fort Covington, New York, in 1919 when the flu hit. Only four years old at the time, she could still recall years later how "everybody in the family was so weak and horribly sick," said her son, Methodist pastor Stephen C. Butler (ret.) "They had a wood-fired kitchen stove, but no one was well enough to chop wood, and there was probably frost or even snow on the ground back then. [This was on the Canadian border.] The only way they survived was their mother was able to prepare milk and bread, then crawled on her hands and knees and pushed a bowl and spoon with the mixture around the room to feed all the family members. By her sheer determination and will that's how she kept the family alive."

Mary O'Meara was 30 and living in New York City at the time of the pandemic. Her granddaughter, Barbara Fisher Coughlin, remembered her pronouncing it as "the influENza!" Back then, O'Meara was working as a seamstress, even making clothes for Teddy Roosevelt's family. Then, one day, "she came home, and saw that her brother Jim had scalded his foot … and that's the last thing she remembered for days," Fisher Coughlin said. "She was so sick that she had this lustrous hair and it fell out." Adding to the horror was that when O'Meara came to, "she could see caskets stacked outside the cemeteries."

Most influenza outbreaks kill the young, the old, or the already weak; in contrast, the 1918 pandemic predominantly struck the young and virile. An infection of the hale and hearty, it caused life expectancy in the United States to drop by twelve years.

What made this particular strain so deadly? Can it come back?

First, it's important to note that the flu, whether you call it Spanish, avian, or Hong Kong, is a virus, with all the characteristics that go with it: it's infinitesimally tiny, it's an infectious agent, and it needs a host to spread. It has no thoughts, feelings, or metabolic activity. Where viruses largely differ is in the way they're spread. The flu is a respiratory disease that spreads outside the body through coughing, sneezing, or instances where someone has touched a place that's been coughed or sneezed on. It is not spread through sex, just as HIV is not spread through sneezing, but both are viruses that need a host to survive.

> **Most flu outbreaks disproportionately kill juvenile, elderly, or already weakened patients. However, the 1918 flu overwhelmingly struck the young and healthy.**

Most flu outbreaks disproportionately kill juvenile, elderly, or already weakened patients. However, the 1918 flu overwhelmingly struck the young and healthy. Those between the ages of 20 and 40 accounted for nearly half of the fatalities. This abnormal result is believed to have been caused by what's known as a "cytokine storm," in which the immune system—which we already know can be bloodthirsty when it comes to invaders—over-responds to the threat of infection. In this case, a young person's strong immune system ravaged their bodies, while those with weaker immune systems were more likely to recover. It was survival of the least fit.

World War I also meant large numbers of troops moving great distances both within and between continents. It uprooted the lives of millions of civilians, especially in Europe. People from places located far apart now came into contact with each other and were more liable to be exposed to any new form of infections, including the flu. When exposed to pandemic influenza after the United States entered the war in 1917, those from rural backgrounds were more likely to die than those who came from cities. Surgeon General William C. Gorgas told one training camp commander, "We know perfectly well that we can control pneumonia absolutely if we could avoid crowding the men, but it is not practicable in military life to avoid this crowding."

Previously isolated populations, such as Alaskans or the Pacific Islanders, were doubly vulnerable when exposed to the 1918 flu. An outbreak in Western Samoa, for instance, killed 22 percent of its people—a high percentage largely because the population had not had any previous exposure to the flu. With many more viruses replicating within so many different populations, a greater scope

FLU AND HUNGER

The 1918 flu affected populations in ways that didn't always involve death. The town of Naas in County Kildare, Ireland, saw most of its gas company workers felled by the flu. This meant gas supplies were cut off, and therefore there was no power in the town for lighting or cooking, which compounded the problems of flu-hit families. In Naas, and in other Irish towns, community kitchens were set up to bring cooked food to families too weak to feed themselves.

existed for the emergence of mutations that could grow and spread more readily in humans.

THE 1918 FLU AND WORLD WAR I

When the flu first appeared on March 11, 1918, it had all the hallmarks of a seasonal flu, albeit a highly contagious and virulent type. One of the first reported cases was a U.S. Army mess cook at Camp Funston, Kansas, named Private Albert Gitchell. Private Gitchell was admitted to the Army hospital with 104-degree fever along with aches and pains and a terrible cough. The previous night, he had been serving dinner to his fellow soldiers.

A few hours after he was admitted, Corporal Lee Drake arrived with almost identical symptoms. Then, it was Sergeant Adolph Hurby. One by one, men with very high fevers and horrendous coughs made their way to the infirmary. By that afternoon, Camp Funston had 107 cases of the flu, a total of 522 reported within the first week alone, and 1,127 by the following month. In the end, 46 of those afflicted at Fort Riley—where Camp Funston was located—died.

Massachusetts's Camp Devens had three divisions activated and training during the war. Approximately 850 soldiers, mostly privates, died at Camp Devens from the flu.

Camp Devens physicians performing autopsies related that the victims' lungs showed "intense congestion and hemorrhage." Surgeon General Gorgas sent epidemiologists Victor Vaughn and Rufus Cole and pathologist Dr. William Henry Welch to investigate what was happening at Camp Devens. They witnessed a flu victim's autopsy, and Cole noted that Welch "turned away from the blue, swollen lungs with wet, foamy, shapeless surfaces [and] became … nervous, saying, 'This must be some new kind of infection or plague.'" Added Cole,

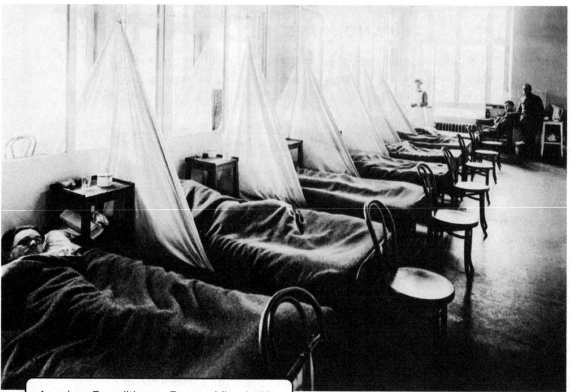

American Expeditionary Force soldiers in Aix-les-Bains, France, rest in a hospital. The tight fighting conditions of trench warfare during World War I helped to spread the flu rapidly among troops.

"It was not surprising that the rest of us were disturbed, but it shocked me to find that the situation, momentarily at least, was too much even for Dr. Welch."

As they investigated Camp Devens, though, the virus kept on moving. Before any travel ban could be imposed, replacement troops left Camp Devens for Camp Upton in Long Island, New York—the Army's debarkation point for France—and carried the flu with them. Throughout April and May 1918, the virus spread like wildfire through England, France, Spain, and Italy. An estimated three-quarters of the French military was infected in the spring of 1918 along with as many as half of the British troops. This was the first wave of the pandemic; the second would be worse.

That wave started in the fall of 1918. At that point, Camp Upton was looking more like a morgue. Of one patient, medical officers recorded that "the patient looked sick and suggested a serious condition … his face was often [bluish], sometimes ashy.… He expressed no pain or suffering. If his mind was

PLAGUES, PANDEMICS AND VIRUSES

clear he expressed a sense of euphoria, or of unnatural realization of his condition, which in particular marked the advanced stages of the disease." As they walked through Camp Upton's pneumonia wards, which contained as many as 900 patients, medical officers experienced "horror at … the magnitude of the catastrophe that had stricken wholesale the young soldiers prepared to face another enemy but helpless before this insidious one."

A FLU BY ANY OTHER NAME

According to John Barry, author of *The Great Influenza: The Story of the Deadliest Pandemic in History,* "because we were at war, the national public-health leaders basically lied to the public." He added:

> They said things like, "This is ordinary influenza by another name." Or, "You have nothing to fear. Proper precautions are taken," so forth and so on. This was echoed by local leaders in many cities, Philadelphia being a prime example. So they had a big Liberty Loan parade scheduled, which they declined to cancel, although all the medical community urged them to. And 48 hours later, just out like clockwork, influenza exploded in the city.
>
> And health results were lethal. Later, they did institute what we call social distancing and closed everything down. Restaurants, churches, services. But it was too late because the virus had already become widely disseminated in the city. And Philadelphia had one of the worst experiences in the pandemic. I think roughly 14,500 people in Philadelphia died. One of the lessons is not just social distancing, but you have to implement these measures early. If you don't, if you wait until a lot of people are sick and it's widely disseminated … it's way too late and it will not have significant impact. But if you do do it early—if you get widespread compliance—these measures do work.

Consider what happened in 2020 not days or weeks but months after COVID-19 arrived. Quotes akin to "This is ordinary influenza by another name" were followed by "This is COVID-19, not COVID-1, folks," according to White House counselor Kellyanne Conway during an appearance on *Fox & Friends.* Similarly, on his February 24, 2020, radio show, Rush Limbaugh said, "Now, I want to tell you the truth about the coronavirus.… I'm dead right on this. The coronavirus is the common cold, folks.… Why do you think this is COVID-19? This is the 19th coronavirus. They're not uncommon." The pandemic was being politicized as part of a different kind of war, one fomenting between red and blue (Republican and Democrat) states. (Note: COVID-19 got its name from the year it was first reported—2019—not because it's the nineteenth coronavirus. As per the WHO's February 11, 2020, report: "Following [our] best practices for naming of new human infectious diseases … WHO has named the disease COVID-19, short for 'coronavirus disease 2019.'")

On the subject of COVID-19, President Donald Trump has alternately called it a "hoax" and then also said "I felt it was a pandemic long before it was called a pandemic" in addition to, "We have it totally under control. It's one person coming in from China, and we have it under control. It's going to be just fine."

Back in 1918, as thousands of his fellow Americans were dying, President Woodrow Wilson said nothing. In 1916, Wilson had run for reelection on the slogan "He Kept Us Out of War," but in January 1917, the Germans sank five American merchant ships, forcing Wilson's hand and America into war on April 6, 1917, and now, he was doing everything in his power to make men keep fighting it.

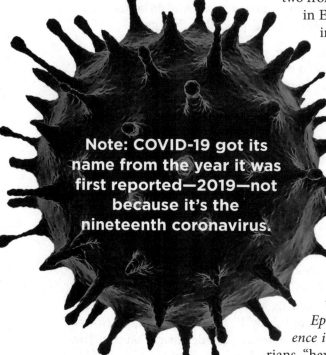

Note: COVID-19 got its name from the year it was first reported—2019—not because it's the nineteenth coronavirus.

Wilson was incapable of waging a war on two fronts—between the one he could see in Europe and the one he couldn't see in the flu. It was easier to ignore the invisible. It was also to his peril and that of millions of others. "Frankly, I don't think Wilson gave much attention to the flu," said John M. Cooper, emeritus professor at the University of Wisconsin–Madison. "From going through his papers, there just isn't much there."

"President Woodrow Wilson had been extraordinarily close-mouthed about the epidemic from the first," wrote Sandra Opdycke in *The Flu Epidemic of 1918: America's Experience in the Global Health Crisis*. Historians "have been unable to find a single occasion on which he mentioned it in public."

PLAGUES, PANDEMICS AND VIRUSES

Others in his sphere followed suit. In the September 17, 1918, edition of *The Philadelphia Inquirer* under the headline "184 Cases Influenza in New York," the unnamed writer reports that then health commissioner Dr. Royal S. Copeland said that "there was no cause for alarm over the presence of the disease."

Reported flu cases dipped in the summer of 1918, offering a glimmer of hope that the virus had run its course, but somewhere in Europe, a mutated strain had just emerged, which not only had the power to kill perfectly healthy young men and women but to do so within 24 hours of the first symptoms.

In late August 1918, military ships departed the English port city of Plymouth, carrying troops infected with this new, far deadlier strain of flu, and as these ships arrived in cities like Brest, France; Boston, Massachusetts; and Freetown, Sierra Leone, the second wave of the global pandemic began.

"The rapid movement of soldiers around the globe was a major spreader of the disease," said James Harris, historian at Ohio State University. "The entire military industrial complex of moving lots of men and material in crowded conditions was certainly a huge contributing factor in the ways the pandemic spread."

British military doctors conducting autopsies on soldiers killed by this second wave of the 1918 flu described the heavy damage to the lungs as akin to the effects of chemical warfare.

From September through November 1918, the death rate from the 1918 flu skyrocketed. This was no ordinary flu. In the United States alone, 195,000 Americans died of the flu just in October, and because thousands of American nurses were working on the front lines in Europe, a severe shortage occurred back home, worsened by the American Red Cross's refusal to use trained African American nurses until the worst of the pandemic had already passed.

During the height of the pandemic, President Wilson met with General Peyton March. The president said, "General March, I have had [messages] sent to me by men whose ability and patriotism are unquestioned that I should stop the shipment of men to France until the epidemic of influenza is under control."

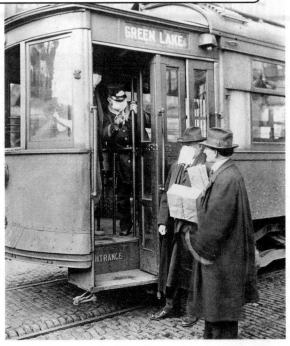

In a scene reminiscent of the events of 2020 with COVID-19, a 1918 Seattle trolley conductor tells customers they can only board if they are wearing masks.

PLAGUES, PANDEMICS AND VIRUSES

1918 WAS MUCH LIKE TODAY

On October 4, 1918, the *Inquirer* reported, "There were six deaths in the temporary hospitals here last night and today from the Spanish influenza or pneumonia produced by it and in consequence of the large number of cases physicians are in constant demand. There is also a shortage of nurses. If the disease does not abate more temporary hospitals will be opened tomorrow. The difficulty is in securing equipment for them." We would be facing these exact same problems 102 years later.

The general responded, "Every such soldier who has died [of influenza] just as surely played his part as his comrade who died in France."

This is what happens when you seek medical advice from an Army officer instead of a medical professional. President Wilson listened to him.

In September 1918, just two days into their trip across the Atlantic, more than 500 soldiers were sick with the flu. By the time the ship reached France, 77 were dead. This would also be the same ship that would bring President Wilson to the Paris Peace Conference on December 4, 1918, and assistant secretary of the Navy Franklin D. Roosevelt to France in January 1919. Both men would contract the 1918 flu.

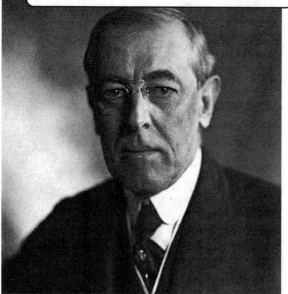

Taking a position rather similar to President Donald Trump, President Woodrow Wilson (pictured) tried to suppress the seriousness of the Spanish flu. In his case, he did so because he felt news of the flu would hamper the war effort.

A NEW WORLD ORDER

In 1892's *Principles and Practice of Medicine*, Canadian physician Sir William Osler wrote, "Almost every form of disease of the nervous system may follow influenza." This was true of the 1918 pandemic strain; Osler himself would die from either the pandemic or an unrelated lung disease in 1919.

In early 1918, President Wilson outlined Fourteen Points that were to be used for peace

BLACK NURSES IN THE MILITARY

When the United States entered World War I in 1917, black nurses tried to enroll in the Army Nurse Corps but were rejected. A few black nurses eventually served, but it was not because the Army Nurse Corps finally saw beyond their color; it was because the flu epidemic had killed so many people that far too few white nurses were still alive. Decades later, after Hitler invaded Poland, the United States began an intense war preparedness program, and the Army Nurse Corps expanded its recruiting process. Thousands of black nurses who wanted to serve their country and earn a steady military income filled out applications and received the following letter:

> Your application to the Army Nurse Corps cannot be given favorable consideration as there are no provisions in Army regulations for the appointment of colored nurses in the Corps.

> The National Association of Colored Graduate Nurses (NACGN)—an advocacy organization founded in 1908 for black registered nurses—challenged the letter. With political pressure from civil rights groups and the black press, 56 black nurses were finally admitted into the U.S. Army Nurse Corps in 1941—all sent to segregated bases in the South.

> On July 26, 1948, President Harry Truman signed an executive order that desegregated the U.S. Armed Forces. This went into effect during the Korean War (1950–1953).

negotiations in order to end World War I. Though the Triple Entente (which included the United States) had primarily fought Germany and Austria-Hungary, Wilson's statement concluded with this:

> We have no jealousy of German greatness, and there is nothing in this programme that impairs it. We grudge her no achievement or distinction of learning or of pacific enterprise such as have made her record very bright and very enviable. We do not wish to injure her or to block in any way her legitimate influence or power. We do not wish to fight her either with arms or with hostile arrangements of trade if she is willing to associate herself with us and the other peace-loving nations of the world in covenants of justice and law and fair dealing. We wish her only to accept a place of equality

among the peoples of the world—the new world in which we now live—instead of a place of mastery.

Though many, including former president Theodore Roosevelt, called it "high-sounding and … meaningless" and said it could be interpreted "to mean anything or nothing," it was nevertheless accepted in total by France and Italy, and Wilson delivered it as a speech ten months before the end of the war, which took place on November 11, 1918.

Wilson caught the flu in April 1919 during the Paris Peace Conference at the most critical part of the postwar negotiations. Before the illness, Wilson was unshakeable in his belief that severely punishing Germany would result in another war, not peace. Just before becoming ill, he was so upset with how the negotiations were proceeding that he threatened to leave Paris without a treaty.

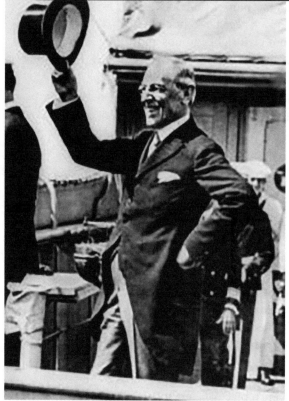

Wilson is shown in this 1919 photo returning from the Versailles Peace Conference. Little did the American public know he had been sick with the flu just a few months before.

Then, he got sick—so sick that many believed that the conference would be canceled. He could barely move. Coughing spasms hit him for days. Then, similar to what Sir William Osler had written regarding a neurological component to the flu, a strange paranoia began to come over Wilson. His staff recalled, for instance, that he became bizarrely protective of the furniture in his hotel room and thought that visitors were going to steal it.

Historians first believed that Wilson had had a stroke in Paris, which would account for his strange behavior, but in 2007, historian John M. Barry, in his book *The Great Influenza*, disagreed, arguing that Wilson's symptoms—high fever, coughing, and exhaustion—were not characteristic of a stroke. They were symptoms of the flu. Wilson's own physician at the time, long before historians added to the record, even diagnosed Wilson with the flu.

After days spent recovering, Wilson insisted on returning to the treaty council's negotiation table despite having low levels of energy and mental acuity. Barry writes, "Then … only a few days after he had threatened to leave the conference … without warning or discussion with any other Americans, Wilson suddenly abandoned principles he had previously insisted upon." He even told the council, "Gentlemen, this is not a meeting of the Peace Commission. It is more a Council of War." This is about as far from the Fourteen Points as one could get, and it happened in only a matter of days.

The result was a treaty about which Wilson told his press spokesman, Ray Baker, "If I were German, I think I should never sign it." Sign it they did, however, and four months later, Wilson's health suffered further after a stroke that left him debilitated. Historians are left wondering what might have been different had Wilson never gotten the flu.

The Germans did sign the treaty, becoming so financially ruined and internationally humiliated by the terms of the conference that it became a huge factor for what would cause World War II less than 20 years later.

THE HIDDEN ENEMY

In the race to develop a vaccine ... actually, no race to develop a vaccine occurred. A microscope that allowed one to see something as small as a virus would not be built until the 1930s. Instead, 1918's top medical professionals were convinced that the flu was caused by a bacterium called *Pfeiffer's bacillus*.

After a global flu outbreak in 1889, German physician Richard Pfeiffer discovered that all of his infected patients carried a particular strain of bacteria he called *Haemophilus influenzae*. When the 1918 flu pandemic hit, scientists believed that the culprit was the same bacteria, but it wasn't. Millions of dollars were invested in state-of-the-art labs to develop techniques for testing for and treating *H. influenzae*, but it would be all for naught.

The first wave of the flu appeared in the spring of 1918, which is in itself unusual because flu season begins in the fall; we're usually hounded at drugstores to get our flu shots around the same time Halloween decorations hit the shelves. However, as far back as the sixteenth century, historical records have shown that deadly cases of the flu can arrive at any time of year, whenever the flu finds an opportunity to latch on to multiple hosts. Remember, viruses know nothing, and they don't have an urge to strike in cold weather. If anything, they're simply opportunists—and with a strain like the 1918 flu, which thrived on healthy people, the virus didn't need to wait to invade once the cold weather suppressed immune systems.

In 1918, epidemiologists were not yet able to link human influenza to avian and swine influenza. Despite similarities to other flu pandemics, many wondered if it was in fact a form of influenza at all. In the 1930s, closely related influenza viruses (now called H1N1 viruses) were isolated from pigs and then from humans. Studies soon linked both of these viruses to the 1918 pandemic. Neither were *the* virus that caused the 1918 flu, but they were related to it.

The 1918 virus may have mutated until the 1950s, when it disappeared altogether. That was as far as they were able to get.

Over time, the desire to learn what constituted the 1918 flu was met with opportunity and technology. A February 1999 paper in the *Proceedings of the National Academy of Science* journal by Drs. Ann Reid and Johan Hultin described their efforts to determine the 1918 virus's hemagglutinin. These surface proteins give a virus the ability to enter and infect a healthy cell (which, in this case, was a healthy respiratory cell).

In the 1999 study, the authors succeeded in sequencing the full length of the 1918 virus's hemagglutinin using RNA fragments of the virus obtained from its victims: a 21-year-old Fort Jackson, South Carolina, service member; "Lucy" from Brevik Mission, Alaska; and a 30-year-old male service member stationed at Camp Upton, New York. Lung tissue from the two soldiers had been preserved after they died; "Lucy" was located beneath permafrost in 1997.

H1N1 VERSUS H2N2

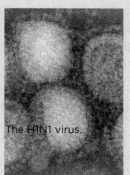
The H1N1 virus.

Hemagglutinin is the "H" of H1N1. "N" stands for neuraminidase, the protein that helps new viruses break free after budding from the membrane of a host cell. Flu vaccines work by targeting a flu virus's unique hemagglutinin and preventing it from binding. Medications like Tamiflu also work by inhibiting the neuraminidase.

H1N1 can infect birds, people, pigs, and horses. H2N2 can only infect people and birds. The Asian Flu Pandemic of 1957 was the first time that people had been infected by H2N2 (which may have been the result of a recombination with H1N1), and since our immune systems had never come across it, 70,000 Americans died. H2N2 then picked up H3 from birds in 1968 to cause the Hong Kong Flu Pandemic, which killed another 30,000 Americans.

Sequencing results implied that an ancestor of the 1918 virus infected humans sometime between 1900 and 1915 before its final mutation into a monster. The 1918 hemagglutinin had a number of mammalian, as opposed to avian, or bird, adaptations. Phylogenetic analysis, which is used to group influenza viruses in accordance with their evolutionary development and diversity—like tracing the genealogy of a virus—placed the 1918 virus's hemagglutinin within the mammalian group. However, researchers believed that the virus most likely obtained its hemagglutinin from avian viruses but had been adapting in a mammalian host for an unknown period of time before emerging in pandemic form.

In October 2005, a *Science* report titled "Characterization of the Reconstructed 1918 Spanish Influenza Pandemic Virus" chronicled the research done by Dr. Terrence Tumpey and his CDC colleagues. To evaluate the 1918 virus's harmfulness, mice were infected with the 1918 virus, and then measures of morbidity (i.e., weight loss, virus replication) were documented. For comparison, other mice were infected with different flu viruses that were designed via reverse genetics in order to have varying combinations of genes from the 1918 virus and the seasonal flu viruses we get today. These viruses were referred to as "recombinant viruses."

The fully reconstructed 1918 virus could replicate extremely quickly. Four days after infection, the amount of 1918 virus found in the lung tissue of infected mice was 39,000 times higher than that from one of the comparison flu viruses.

THE WORK OF DR. JOHAN HULTIN

In 1951, Dr. Johan Hultin tried to isolate the 1918 influenza virus from victims who had been buried in the Alaskan permafrost of a town called Brevig Mission, which is about 65 miles northwest of Nome. During the pandemic, 72 of the town's 80 residents died of the flu. Dr. Hultin, with permission of the surviving residents of the town and their descendants, found the bodies but, even with permafrost conditions, no live viruses. Then, in July 1997, Dr. Hultin read an article in *Science* by Dr. Jeffrey Taubenberger, who was seeking samples of the 1918 flu. Now 72, Dr. Hultin offered his services and, paying his own way, returned to Brevig Mission after 46 years. Again, he received permission to dig for flu victims, and he unearthed the remains of an obese woman, roughly 30 years old. The fat had protected her lungs—and therefore the virus—from decaying. Dr. Hultin had found his samples. He named her "Lucy."

Dr. Tumpey determined that the eight genes of the 1918 virus played particularly important roles in its infectiousness and severity, so it was not any single component of the 1918 virus but a unique combination of all of its genes that made it so particularly dangerous.

Tumpey and his colleagues wrote that "the constellation of all eight genes together make an exceptionally virulent virus." No other human flu viruses tested were as shockingly lethal, so what made the virus so deadly? Nature, evolution, and the intermingling of people and animals. It showed that nature's ability to produce pandemics did not stop with the Black Death.

THE PHASES OF THE FLU

Pandemics can pose a problem for viruses. Once they've swooped in and killed a wide swath of people, the population that's left may either be naturally immune or have built up an acquired immunity, so the virus, in the form that it's in, needs to mutate, or it, too, shall die. The 1918 flu is a perfect case study. It came in three waves, like tidal waves: Phase 1 was the least fatal and had done all the damage it could. A ferocious Phase 2 of the virus arrived shortly after, followed by a nearly equally deadly Phase 3. While Phase 3 did coincide with the wintry climates of the Northern Hemisphere, it had less to do with the weather and more to do with the virus's mutation.

The phases of the 1918 flu are difficult to understand. Even working under the assumption that the war caused people who would never normally meet to not only meet but be sharing bunkers and trenches. Why would such a fast viral evolution occur? Could the explanation be that the virus just happened to mutate terribly profoundly almost simultaneously around the world in such a short frame of time coinciding with a world war?

Normally, to acquire superviral status, the 1918 flu would have needed years of global infections, not weeks of local ones, and, having taken a foothold, such viruses would then usually take several months to swoop around the world.

Even by pandemic standards, three waves over the course of one year, with barely a break in between, is blessedly rare, but viral evolution is not. The reason we're still getting flu shots is because flu viruses are mutating as we speak.

These mutations are crucial to the recurrence and strength of the flu virus and could be the reason COVID-19 became a pandemic. (Note that many flu viruses coexist right now, not just "a" flu virus wreaking havoc.) Without such changes, the flu would disappear once the human population hit an immunity point that would be impossible for the virus to overcome.

Due to its virulence, the 1918 flu is still being studied today—not just the virus itself, as seen previously, but its effect on individuals and the world as a whole. According to the *Journal of Developmental Origins of Health and Disease*, Americans who were *in utero* when the pandemic was at its peak ended up having a higher risk of a heart attack in adulthood than those who were born before or after the pandemic. Specifically, of the 100,000 Americans studied who were born in the years 1915–1918 and 1920–1922, the rate of heart attacks—about 200 for every 1,000 people—were the same, but for those born between October 1918 and June 1919, when the pandemic was at its peak, the number of heart attacks increased more than 20 percent.

The reason we're still getting flu shots is because flu viruses are mutating as we speak.

Also, U.S. Army enlistment data taken from those born between 1915 and 1922 found that men born in 1919 were 0.05 inches shorter than the average height of other enlisted men. Furthermore, children born just after flu pandemics had higher rates of physical disabilities, performed worse in academic tests, and earned a lower income compared to those born before or after the pandemic. Dr. Ellen Harrison, director of obstetrical medicine at Montefiore Medical Center, believes that a link exists between an expectant mother having the flu and a child's cardiac health, height, and/or risk of mental illness (e.g., schizophrenia).

After it vanished, the 1918 flu quickly faded from public memory, which is why historians call it the "forgotten pandemic." This might be due to limited media coverage—first for public morale reasons, as a war was also going on at the time, and second, because of the war, people's attention was diverted; the short duration of the pandemic might have also played a role. Its timing made the flu an extension of the war, with people not sure where one ended and the other began. It's difficult to believe that with all the destruction this pandemic wrought and how relatively recent it was compared to the Black Death, people struggled so much to describe it. Its spread was overshadowed by the deadliness of World War I and covered up by news blackouts and poor record keeping.

In *Pale Rider: The Spanish Flu of 1918 and How It Changed the World*, Laura Spinney noted, "There are very few cemeteries in the world that, assuming they are older than a century, don't contain a cluster of graves from the autumn of 1918—when the second and worst wave of the pandemic struck—and people's memories reflect that. But there is no cenotaph, no monument in London, Moscow, or Washington, D.C. The Spanish flu is remembered personally, not collectively." This is true even less so now since most people who lived through it are no longer here.

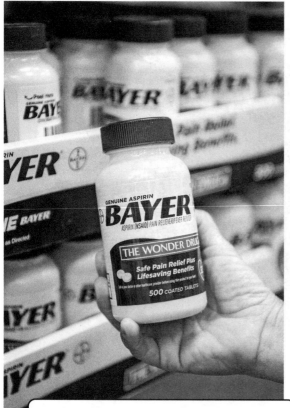

A ludicrous conspiracy theory about the 1918 pandemic was that Bayer aspirin, which was and is produced by a German company, somehow infected people with the virus.

1918 Conspiracy Theories

We can't have a pandemic without a conspiracy theory, right? Whether it's Jews who poisoned Gentile wells, causing the Black Death; a government conspiracy that caused HIV/AIDS; or, in this case, because we'd been fighting Germany, the flu was therefore a German biological weapon. The U.S. government suggested that aspirin, then a popular new "wonder drug," and its German manufacturer, Bayer, were to blame. Ironically, aspirin was one of the few treatments that actually helped flu victims feel better.

WHAT WE LOST AND WHAT WE GAINED

Thomas Wolfe, one America's greatest novelists, wrote in a May 1923 letter to his mother, Julia, about the impact his brother's death had on him. "This is why I think I'm going to be an artist. The things that really mattered sunk in and left their mark … [including] sometimes death.…"

Ben Wolfe had died in 1918 of the flu pandemic and inspired Thomas's most famous novel, the semiautobiographical *Look Homeward, Angel*, which was about a young writer trying to break free of his suffocating, small-town life. It includes an account of his brother's death (who is also named Ben in the novel):

> Ben drew upon the air in a long and powerful respiration; his gray eyes opened. Filled with a terrible vision of all life in the one moment, he seemed to rise forward bodilessly from his pillows without support a flame, a light, a glory joined at length in death to the dark spirit who had brooded upon each footstep of his lonely adventure on earth; and, casting the fierce sword of his glance with utter and final comprehension upon the room haunted with its gray pageantry of cheap loves and dull consciences and on all those uncertain mummers of waste and confusion fading now from the bright window of his eyes, he passed instantly, scornful and unafraid, as he had lived, into the shades of death.

If Ben Wolfe had lived, perhaps the world would not have had the pleasure of reading Thomas Wolfe. It's not known for sure whether the author would have given up his literary fame for his brother's recovery; being that Ben was not only his brother but the person he was closest to, the answer would most likely be "absolutely." Sadly, Thomas Wolfe would die young as well from tuberculosis.

Of Time and the River and *You Can't Go Home Again*, also part of Wolfe's work, are the things we gained from the pandemic. Willa Cather's Pulitzer Prize-winning *One of Ours* and Katherine Anne Porter's *Pale Horse, Pale Rider* both had the flu as the main theme.

We nearly lost some important people to the 1918 flu. Franklin Delano Roosevelt, known for having polio as well as for being president of the United States during World War II, caught the flu during World War I. In September 1918, FDR, then the assistant secretary of the Navy, had just inspected U.S. troops in Europe and, either before leaving France or on board the transport, he came down with the flu and had to be carried off the troopship *Leviathan* by stretcher.

Edvard Munch painted "Self-Portrait after the Spanish Flu" in 1919, in which he is gazing as if in a daze at the viewer. (Since Munch's early years, sickness and sadness were important subjects partly because he lost his mother and sister to TB and partly because of his own fragile health. To quote the man whose most famous work is 1893's "The Scream": "The angels of fear, sorrow, and death stood by my side since the day I was born.") David Lloyd George, the prime minister of Great Britain, along with prominent authors and artists such as Franz Kafka and Georgia O'Keeffe, caught the flu but survived. However, Austrian painter Gustav Klimt, his protégé Egon Schiele, and French poet Guillaume Apollinaire all died.

A public-health system was still being developed when the flu began, but it spurred the development of public-health systems across the developed world.

In Washington, D.C., in October 1918, local health officials banned public gatherings in order to tamp down the spread of infections. Across the city, schools and colleges closed, while Congress and the Supreme Court adjourned. De facto hospitals opened across the city as health-care officials cared for the constant stream of the sick and dying.

A public-health system was still being developed when the flu began, but it spurred the development of public-health systems across the developed world.

Other parts of the world, however, did not have anything close to a public-health system—or barely any kind of health system, for that matter. In British-ruled India, most of the doctors were off fighting the war, and the infrastructure Great Britain was tasked with upholding and improving was in tatters and not equipped to deal with a pandemic. The Ganga River was overflowing with bodies.

The 1918 flu would claim between 10 to 25 million lives in India—almost one-fifth of the global death toll and 4 percent of the population as per the 1911 census.

Mahatma Gandhi, leader of what would eventually be a successful campaign for Indian independence, caught the flu. In a letter to a friend, he wrote: "Our ancestors could build such tough bodies in the past. But today we are reduced to a state of miserable weakness and are easily infected by noxious germs moving about in the air. There is one and only one really effective way by which we can save ourselves from them even in our present broken state of health. That way is the way of self-restraint.... I request you all, therefore, to keep to your beds for some days."

Laura Spinney, author of *Pale Rider*, said: "People were dying in droves and in the absence of any British doctors.... That vacuum during a medical emergency brought Indians together to fight the deadly disease.

"The people who stepped into that breach tended to be the militants, the grassroots militant activists for independence who had already worked out how to cross caste barriers and work together for a different goal, i.e. independence," Spinney says. "Once the pandemic passed, emotion against the British was even higher than it had been before. And secondly, those people were far more united than they had been. And now they came together behind Gandhi. He found that he suddenly had the grassroots support that he had been lacking until then."

For a different kind of story, imagine a world without Disney World—or, indeed, without Disney. Many beloved films, TV programs, and amusement park attractions would not exist today, as well as iconic cartoon characters and memorable music.

This isn't even taking into consideration franchises and all that go with them, like *Star Wars*, *The Muppets*, and *Pirates of the Caribbean*—and we haven't even begun to talk about Mickey Mouse.

The shape of entertainment would be unrecognizable without the man who began it all—Walt Disney—a man who nearly died of the 1918 flu.

On September 1918 during World War I, Walt Disney, aged 17, lied about his age in order to join the Red Cross Ambulance Corps. Assigned first to a training facility on the south side of Chicago, Disney immediately came down with the flu. He returned home a very sick man, who was luckily nursed back to health by his mother, who did not get sick with the flu. Ten years later, Disney cocreated Mickey Mouse.

Disneyland, Disney World, Epcot Center, Tokyo Disney, and Disneyland Paris were closed during COVID-19 along with Disney hotels, cruises, and resorts.

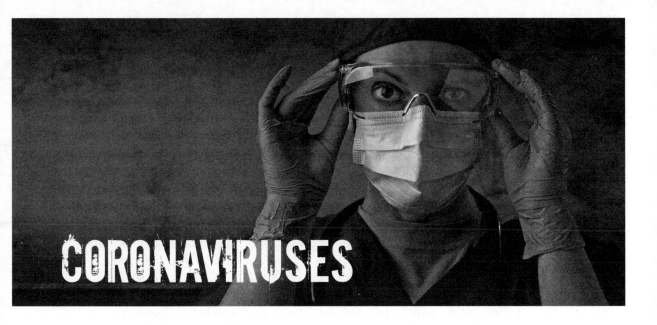

CORONAVIRUSES

A virus is "simply a piece of bad news wrapped up in protein," biologists Jean and Peter Medawar wrote in 1977.

Coronaviruses are not new, though researchers believe that the virus's most recent common ancestor existed about 10,000 years ago, which, in viral terms, makes it relatively young.

The coronavirus gets the *corona* part of its name from the Latin word for "crown" or "halo" or from the Greek word *korónē?* for "wreath"—all of which describe the circle that appears on the virus when you look at it under a microscope, like the light that emanates from the sun and stars. In the coronavirus family tree, we can reach way back to its realm: *Riboviria*. This realm is strictly for viruses that replicate through RNA instead of DNA. Next is phylum, which is *Incertae sedis*, a Latin phrase meaning "of unknown placement," meaning that no consensus exists among researchers as to how the coronavirus, at this level in the family tree, relates to other viruses.

We start to enter a recognizable place in the order: *Nidovirales*. Members of *Nidovirales* include the families *Roniviridae*, which infects crustaceans (yes, shrimp get sick, too!) and *Coronaviridae*. In 2003, a *Nidovirales* symposium was nearly cancelled due to lack of interest. Then, the coronavirus known as SARS emerged, and the symposium sold out.

"Coronavirus" is the common name for *Coronaviridae*, which is the family it belongs to. Coronaviruses cause diseases in mammals and birds. According to epidemiologist Anita Ghatak, "There are hundreds of coronaviruses but only seven have been known to infect humans. Four of the seven are known

NIDOVIRALES SYMPOSIUM

The 2020 Nidovirales symposium, whose logo is a wave cresting over a virus made to look like the sun, offered attendants "the chance to interact with old friends and collaborators, and meet new people to broaden your nidovirus horizons and beyond. Present your latest research to a dedicated audience of around 200 participants, and learn about the most recent and groundbreaking scientific insights in the nidoviral molecular biology.… Feel welcome at the conference venue, your 'holiday-feel' place to stay Hotel Zuiderduin, beautifully refurbished (for those who remember the NIDO 2003 edition), with in-house swimming pool, spa/wellness area, bar and bowling alley, and only a mere 350 meters away from the white sand of the spacy and broad Egmond beach, with its numerous restaurants, terraces and bars looking out over the stunning North Sea." Scheduled to take place in the Netherlands in May 2020, it was postponed until June 2021 because of COVID-19.

to cause the common cold, while the remaining three cause much more serious respiratory infections—SARS, MERS, and COVID-19."

As mentioned, the genetic material in coronaviruses is RNA, while for other viruses, it's DNA. Far more DNA than RNA viruses exist, and they cause diseases that can last a lifetime, like herpes, chicken pox (which comes from a herpes virus) and hepatitis B (though hepatitises A and C are RNA viruses).

RNA viruses have simpler structures than DNA viruses and mutate rapidly. They also tend to cause epidemics, such as measles, HIV/AIDS, Ebola, Zika, SARS, and COVID-19. Paul Turner, a Rachel Carson Professor of Ecology and Evolutionary Biology at Yale University, told *The New Yorker*, "They're the ones that surprise us the most and do the most damage."

Scientists first saw the coronavirus in the 1950s while researching why chickens were catching bronchitis, but coronaviruses have been replicating and growing as a family for thousands of years. Bats and viruses make the perfect team: Multiple strains of coronaviruses can infect one bat at the same time, then combine and replicate inside them to create even more strains. These viruses then jump to different species, like humans—just as we've seen with viruses like smallpox and HIV. (In terms of design and methods of replication, the coronavirus resembles HIV: round, with protruding receptors, containing RNA—though here is where the comparisons largely end because HIV infects the immune system

PLAGUES, PANDEMICS AND VIRUSES

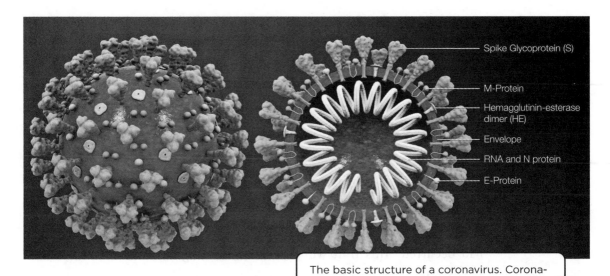

The basic structure of a coronavirus. Coronaviruses include SARS, MERS, and COVID-19.

and is with a patient for life, while coronaviruses infect the respiratory system as well as the heart, brain, and other organs.)

Coronaviruses similar to the one that made chickens sick were then found in diseased pigs and cows, and in the 1960s, two strains were discovered that caused the common cold in people. These strains may have jumped from animals to humans thousands of years ago, but since colds don't normally lead to death, research on them and other coronaviruses essentially ceased.

To become infected by a coronavirus, you have to come into contact with someone who had it and be exposed to respiratory secretions (i.e., sneezing or coughing), physical contact with them, or touching a surface that the virus is on and then touching your nose or eyes—entrances into your body that you touch all the time without knowing it. The first symptoms are mild and reminiscent of those of a cold: coughs, aches, and a fever. Some victims also lose their sense of smell and, as a consequence, their sense of taste (taste depends on smell), but the symptoms can develop into something worse.

Before COVID-19, the coronavirus that had made the most recent headlines was Middle East respiratory syndrome (MERS).

MERS

MERS was first reported in 2012 after scientists sequenced the genome of a virus taken from a person who was sick with what had seemed like the flu—but this was a new kind of flu. A second case was discovered later in 2012 when a 49-year-old Qatari man showed similar flulike symptoms; the viral sample taken from him showed a pathogen nearly identical to that of the earlier case. By November 2012, more cases were appearing in Qatar and Saudi Arabia. This is when rapid research and monitoring of the then unknown coronavirus began.

MERS-CoV, the virus that causes MERS, attacks cells in the lungs. It's able to avoid a person's innate immune system (as opposed to their acquired immune system) and silences the proteins that would normally alert the immune system to an invader. (It is also possible for silent MERS to occur, where a patient is infected but "asymptomatic," or without symptoms. Early research has shown that up to 20 percent of those who had MERS had no symptoms but had MERS antibodies in their blood—which meant that a MERS infection had occurred. This trait will become critical again when learning about COVID-19.)

Research by epidemiologist Ian Lipkin of New York's Columbia University showed that a virus isolated from an Egyptian tomb bat seemed to match the virus that causes MERS. However, the animal that was largely getting humans sick was unknown until August 9, 2013, when a report in the journal *The Lancet Infectious Diseases* revealed that in the blood tests of Omani camels, 50 out of 50 had antibodies against MERS. Blood serum taken from European sheep, goats, cattle, and other types of camels had no such antibodies.

To date, the evidence available suggests that this virus—one type of virus among many in bats—had been in bats for some time and had spread to camels, recombined within the camel, and caused a camel coronavirus by the mid-1990s. The virus then spread from camels to humans by the early 2010s. The original bat host species and the time of initial infection have yet to be determined. We do know that MERS has evolved into three clades—or groups—differing in host and geographic distribution.

By 2015, MERS cases had been reported in more than 20 countries, including Saudi Arabia, Qatar, Egypt, the UAE, Kuwait, Turkey, Oman, Algeria, Bangladesh, Austria, the United Kingdom, mainland China, Thailand, and the Philippines. According to the CDC, "MERS represents a very low risk to the general public in this country. Only two patients in the U.S. have ever tested positive for MERS-CoV infection—both in May 2014—while more than 1,300 have tested negative."

MERS-CoV is not as easily transmittable as other coronaviruses. You need to be in close contact with an infected person to become infected yourself.

PLAGUES, PANDEMICS AND VIRUSES

Graphs comparing the MERS outbreak with SARS worldwide.

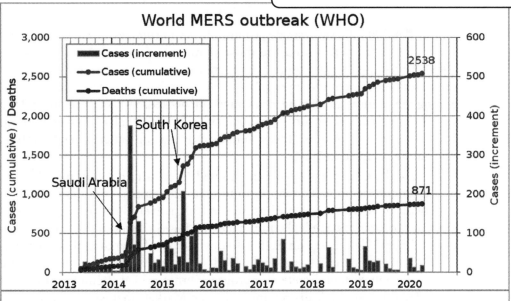

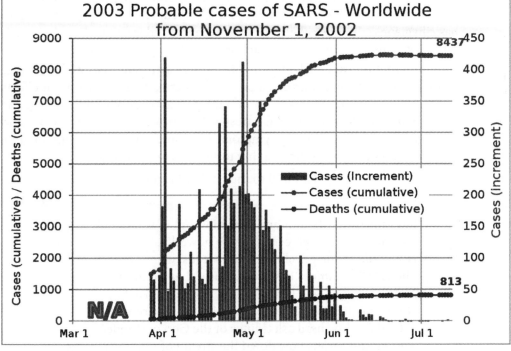

The risk to the global population is currently deemed to be fairly low by the WHO.

SARS

In 2003, China was devastated. Severe acute respiratory syndrome (SARS) had caused the most significant sociopolitical crisis since 1989's Tiananmen Square protest. Its economy was poised for a serious downturn. Hesitation about the appropriate message to share spawned fear and panic among the Chinese and let the virus travel unchecked. SARS spread around the world—often carried by airline passengers—and eventually killed more than 800 people in 37 countries. It was contained by placing patients in quarantine. The outbreak ended in 2004.

So, the Chinese government wanted to ensure that nothing like that would happen again, but at the same time, exotic animals being sold as food and medicine was (and is) a big business in China. Everything from cats to wolf pups to porcupines were locked up cheek by jowl in cages, biting, scratching, urinating, and defecating on each other, while people handled them without any form of protection. The country's food-safety standards and sanitation were practically nonexistent despite numerous government-led attempts to improve them. Food poisoning is distressingly regular. Markets that weren't licensed to trade in live species nevertheless did so unchecked. Workers weren't trained in basic hygiene techniques like glove wearing and hand washing. Dangerous additives were used to increase production. Health inspectors were bribed.

SARS first appeared 44 years after then Chairman Mao Zedong wrote "Farewell to the God of Plague," a poem celebrating China's successful efforts to wipe out schistosomiasis from certain populations who lived along the Yangtze River. (Schistosomiasis is a freshwater parasite that grows in snails and then moves to humans, causing symptoms like cholera, while their eggs migrate to the central nervous system, leading to seizures or paralysis.)

"Farewell to the God of Plague"

I

So many green streams and blue hills, but to what avail?
This tiny creature left even Hua To powerless!
Hundreds of villages choked with weeds, men wasted away;
Thousands of homes deserted, ghosts chanted mournfully.
Motionless, by earth I travel eighty thousand li a day,
Surveying the sky I see a myriad Milky Ways from afar.
Should the Cowherd ask tidings of the God of Plague,
Say the same griefs flow down the stream of time.

PLAGUES, PANDEMICS AND VIRUSES

II

The spring wind blows amid profuse willow wands,
Six hundred million in this land all equal Yao and Shun.
Crimson rain swirls in waves under our will,
Green mountains turn to bridges at our wish.
Gleaming mattocks fall on the Five Ridges heaven-high;
Mighty arms move to rock the earth round the Triple River.
We ask the God of Plague: "Where are you bound?"
Paper barges aflame and candle-light illuminate the sky.

After the initial discovery, the first question was whether this new virus had arisen from a virus that humans had previously encountered but had become more virulent due to mutation or it was a virus newly introduced into the human population from an animal—a spillover event.

Not just one but several studies revealed a higher-than-normal prevalence of SARS cases among wild animal traders. One found that 40 percent of wild animal traders who worked in a Guangdong food market in 2004 had SARS antibodies compared to 5 percent of vegetable traders from the same market. Serum samples analyzed in May 2003 from workers in three live animal markets in Guangzhou revealed that of the 508 animal workers analyzed, 13 percent had SARS antibodies and, of those, 72 percent had handled Asian palm civets, an animal related to the mongoose and native to Asia, where it's eaten, whose musk was once an ingredient in Chanel No. 5.

SARS first occurred in China's Guangdong Province in November 2002 and moved to Hong Kong on February 21, 2003....

Also, the early-onset cases were more likely to have lived within walking distance of animal markets than the late-onset cases. SARS was also discovered in smaller amounts in the raccoon dog (which is neither a raccoon nor a dog; it's more like a fox). This evidence showed that SARS came from animals—possibly these animals.

SARS first occurred in China's Guangdong Province in November 2002 and moved to Hong Kong on February 21, 2003, when Liu Jianlun, a Guangdong doctor who arrived in February and stayed on the ninth floor of the Metropole Hotel in Kowloon, infected sixteen of the hotel visitors. Those visitors, without knowing they had the disease, then traveled to Singapore, Taiwan, Vietnam, and Canada.

SARS in Canada

Needless to say, Canada was caught unprepared for a never-before-encountered flulike virus that looked like it could grow into a pandemic. Healthcare workers (HCWs) were caught in the crossfire, trying to treat patients without getting sick themselves.

On March 28, 2003, Ontario's Provincial Operating Centre (POC) published a set of SARS-specific recommendations to guide HCWs on best practices to avoid catching and transmitting SARS. Training had to be completed, including video sessions and lessons equipping HCWs for safe interactions with SARS patients. Unfortunately, little of this training was done before HCWs began to treat SARS patients. More than one-third of HCWs never received *any* type of formal training, and half of those received their formal training only after they'd begun working with SARS patients. At the same time, many of the HCWs who'd had training received it from another HCW, allowing for errors in communication. Aside from this type of training (or lack thereof), many HCWs complained that most efforts—which included only posting informational posters in the wards—were inadequate.

A study published in 2006 suggested that these guidelines were not fully practiced or enforced, causing many HCWs to become infected. The study followed seventeen HCWs in Toronto hospitals who had developed the disease and interviewed fifteen of them regarding the amount of training they'd received on dealing with SARS cases and how often they used protective equipment. The study concluded that HCW practices did not fully meet the recommendations set forth by the POC, providing greater evidence that this was the main cause of SARS infections within HCWs.

The End of SARS

Dr. Carlo Urbani, a microbiologist from Italy, is largely the person to be thanked for helping to bring about a swift end to an outbreak that could have been far worse. In February 2003, Dr. Urbani was called into the Hanoi French Hospital to look at a patient named Johnny Chen, an American businessman who had become ill with what doctors first thought was a bad case of influenza. Now, they weren't so sure. Urbani realized that Chen's symptoms were probably due to a new and highly contagious disease. He immediately notified the WHO, triggering a response to the epidemic—mainly isolation and quarantine measures—that would end it within five months. He also persuaded the Vietnamese Health Ministry to begin isolating patients and screening travelers, thus slowing the early pace of the epidemic.

On March 11, 2003, as Dr. Urbani flew from Hanoi to a conference in Bangkok, Thailand, where he was to talk on the subject of childhood parasites, he started feeling feverish on the plane. A colleague who met him at the airport called an ambulance. Urbani had contracted SARS while treating patients in Hanoi. His Bangkok hospital room became an improvised isolation ward, and as his lungs weakened, he was put on life support. During a moment of consciousness, Urbani asked for a priest to give him the sacrament of last rites and asked for his lung tissue to be donated for scientific research. Urbani died on March 29, 2003. SARS-CoV Urbani strain later became the reference variant of this outbreak.

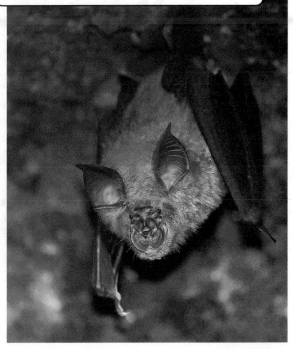

Horshoe bats like this one live in Asia and often carry diseases that are not transmitted directly but, rather, give viruses to animals such as civets, which then pass it along to humans.

Chinese scientists—led by Shi Zheng-Li and Cui Jie of China's Wuhan Institute of Virology—were determined to trace the source of the outbreak and stop it before it started again. Scientists initially suspected that Asian palm civet cats sold in Chinese markets were the source of the virus, but they later turned their attention to bats.

In one study conducted between March–December 2004, blood, fecal, and throat swabs were collected from 408 bats within four locations in China. Three cave-dwelling species belonging to the genus *Rhinolophus*—the horseshoe bat—had a high number of SARS antibodies. Genome-sequence analysis indicated that the SARS-like coronaviruses in these bats were genetically almost identical to the ones isolated from humans and civets. SARS was coming from bats.

Horseshoe bats are insect-eating cave dwellers in a part of the world—southern China—that offers quite a wide variety of caves. The three species spreading SARS were Pearson's horseshoe bat, the big-eared horseshoe bat, and—last but not least—the least horseshoe bat.

What fecal samples also revealed was that several different strains of this virus existed, meaning that this particular strain of the coronavirus had been mutating within bats for years. When the bats' SARS-like viruses combined with the civets', the civet became an amplifier host, leading to the outbreak in humans. The civet isn't the only mammal capable of hosting a SARS virus, though. As David Quammen wrote in his book *Spillover*, "You could kill every civet in China and SARS would be among you.... Susceptible animals might include ... ferret dogs, raccoon badgers, who knows what. So many different candidates pass through the wildlife supply chain."

During the peak of China's SARS outbreak, most animal traders handled several animal species, providing countless opportunities for animal-to-animal contact: while transporting them, where animal cages are often piled one on top of the other, or in the market, where a vast number of different animal species were housed under a single roof at the same time. Wholesale animal markets or warehouses brought forth the possibility of long-term interspecies contact because animals can be kept together for a long time before being sold individually. The notion of interspecies transmission in markets is supported by finding SARS antibodies in civets and raccoon dogs in the market—not in the farms that claimed to have supplied the animals—so not only were humans catching SARS in markets, but animals were giving it to each other as well.

> In a perfect world, we would take the lessons we learned from SARS and reapply them to either prevent another wide-ranging outbreak or be prepared if one emerges.

Three separate surveillance studies showed that SARS infections occurred readily

PLAGUES, PANDEMICS AND VIRUSES

within the civet wildlife market populations: people were getting sick after eating them. As a result, thousands of civets in captivity were butchered, electrocuted, smothered, and drowned.

The identification of bats as the natural reservoir of SARS played an important role in understanding how to combat it. Bats have also been identified or implicated as the natural reservoir host for an increasing number of new and often deadly zoonotic viruses. In 2006, the WHO reported that the "SARS episode has underscored the importance of changing animal husbandry practices or more viruses are likely to emerge from the animal world. Old and unhygienic veterinary practices must be discarded or the public health risk from zoonotic diseases will always be with us." However, memories are short-lived, and although a terrifying outbreak suppressed the wildlife markets, they went underground until the outbreak ended, then were back on the streets unregulated.

In a perfect world, we would take the lessons we learned from SARS and reapply them to either prevent another wide-ranging outbreak or be prepared if one emerges. This opportunity presented itself in 2019 with the novel coronavirus.

COVID-19

SARS is closely related to COVID-19. COVID-19 is the respiratory illness that is caused by the virus SARS-CoV-2, or *Severe Acute Res-*

SARS CONFINEMENT IN CHINA

Confinement in China during SARS led to one unexpected development—the explosion of online shopping. Afraid to leave home for anything but the essentials, many Chinese began using their computers to take up the slack; the outbreak also happened to coincide with the beginning of high-speed connectivity at home. As a result, online retail companies like Alibaba exploded. Now, Alibaba is the world's largest retailer and e-commerce company, is one of the largest internet companies and artificial intelligence companies, one of the biggest venture capital firms, and one of the biggest investment corporations in the world. Not bad for a company that was cofounded in 1999 by Jack Ma, who today is a business magnate but as a youth took four years to pass the Chinese entrance exam to get into college and admitted that he applied for 30 jobs and was turned down by all of them.

piratory *Syndrome Coronavirus 2*, though in order to avoid confusion with SARS, both the virus and the disease are often referred to as COVID-19.

COVID-19 is a novel—meaning new—coronavirus that was first identified during an investigation into an outbreak in Wuhan, China, in 2019. The name is an acronym that stands for *Coronavirus Disease of 2019*—not, as some have speculated, the nineteenth occurrence of the coronavirus.

The viruses that cause SARS and COVID-19—SARS-CoV and SARS-CoV-2, respectively—share 79 percent of the same genomic sequence. They both belong to the coronavirus family, as do rhinoviruses, the branch of the coronavirus family that causes the common cold. That scratchy throat and runny nose mean that you have an infection in your upper respiratory tract. SARS-CoV-1, the virus that causes SARS, infects the lungs, which are your lower respiratory system. A sore throat and runny nose are irritating, but a lung infection can be fatal: SARS has a mortality rate of about 7 percent.

SARS was called "the first pandemic of the 21st century" in the early 2000s because it spread quickly from continent to continent.

When you cough or sneeze, thousands of tiny droplets of moisture travel several feet into the surrounding air. If you are sick with a bacteria or virus, these microorganisms can be carried along with the droplets and reach another person, infecting them.

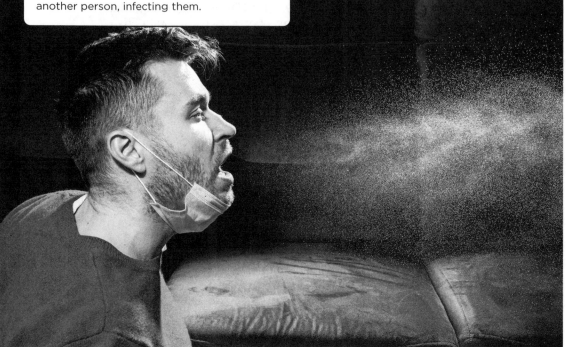

PLAGUES, PANDEMICS AND VIRUSES

Over the course of eight months in 2003, SARS infected 8,098 people, with 774 deaths.

However, SARS-CoV-2 spreads much faster. Within two months of the COVID-19 outbreak, more than 82,000 people had become infected, leading to almost 3,000 deaths. "That's why it is so bad," said Stanley Perlman, a professor of microbiology and immunology. "It has the lower-respiratory severity of SARS and MERS coronaviruses, and the transmissibility of cold coronaviruses."

In other words, during most winters, it seems inevitable that you'll catch at least one cold—you're around people who are coughing, sneezing, and leaving viruses all over the place. Now, picture that inevitability coupled with a potentially fatal infection rather than merely an aggravating one, and you have COVID-19.

Analyses of the SARS-CoV-2 genome does indeed show a spillover event. Any animal that may have been infected by bats before it then infected a human will probably remain a mystery, as the Huanan Seafood Market in Wuhan, China—where the disease may not have started but definitely propagated—was cleaned and the animals destroyed before officials arrived. Pangolins, which are among the most trafficked animals in the world and which also tested positive for the virus while in confinement (though not in the wild), was the most popular guess; part of its coronavirus genome is virtually identical to SARS-CoV-2. However, no one has yet found concrete evidence that pangolins were at the Huanan Seafood Market or even that its vendors trafficked pangolins.

How It Spreads

Say that somebody is standing next to you, and they're infected with COVID-19. They then sneeze or cough. One droplet from that sneeze contains millions of viruses, which can then infect you. This is what "viral shedding" means—and SARS-CoV-2 happens to be a brilliant shedder, making COVID-19 highly transmittable.

Once in the body, SARS-CoV-2 travels to the cells in the upper and lower respiratory systems. It binds to a cell receptor called ACE2; ACE2 receptors are found on cells throughout the body, but coronaviruses tend to focus specifically on the respiratory system because its ACE2 receptors are easiest to bind to. So, to understand it from the virus's perspective, it's not that the virus is looking to give you a respiratory infection. It's only programmed to replicate. If a virus has a "want," that's it, and the place this virus can do that in the most effective way possible is in our respiratory cells—and when SARS-CoV-2 binds, it really grabs hold.

GASTROINTESTINAL INFECTION

Cells with ACE2 receptors also live in the gastrointestinal tract and, as such, SARS-CoV-2 has been found in stool samples. A significant portion of COVID-19 patients have reported diarrhea, nausea, vomiting, and/or abdominal pain as initial symptoms before the onset of respiratory symptoms. A study done at Sun Yat-sen University in Guangdong Province, China, revealed that the virus remained in stool samples for one to twelve days. Furthermore, the stool of seventeen of these patients (or 23.3 percent) tested positive for SARS-CoV-2 even after respiratory samples tested negative.

The virus infects epithelial cells in the lungs as well as in the rectum. People with COVID-19 who use the bathroom, get fecal matter on their hands, then don't wash their hands could spread the virus to others. At the same time, people who don't have COVID-19 who use the bathroom and then don't wash their hands could contract the virus from bathroom surfaces. In short: another reason to wash your hands.

Spike proteins (or "S" proteins, compared to H1N1's "H" proteins) are the segments of the virus that jut out, giving it that coronalike appearance. These proteins orchestrate the binding of the virus to the cell and the subsequent fusion to the cell membrane. The virus that causes SARS has them. The virus that causes COVID-19 has them as well, though they bind at least ten times tighter than other coronaviruses.

Affinity plays a crucial role in various aspects of our lives. It determines how a foot best fits in a shoe or which two people would make a good couple. Affinity is also crucial in disease. SARS-CoV-2 has a higher affinity, or attraction, to ACE2 than SARS-CoV. That higher affinity, or attraction, between the spike protein and ACE2 is part of what causes the significant spread of the virus. After it attaches to the ACE2 receptor, the spike protein splits into two parts: S1 and S2. S1 helps the virus bind to ACE2. S2 then helps the virus fuse to the cell. Once inside, it targets the cell's ribosomes, which use the virus's RNA to rapidly replicate. Because the virus can replicate quickly in our lungs, it can reach enormous levels before the immune system realizes what's hit us. This can cause the immune system to go into overdrive (that cytokine storm that was mentioned earlier) and set everything to attack mode since it has yet to develop antibodies

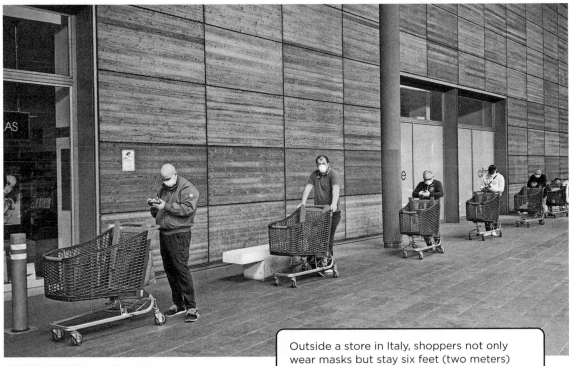

Outside a store in Italy, shoppers not only wear masks but stay six feet (two meters) apart to help maintain a safe distance, making it less likely to come in contact with COVID-19.

to fight these new invaders (antibodies would recognize SARS-CoV-2 from its spikes). This can often do more harm than good.

The basic CDC recommendations to help prevent the spread of COVID-19 are:

- Staying home when sick
- Washing hands often with soap and water for at least 20 seconds
- Wearing masks in public places
- Staying at lest 6 feet (2 meters) away from other people
- Avoiding touching eyes, nose, and mouth with unwashed hands

Pneumonia and COVID-19

COVID-19 has been called a flu, though it's more like a highly contagious pneumonia.

When we breathe, air travels through the large windpipe all the way to tiny sacs at the fingertiplike end of our lungs called alveoli. Breathe in, and the sac inflates. Exhale, and the sac deflates, like letting the air out of a balloon. Small blood vessels called capillaries surround these sacs. The oxygen you inhale passes into these capillaries, which then expel carbon dioxide, which travels into the sacs and then the lungs, where it's exhaled.

Mucus in your airways catch most of the viruses that pass through. Cilia, which is often described as hairlike, pushes this germy mucus out of your airways, where you might get rid of it by coughing. If viruses happen to get past the mucus, they're most likely to be caught and devoured by your immune system.

COVID-19 can wear down your immune system to the point that the viruses that get past the mucus traps begin to overwhelm your lungs, and those alveoli sacs become inflamed. The sacs fill with fluid, and it's tougher for your body to get oxygen. This is what can lead to pneumonia and its symptoms—difficulty breathing, chest pain, coughing, fever, chills, headaches, muscle pain, and exhaustion.

Respiratory failure occurs when you can no longer breathe on your own and need help from a ventilator.

THE H1N1 LESSON

H1N1 was the 2009 flu pandemic that many had forgotten or never knew happened. The virus appeared to be a new strain that resulted from bird, swine, and human flu viruses combined with a Eurasian pig flu virus, leading it to be called swine flu; this was a different H1N1 strain from the 1918 flu. The first human infected was reported in California on April 15 (although other reports have said it was Mexico). Some studies estimated that 11 to 21 percent of the global population at the time—or around 700 million to 1.4 billion people—contracted the illness. It was more than the number of people infected by the 1918 flu pandemic, but it had a much lower mortality number: 284,000. By comparison, the WHO estimates that 250,000 to 500,000 people die of seasonal flu annually.

As to where it came from, gene sequencing didn't reveal the immediate source of the virus; however, the consistent link with pig viruses suggests that human/farm activity was involved. A vaccine was manufactured, but when it was made available, the virus was well past its peak, and government leaders were actually turning it down. In August 2010, the WHO declared the swine flu pandemic officially over.

The odds of you catching COVID-19 and how sick you get depends on a variety of factors: age, gender, and overall health, just to name a few. COVID-19 is particularly fatal for the elderly, though unlike the 1918 flu, it does not hit children or young adults as hard. That doesn't mean they don't get sick, but it appears that they don't usually get *as* sick as someone who's over 65.

People who have conditions like heart disease, asthma, or diabetes are also at higher risk. Because minority populations such as blacks and Latinx are more likely to have these underlying conditions and less likely to have insurance or access to adequate health care, they are often even more at risk than other populations. (These factors are often based on a person's socioeconomic place in the world, as we'll soon see.)

Viral Shedding

A study by German researchers published in March 2020 reported that SARS-CoV-2 can actively shed both before and after symptoms start. Scientists also estimated that infected people with mild symptoms are nonetheless 55 percent as contagious as those with severe cases. In the most severe cases, patients were capable of shedding the virus for almost six weeks.

The virus can linger on copper for four hours, on a piece of cardboard for a day, and on plastic or stainless steel for up to three days. Scientists also found that the virus can survive in the air for three hours, going from person to person via those tiny droplets an infected person breathes, sneezes, or coughs. On the plus side, droplets that hover in the air or linger on surfaces lose their potency right away—the infection window is greatest in the first ten minutes.

Researchers at the University of North Carolina–Chapel Hill had been studying antiviral treatments to locate something that

> The more virulent strains might burn out (which, however, means many awful deaths), while the remaining hosts—meaning us—might build up some immunity.

PLAGUES, PANDEMICS AND VIRUSES

worked not just against SARS and MERS but for a novel coronavirus that they knew would inevitably arrive. They did much of the early research into the drug now known as remdesivir, which was developed through a partnership between the university and the pharmaceutical company Gilead. Remdesivir, in animal models, was able to bypass, avoid, or block the coronavirus's proofreading function, which helped stop the virus from replicating successfully in the body.

The more virulent strains might burn out (which, however, means many awful deaths), while the remaining hosts—meaning us—might build up some immunity. More immediately, the virus's stability—how much it is thriving among us right now and mutating only minimally—bodes well for the performance of antiviral drugs and, eventually, a vaccine. If the growing number of mitigation measures—this unprecedented international shutdown—are held in place for enough time, the speed at which the virus is spreading should slow, giving hospitals and health-care workers some relief.

COVID-19 Testers

Greg Galvin, Ph.D., is the president of Rheonix, a molecular diagnostic firm based in Ithaca, New York. They're one of many private-sector companies working to fill the COVID-19 tester gap by developing their own. How does a tester work? "Here's a very high-level description," says Dr. Galvin. "We take a cell from a nasal swab, bust it open and take RNA out, purify it, and use a polymerase change reaction to make millions of copies of genetic material and react that against a known set of assays." (An assay is a test that identifies a pathogen—in this case, SARS-CoV-2.) Dr. Galvin continues:

> The RNA of a virus is a very long stream of nucleotides of which there are four letters. It's like taking a sentence and removing all the punctuation—looking at the whole list is a very cumbersome way of genome sequencing. But usually you can identify the RNA strands of coronavirus within a more reasonable length.

> When the coronavirus first emerged, the CDC published two segments—N1 and N2—that they deemed to be accurate enough. If you found those two segments, then you've found it. Then the FDA actually reduced it to N1 as the only one you need. So we have probes, which are short segments of genetic material that will bind to N1 if it's present. Three dots will light up. If there's nothing present it won't light up. Specificity and sensitivity are most important: How accurately does it identify the presence or

PLAGUES, PANDEMICS AND VIRUSES

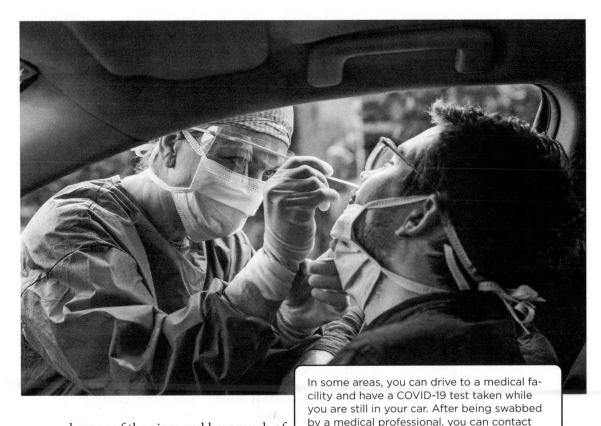

In some areas, you can drive to a medical facility and have a COVID-19 test taken while you are still in your car. After being swabbed by a medical professional, you can contact your doctor later for results.

absence of the virus and how much of the virus needs to be present in order to get a positive result.

These tests aren't for home use, however:

The U.S. was very slow to roll out testing, and part of that was originally the only lab allowed to analyze the tests was the CDC. So everyone had to send their tests to Atlanta. Then the FDA allowed state public health labs and third party labs like Quest Diagnostics to run the tests. But they're still taking days or more than a week to get results back due to the transit time. We can deploy our system to upstate hospitals in Syracuse or Rochester and have testing done in [these communities]. The testers that are making news at the moment are the same basic molecular testing that we're talking about, but they're at a state health department lab.

In February, the CDC rolled out a three-step diagnostic test and distributed testing kits—each of which could run about 800 tests—to state and local health laboratories. It was reported that many of the tests were broken, leading to a logjam in testing and more people going undiagnosed, but that wasn't the entire story. According to Dr. Galvin, "That was the media not quite getting it right. CDC first had three coronavirus identifiers—N1, N2, and N3. N1 and N2 were for SARS-CoV-2, and N3 was more a generic coronavirus identifier. Due to lack of quality control in the manufacturing of the test, it was unreliable for N3, but the N3 test is irrelevant and no one is testing for N3 now. So it really didn't impact anything."

Antibodies

The presence—or lack—of antibodies is critical in determining whether or not someone has had or still has a particular infection. Because the characteristics of COVID-19 can include a long incubation period or mild to no symptoms, it can at times be impossible to establish whether a person is contagious and can infect someone else or has already recovered from COVID-19 without knowing it.

IS COVID-19 SEASONAL?

No one knows if the "seasonality" seen in flu outbreaks will apply to COVID-19. Seasonality itself is not an entirely well-understood phenomenon. It could be that our respiratory systems are more at risk from the dry, cold air than the more humid air or that these viruses survive better in colder and darker weather. According to epidemiologist Anita Ghatak, "A virus can be inactivated by heat and/or light. However, this is not the underlying explanation of why flu season is cyclical in the colder months in the United States. The most popular theories include:

"During the winter, people spend more time indoors in closer proximity and/or surrounded by the same ambient air as an infected individual, so they may be more likely to contract the virus.

"Shorter winter days have less sunlight and will inherently lower one's level of vitamin D and melatonin, compromising the human immune system and therefore its ability to fight the virus.

"The influenza virus has been observed to survive better and longer in colder, drier climates and, therefore, is able to infect more people."

An antibody test is different from a COVID-19 test. A COVID-19 test is a diagnostic test used to diagnose whether or not a person is currently infected with SARS-CoV-2. A swab goes deep into the nasal cavity or down the throat, and the sample is sent to a lab, where technicians then determine if SARS-CoV-2 is present. (However, collecting specimens can cause sneezing or coughing, which poses additional hazards for health-care workers.) The COVID-19 test can also tell how much of the virus is present—what's been referred to as the "viral load." It's been suggested that the higher the viral load, the sicker a patient will become.

An antibody test, also known as a "serology test," could indicate a past infection and some degree of protection against getting COVID-19 again: it just requires taking blood from a finger. Simple, right? Well, nothing is simple when it comes to COVID-19, but much of that has to do with the fact that this is, indeed, still a novel coronavirus.

Some factors to consider with a serology test:

- Because it takes the body several days after being infected to develop antibodies, a serology test given too early could come back negative, even if a patient has the virus.

- If the test does come back positive, the patient can still have the virus and still be contagious; it just means their immune system is in the process of fighting it off.

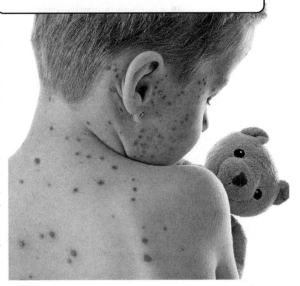

The virus that causes chicken pox is one case in which the human body develops antibodies that, for most people, defend against a recurrence all their lives. Not all viruses are so easily defended against, however.

- The number of antibodies does not absolutely reflect how sick or healthy a COVID-19 patient is.

- The length of immunity is unknown in a person who has recovered from COVID-19.

Let's expand on that last point. With illnesses like chicken pox, once you get it, you'll probably never get it again, but step on a nail as a kid, and you'll need a shot that'll prevent you from getting tetanus. Step on one again a year later, and you're unlucky but safe from tetanus. But step on one 20 years later as an adult, and you're unlucky and will need another shot. That's because we know that people are only immune to the bacteria that causes tetanus for about ten years. COVID-19 is too new for us to judge how long immunity will last.

What we can only do right now is compare COVID-19 to the immunity of other coronaviruses. You may not know it, but after a bout with the common cold, you're immune to it until your immunity starts declining after about two weeks. However, studies of SARS-CoV—which is genetically quite similar to SARS-CoV-2—shows that immunity peaks at around four months but offers protection for roughly two to three years.

Despite this, genetically quite similar doesn't mean identical. The viral load of both SARS-CoV and MERS-CoV peaks during the onset of symptoms, so while you're clearly getting sick, you're also at your most contagious, so you know to self-quarantine and people will know to stay away from you.

The high viral load that's present right away with SARS-CoV-2 before the onset of symptoms is one of the reasons why it may be transmitted so easily within families, at the office, or at religious gatherings, just to name a few.

However, it must be stressed that this virus is so new to us and that studies have been done with so many kinds of variables—country, age, gender, preexisting conditions, blood type, how sick someone is with COVID-19, how healthy they are despite having COVID-19—that the only thing we can be sure about COVID-19 is that it's an emerging infection full of unknowns. Results can show that high antibody levels correlate to getting better, or, as is the case with a study published in *The Lancet*, results can show that antibody levels do not correlate at all with the virus's severity. In fact, one patient who had had an excellent early antibody response after the onset of symptoms nevertheless became quite sick from COVID-19. Also, within this study, patients who died of COVID-19 had developed faster peak antibody responses compared to those who recovered but were left with a lower number of antibodies.

China and COVID-19

In China, politics and censorship often block legislation that can help its people. In 2006, author Zhou Qing wrote about this in a groundbreaking exposé, *What Kind of God*, regarding the Chinese food industry; two-thirds of the book was removed before publication, and its success forced him into exile.

The Chinese government's knee-jerk reaction to COVID-19 was to put denial above the safety of its people. By not initially taking aggressive measures to warn the public and medical professionals, public-health experts say that the Chinese government lost one of its best chances to prevent the coronavirus from becoming an epidemic.

SARS had killed 800 people only fifteen years earlier, but to quarantine patients would be to admit a problem. China did not want to admit that it had a severe problem on its hands, particularly at a time when its local officials prepared for their annual congresses and the New Year celebrations were around the corner.

The first COVID-19 symptoms appeared in early December 2019, when medical staff were puzzled as to why a group of patients who seemed to have pneumonia did not respond to the usual treatments. These patients had something else in common: they all worked at Huanan Seafood Market.

The first COVID-19 symptoms appeared in early December 2019, when medical staff were puzzled as to why a group of patients who seemed to have pneumonia did not respond to the usual treatments.

Huanan Seafood Market's name was a bit of a misnomer: it also sold beavers, chickens, crocodiles, dogs, koalas, otters, pigs, porcupines, rats, turtles, and … bats and civets. It took up over a block in a part of the city that was home to a growing middle class. The market had cages with dogs next to cages with civets, which were put on top of cages with porcupines, which were on top of cages with chickens. They also sold wild game and live reptiles, which are considered delicacies. These animals urinated and defecated on each other, were crammed into tight spaces, and were handled by people who lacked any kind of safety training, surrounded by garbage and little ventilation. Virus-laden fluids and secretions mixed, creating brand new viruses, especially when the animals were slaughtered right in front of customers.

Christian Walzer, executive director for health at the Wildlife Conservation Society, told *The New York Times*, "If you planned it and thought, 'I am going to make new viruses,' that is exactly how you would do it."

The markets may have produced outbreaks in the past that burned out locally. Now, with exploding populations and access to cheap airlines and fast trains, bat viruses from the depths of jungles or the deep interiors of caves can spread to every corner of the globe within days.

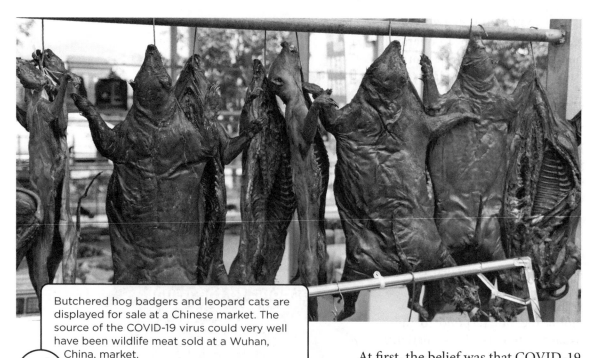

Butchered hog badgers and leopard cats are displayed for sale at a Chinese market. The source of the COVID-19 virus could very well have been wildlife meat sold at a Wuhan, China, market.

At first, the belief was that COVID-19 began at the Huanan Seafood Market, spreading from animal to human. As of now, this has not been proven, but it did at least begin around there and mushroomed from there.

For the next seven weeks, the Chinese government threatened doctors in order to keep them quiet and censored the press. Meanwhile, Wuhan's 11 million residents—in addition to the tens of thousands who traveled through the city's transportation hub each day—were unaware of the presence of a deadly virus all around them.

Then, the Huanan Seafood Market was shut down, with workers in hazmat suits washing out stalls and spraying disinfectants. This was the first visible government response to the disease. The day before, on December 31, 2019, Chinese authorities had alerted the WHO's Beijing office of an outbreak. Wuhan's Health Commission, the agency that oversees public health and sanitation, announced that 27 people were suffering from pneumonia of an unknown cause, but its statement also said not to worry because "the disease is preventable and controllable."

The annual meeting of People's Congresses took place on January 7, 2020, a time when the Communist Party-run legislatures praise themselves in the spirit of the new year. No one was in the mood to hear about a coronavirus.

When Zhou Xianwang, the mayor of Wuhan, gave his annual report, he promised elite medical schools and a futuristic industry park for medical companies. Not once did he or any other leader mention an outbreak.

The Whistleblower

Lu Xiaohong, the head of gastroenterology at City Hospital No. 5, told the newspaper *China Youth Daily* that she had heard on December 25, 2019, that the disease was spreading among health-care workers ... three weeks before the authorities would acknowledge it.

Dr. Li Wenliang, an ophthalmologist, was also one of the first to sound the alarm. In an online medical chat room through WeChat, he wrote the following on December 30, 2019:

> (CST 17:43)
>
> Li: There are 7 confirmed cases of SARS at Huanan Seafood Market.
>
> Li: (Picture of diagnosis report)
>
> Li: (Video of CT scan results)
>
> Li: They are being isolated in the emergency department of our hospital's Houhu Hospital District.
>
> (CST 18:42)
>
> [Unknown Writer]: Be careful, or else our chat group might be dismissed.
>
> Li: The latest news is, it has been confirmed that they are coronavirus infections, but the exact virus is being subtyped.
>
> Li: Don't circulate the information outside of this group, tell your family and loved ones to take precautions.

Screenshots of the WeChat messages were leaked, and four days later, on January 3, 2020, police from the Huanan Public Security Bureau interrogated Dr. Li, reprimanding him for "making false comments on the Internet." He was then forced to write a retraction. The police warned him that if he continued to violate the law, he would be prosecuted.

On January 10, he resumed his practice and treated a woman for glaucoma. He did not know that she had already been infected with SARS-CoV-2, probably from her daughter. She and her daughter both became sick. So did Dr. Li. In the days before his death, Dr. Li told *The New York Times*, "If the officials had disclosed information about the epidemic earlier I think it would have been a lot better.... There should be more openness and transparency."

Nine days after the market closed, a 61-year-old man who had been a regular customer at the Huanan Seafood Market became the first official coronavirus fatality, according to a report by the Wuhan Health Commission. The authorities didn't disclose his death until two days after it occurred and also omitted the fact that his wife had developed symptoms after he did, but she'd never been to the Huanan Seafood Market.

Several days earlier and about 20 miles from the market, scientists at the Wuhan Institute of Virology—including Zheng-Li Shi, who had helped determine SARS's origin—were studying patient samples in order to determine where this new form of coronavirus was coming from. While the public was still in the dark, the virologists quickly determined that the new outbreak was related to SARS, and, like SARS, they believed that bats were the initial host, just as SARS spread when the virus jumped from bats to civets to humans.

Officially, however, the government's efforts to provide the least amount of knowledge persisted. "If there are no new cases in the next few days, the outbreak is over," Guan Yi, a professor of infectious diseases at the University of Hong Kong, said on January 15, 2020. Even the WHO echoed these sentiments.

Soon after this, Thailand reported the first confirmed case outside China, which had occurred on January 13.

China Comes Clean

On January 20, more than a month after the first symptoms spread, epidemiologist Dr. Zhong Nanshan, who was instrumental in the fight against SARS, announced on state television that this type of coronavirus spread through human contact. He even used the example of how one patient had infected at least fourteen health-care workers. The secret was out.

Three days later, Wuhan announced that it was closing down—and those still in the city would be quarantined. This was an unprecedented move that had finally been approved by the Chinese government. Once the coronavirus had breached China's borders, it became too large to be contained, and because the crisis went from 0 to 60 seemingly within seconds, residents who had believed that this was nothing more than a bad cold panicked. Crowds raced to leave before the deadline of January 23.

Wuhan's mayor, Zhou Xianwang, took responsibility for the delay, but he said that his hand was forced by the national law on infectious diseases, which allows provincial governments to declare an epidemic only after receiving central government approval. During an interview on China's national TV on January 27, Zhou admitted, "After I receive information, I can only release it when I'm authorized." He then offered to resign. His resignation was denied.

Wuhan's mayor, Zhou Xianwang, took responsibility for the delay, but he said that his hand was forced by the national law on infectious diseases....

On February 2, health officials said that a 44-year-old man in the Philippines died of the coronavirus, making him the first known death outside of China. The man, a resident of Wuhan, died on February 1 after developing what officials called "severe pneumonia."

"This is the first known death of someone with 2019-nCoV outside of China," the WHO's office in the Philippines said in a statement. "In his last few days, the patient was stable and showed signs of improvement," said the Philippines health secretary, Francisco Duque III. "However, the condition of the patient deteriorated within his last 24 hours, resulting in his demise." (Under Duque's direction, as of April 9, 2020, the Philippines was only able to perform 1,000 tests per day for the 105 million Filipinos nationwide.)

Bats

The detective work continued since to know how this virus came to be would help put it to an end. It was now common knowledge that COVID-19 was found in those associated with the Huanan Seafood Market—not only people who handled the animals but also those who touched surfaces, shopped, or even just walked through. However, the first reported cases of COVID-19 might have been in people who were not associated with the market. People may have contracted the disease from animals at another food market or somewhere else and then passed it on to other people.

ARE BATS THE PROBLEM?

Although the Wuhan outbreak is the sixth one caused by bat-borne viruses in the past 26 years—the other five being Hendra in 1994, Nipah in 1998, SARS in 2002, MERS in 2012, and Ebola in 2014—it's not the bats that are the problem; they help their ecosystems by eating insects and pollinating plants. The problem is when we come into contact with them and/or take over their habitat. Only months before the coronavirus outbreak, *MDPI*, a Swiss academic magazine, published an article by Chinese researchers who wrote that "it is generally believed that bat-borne [coronaviruses] will re-emerge to cause the next disease outbreak." They added, "In this regard, China is a likely hot spot."

In a 2017 report in *Nature*, Dr. Peter Daszak, Kevin J. Olival, and other colleagues from EcoHealth Alliance reported that "bats are host to a significantly higher proportion of zoonoses [at least 60] than all other mammalian orders." In addition, they estimate that about seventeen zoonoses (diseases that can spread from animals to humans) have yet to be discovered in *every* bat species.

Bats' tolerance toward viruses, which is far greater than that of any other mammal, is just one characteristic that sets them apart—they're also the only mammals that can fly. They also eat tons of disease-carrying insects and play a critical role in pollinating fruit like bananas and mangoes. About a quarter of all mammalian species are bats.

How bats can carry so many viruses is still an unanswered question. Researchers believe that the ability to fly may contribute to a lower immune response to viruses—inflammation may hamper the ability to fly—and therefore cause a lower rate of virus replication overall. Not only do bats survive, but they survive for long periods of time—they're remarkably long-lived for small mammals. The United States's big brown bat can live for nearly 20 years in the wild. Others live to 40. One Siberian bat lived to be at least 41. Other small mammals, like house mice, live for about two years.

Are viruses just attracted to bats? How come they carry so many? The answer is long life spans and close quarters. Bats often cluster in huge colonies within caves, where crowded conditions are ideal for passing viruses back and forth. It's also their ability to live long and healthy lives while loaded with more viruses than even the rat—viruses that can kill animals, such as humans. When we eat bats, handle them, and invade their habitat, the consequences can be devastating. For example, many bat species now have to roost in attics from where they can get to other parts of a house, bringing them into contact with humans and potentially spreading viruses—and for many of these bat-hosted viruses, no known cure or vaccine exists.

Indeed, scientists conclude that the rapid spread of people into once remote regions have put us in ever-closer proximity to virus-carrying animals. Countless pathogens jump across animal species on a daily basis—most of the time with no visible effect—but increasingly, these pathogens are taking advantage of the new opportunities that humans have created as they reshape the natural environment.

Many viruses, such as smallpox and polio, specialize in a single host—us—but other viruses can infect a range of species in what scientists call spillover events. Increasing human encroachment into previously wild areas creates ample opportunities for pathogens to test their mettle against a new species. Infectious diseases from AIDS to Zika started out this way, and researchers have no idea how many other viruses lurk. We're only a few mutations and a lucky break away from causing the next pandemic.

That's more people coming into contact with more animals that are carrying more diseases. David Quammen wrote in his 2012 book, *Spillover: Animal Infections and the Next Human Pandemic*, "You go into a forest and you shake the trees—literally and figuratively—and viruses fall out."

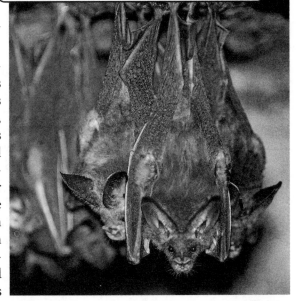

One reason bats tend to carry viruses is that they often sleep in large groups together, spreading viruses among themselves.

In 2020, researchers at University of California–Berkeley note that disrupting a bat's habitat seems to cause them stress, which makes them shed even more virus into their saliva, urine, and feces that can infect other animals and humans. "Heightened environmental threats to bats may add to the threat of zoonosis," said Cara Brook, a postdoctoral Miller Fellow at UC Berkeley and the first author of the study. She's part of a bat-monitoring program funded by the U.S. Defense Advanced Research Projects Agency (DARPA) that is currently underway in Madagascar, Bangladesh, Ghana, and Australia. The project, Bat One Health, explores the link between the loss of a bat's habitat and the spillover of bat viruses into other animals and humans.

This is the case in the southern Chinese province of Yunnan, where a cave may hold the origins of the deadly coronavirus. Its location is being kept a secret, but researchers found it after searching for caves once they knew that this is a bat-borne disease but not finding many bats in wildlife markets. As it turned out, people were hunting them and selling them directly to restaurants.

Researchers at the Wuhan Institute of Virology found that SARS-CoV-2 is more than 96 percent genetically identical to a bat virus found in that cave. They published the results in the journal *Nature* on February 3, 2020. Another study published in the January 22, 2020, edition of *Medical Virology* asserted that the SARS-CoV-2 "appears to be a recombinant virus between the bat coronavirus and an origin-unknown coronavirus. The recombination occurred within the viral spike glycoprotein, which recognizes cell surface receptor." This means that the bat coronavirus combined with this new coronavirus gave it the receptors needed to infect human cells. This would've been something that this particular bat coronavirus was unable to do before the recombination happened.

This recombination is not surprising given that coronaviruses are particularly adaptable. The coronavirus is up there in the Darwinian survival of the fittest—particularly impressive given that we're still not sure whether or not viruses are alive. Coronaviruses in particular mutate constantly through repeated mistakes that occur in their genome during replication. These mistakes—misread DNA or RNA code—actually benefit the virus by allowing such things as recombination to occur.

COVID-19 Links and the United States

On January 31, U.S. secretary of Health and Human Services Alex Azar declared a public-health emergency at a White House press briefing. U.S. citizens returning from Hubei Province in the previous fourteen days would be subject to up to a fourteen-day quarantine. Foreign nationals, other than immediate family members of U.S. citizens, who had traveled to China in the previous fourteen days, would be denied entry into the country. The temporary measures took effect on February 2 at 5 P.M.

Meanwhile, California health officials reported a third confirmed case of coronavirus in the state, in a man who'd traveled to Wuhan and became ill after returning home. At that point, seven cases had been confirmed in the United States—six in travelers and one a human-to-human transmission between a husband and wife.

"It's very, very transmissible, and it almost certainly is going to be a pandemic," said Dr. Anthony S. Fauci, director of the National Institute of Allergy and Infectious Diseases. "But will it be catastrophic? I don't know."

The Chinese government, in a sudden about-face, built a hospital for coronavirus patients in ten days. A second facility in Wuhan, with 1,500 beds, was completed soon after.

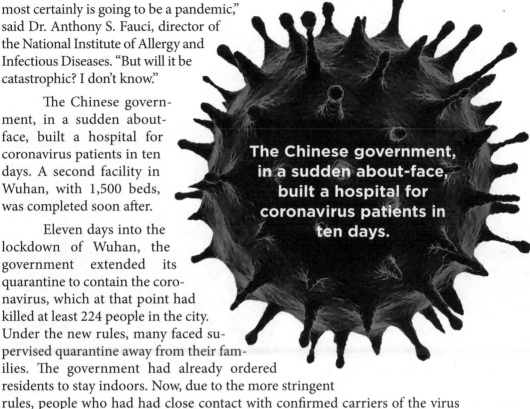

The Chinese government, in a sudden about-face, built a hospital for coronavirus patients in ten days.

Eleven days into the lockdown of Wuhan, the government extended its quarantine to contain the coronavirus, which at that point had killed at least 224 people in the city. Under the new rules, many faced supervised quarantine away from their families. The government had already ordered residents to stay indoors. Now, due to the more stringent rules, people who had had close contact with confirmed carriers of the virus would be "sent to centralized isolation and observation points."

The regulation did not specify where people would be kept for observation, but it warned that people would have no choice.

"Those who refuse to cooperate will be compelled under the law by assisting public security offices," the order said. "During isolation, each district will provide free room and board, as well as medical observation and treatment."

The next death outside of mainland China occurred on February 4, two days after the death in the Philippines. At this point, the death toll from the coronavirus exceeded that of the SARS outbreak.

On January 30, two weeks after the Wuhan lockdown began, the quarantine radius grew from the 11 million people in the city of Wuhan to about 50 million in the entire Hubei Province. A quarantine of this size had never been done before. Some experts believed that quarantine would help; others maintained that it was already too late.

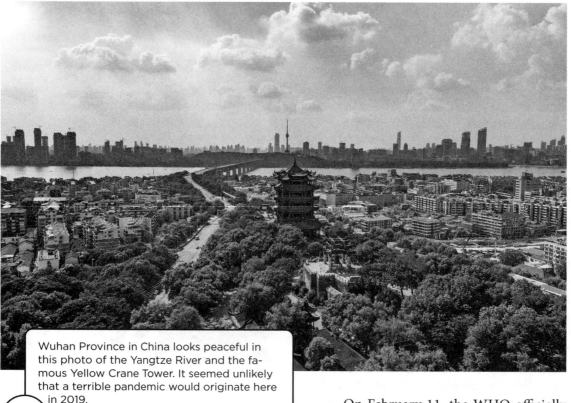

Wuhan Province in China looks peaceful in this photo of the Yangtze River and the famous Yellow Crane Tower. It seemed unlikely that a terrible pandemic would originate here in 2019.

On February 11, the WHO officially named the new coronavirus SARS-CoV-2, and the disease that resulted from it was named COVID-19.

The Chinese government also temporarily banned wildlife trade until the epidemic passed.

At a press conference held on February 13, Japan announced its first COVID-19 death: an 80-year-old woman who, unlike the two other deaths, had not been to mainland China. Japanese officials also said that dozens of new cases had been confirmed, including 44 who had been on board a cruise ship quarantined off Yokohama, south of Tokyo. "We don't know what's going on, we've been floating around for about two weeks now," said one passenger. "We're all a bunch of human beings that have lives outside this cruise ship that need us." The cruise ship, the *Diamond Princess*, arrived in Yokohama on February 3. Passengers were to go home the next day, but after discovering that an 80-year-old man who had disembarked in Hong Kong had tested positive for COVID-19, the Japanese government quarantined all 3,711 people aboard. The infected included at least 138 people from India (including 132 crew members and six passengers), 35 Filipinos,

32 Canadians, 24 Australians, 13 Americans, four Indonesians, four Malaysians, and two Britons. Home countries arranged to evacuate their citizens and quarantine them further in their own countries. By March 1, all aboard, including the crew and the captain, had disembarked. By April 14, fourteen of those who were on board died of the disease.

U.S. Leadership

American leaders, unfortunately, have viewed this pandemic as more of a political issue than a medical one, and their actions have reflected this. The scarcity of tests nationwide and delay in testing cases has also led experts to warn that it's impossible to even know where all the hot spots are in the United States. For starters, limited tests were available that could only be handed by the CDC in Atlanta, so all tests in the United States had to be sent to Atlanta for processing. Then, third-party companies like Quest Diagnostics were given the green light when the CDC got overwhelmed, but even this requires tests to be mailed, pro-

---

WHY WAS ITALY SO VULNERABLE?

❝Italy should be a warning to everybody, everywhere," said Professor Massimo Galli, who specializes in infectious diseases at the University of Milan. Speaking to RTÉ News from his office in Milan, he said the initial measures being taken by Italy were the "minimum necessary." Asked to explain the prevalence of the coronavirus in Italy, Professor Galli said the country was unfortunate to experience infection early, before a high degree of awareness existed among the public or medical professionals. "We have an epidemic because of one person who returned with an infection in an asymptomatic phase and it spread underground in the 'red zone,'" he said, referring to the Lombardy region in the north of Italy. "The fire spread in a large part of our region…. What happened in Italy could happen everywhere in Europe…. Maybe we are particularly unlucky."

Also, Italy has the second-oldest population in the world, making the country extra vulnerable to COVID-19. Its measures, in retrospect, have been seen as less than proactive in the face of a pandemic, though the Italian government did make huge steps as far as quarantining and isolating. Videos of Italians singing from their windows while quarantined went viral.

---

cessed, and mailed back. Thankfully, this process has become more streamlined, but not before untold lives could've been spared or suffering avoided.

On January 22, when asked by a CNBC reporter if he had "worries about a pandemic," the president answered, "No, not at all. We have it totally under control. It's one person coming in from China, and we have it under control. It's going to be just fine."

The United States remained relatively silent on the issue for the next month. On February 4, during his State of the Union Address, President Donald Trump spent 20 seconds of the 75-minute speech covering COVID-19. President Trump said that he was working with Beijing "on the coronavirus outbreak in China." The president did not mention that U.S. intelligence agencies had already sent warnings to the White House about what was then already a growing epidemic.

On February 6, President Trump and Chinese president Xi Jinping spoke that day, with Trump reporting that Xi was "strong, sharp and powerfully focused" and said that the virus would die off in the spring. He also said that China was "professionally run" and that "they have everything under control," consistent with his past statements, like this tweet from January 24: "China has been working very hard to contain the Coronavirus. The United States greatly appreciates their efforts and transparency. It will all work out well. In particular, on behalf of the American People, I want to thank President Xi!"

On February 4, during his State of the Union Address, President Trump spent 20 seconds of the 75-minute speech covering COVID-19.

All was relatively quiet as far as COVID went for the rest of the month except for a few sound bites from the president. On February 26, after the country's first reported COVID-19 cases, Trump said, "We're going to be pretty soon at only five people. And we could be at just one or two people over the next short period of time. So we've had very good luck."

On February 27 at a White House meeting: "It's going to disappear. One day, it's like a miracle, it will disappear."

In a South Carolina campaign rally on February 28, President Trump compared the Democrats' criticism of his COVID-19 response to their efforts to impeach him, saying that "this is their new hoax" used to try to oust him from office. "The Democrats are politicizing the coronavirus. They're politicizing it," President Trump said. "They don't have any clue.... One of my people came up to me and said, 'Mr. President, they tried to beat you on Russia, Russia, Russia.' That did not work out too well. They could not do it. They tried the impeachment hoax."

Then, Trump called the coronavirus "their new hoax," though earlier in the week, President Trump congratulated himself for shutting down flights between the United States and China and forming a Coronavirus Task Force, which was led by Vice President Michael Pence. Overall, however, February has been called the "lost month" in terms of presidential action taken to combat the virus.

In February 2020, President Donald Trump assured Americans that the COVID-19 virus would miraculously disappear and there was nothing for U.S. citizens to fear.

It wasn't until the president's March 11 televised speech from the Oval Office that he acknowledged the severity of the situation.

> My fellow Americans: Tonight, I want to speak with you about our nation's unprecedented response to the coronavirus outbreak that started in China and is now spreading throughout the world.

> Today, the World Health Organization officially announced that this is a global pandemic.

> We have been in frequent contact with our allies, and we are marshalling the full power of the federal government and the private sector to protect the American people.

> This is the most aggressive and comprehensive effort to confront a foreign virus in modern history. I am confident that by counting and continuing to take these tough measures, we will significantly reduce the threat to our citizens, and we will ultimately and expeditiously defeat this virus.

From the beginning of time, nations and people have faced unforeseen challenges, including large-scale and very dangerous health threats. This is the way it always was and always will be. It only matters how you respond, and we are responding with great speed and professionalism.

Our team is the best anywhere in the world. At the very start of the outbreak, we instituted sweeping travel restrictions on China and put in place the first federally mandated quarantine in over 50 years. We declared a public health emergency and issued the highest level of travel warning on other countries as the virus spread its horrible infection.

And taking early intense action, we have seen dramatically fewer cases of the virus in the United States than are now present in Europe.

The European Union failed to take the same precautions and restrict travel from China and other hotspots. As a result, a large number of new clusters in the United States were seeded by travelers from Europe.

After consulting with our top government health professionals, I have decided to take several strong but necessary actions to protect the health and wellbeing of all Americans.

To keep new cases from entering our shores, we will be suspending all travel from Europe to the United States for the next 30 days. The new rules will go into effect Friday at midnight. These restrictions will be adjusted subject to conditions on the ground.

There will be exemptions for Americans who have undergone appropriate screenings, and these prohibitions will not only apply to the tremendous amount of trade and cargo, but various other things as we get approval. Anything coming from Europe to the United States is what we are discussing. [Note: The president misspoke— he meant people coming from Europe, not shipments of goods.] These restrictions will also not apply to the United Kingdom.

At the same time, we are monitoring the situation in China and in South Korea. And, as their situation improves, we will reevaluate the restrictions and warnings that are currently in place for a possible early opening.

Earlier this week, I met with the leaders of health insurance industry who have agreed to waive all copayments for coronavirus treatments, extend insurance coverage to these treatments, and to prevent surprise medical billing.

We are cutting massive amounts of red tape to make antiviral therapies available in record time. These treatments will significantly reduce the impact and reach of the virus.

Additionally, last week, I signed into law an $8.3 billion funding bill to help CDC and other government agencies fight the virus and support vaccines, treatments, and distribution of medical supplies. Testing and testing capabilities are expanding rapidly, day by day. We are moving very quickly.

The vast majority of Americans: The risk is very, very low. Young and healthy people can expect to recover fully and quickly if they should get the virus. The highest risk is for elderly population with underlying health conditions. The elderly population must be very, very careful.

In particular, we are strongly advising that nursing homes for the elderly suspend all medically unnecessary visits. In general, older Americans should also avoid nonessential travel in crowded areas.

My administration is coordinating directly with communities with the largest outbreaks, and we have issued guidance on school closures, social distancing, and reducing large gatherings.

Smart action today will prevent the spread of the virus tomorrow.

Every community faces different risks and it is critical for you to follow the guidelines of your local officials who are working closely with our federal health experts—and they are the best.

For all Americans, it is essential that everyone take extra precautions and practice good hygiene. Each of us has a role to play in defeating this virus. Wash your hands, clean often-used surfaces, cover your face and mouth if you sneeze or cough, and most of all, if you are sick or not feeling well, stay home.

To ensure that working Americans impacted by the virus can stay home without fear of financial hardship, I will soon be taking emergency action, which is unprecedented, to provide financial relief. This will be targeted for workers who are ill, quarantined, or caring for others due to coronavirus.

I will be asking Congress to take legislative action to extend this relief.

Because of the economic policies that we have put into place over the last three years, we have the greatest economy anywhere in the world, by far.

Our banks and financial institutions are fully capitalized and incredibly strong. Our unemployment is at a historic low. This vast economic prosperity gives us flexibility, reserves, and resources to handle any threat that comes our way.

This is not a financial crisis, this is just a temporary moment of time that we will overcome together as a nation and as a world.

However, to provide extra support for American workers, families, and businesses, tonight I am announcing the following additional actions: I am instructing the Small Business Administration to exercise available authority to provide capital and liquidity to firms affected by the coronavirus.

Effective immediately, the SBA will begin providing economic loans in affected states and territories. These low-interest loans will help small businesses overcome temporary economic disruptions caused by the virus. To this end, I am asking Congress to increase funding for this program by an additional $50 billion.

Using emergency authority, I will be instructing the Treasury Department to defer tax payments, without interest or penalties, for certain individuals and businesses negatively impacted. This action will provide more than $200 billion of additional liquidity to the economy.

Finally, I am calling on Congress to provide Americans with immediate payroll tax relief. Hopefully they will consider this very strongly.

We are at a critical time in the fight against the virus. We made a life-saving move with early action on China. Now we must take the same action with Europe. We will not delay. I will never hesitate to take any necessary steps to protect the lives, health, and safety of the American people. I will always put the wellbeing of America first.

If we are vigilant—and we can reduce the chance of infection, which we will—we will significantly impede the transmission of the virus. The virus will not have a chance against us.

No nation is more prepared or more resilient than the United States. We have the best economy, the most advanced healthcare, and the most talented doctors, scientists, and researchers anywhere in the world.

We are all in this together. We must put politics aside, stop the partisanship, and unify together as one nation and one family.

As history has proven time and time again, Americans always rise to the challenge and overcome adversity.

Our future remains brighter than anyone can imagine. Acting with compassion and love, we will heal the sick, care for those in need, help our fellow citizens, and emerge from this challenge stronger and more unified than ever before.

God bless you, and God bless America. Thank you.

That speech came on the heels of an announcement that married actors Tom Hanks

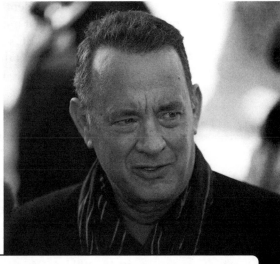

Funny how Americans take notice when a celebrity speaks up. When actor Tom Hanks announced that he and his wife had contracted the coronavirus, many in denial about the pandemic finally took notice.

and Rita Wilson had tested positive for COVID-19 and that the NBA and NHL would be suspending their seasons. It marked a turning point in how Americans began to see the virus.

Spring Ahead

On March 16 in the White House briefing room, the president predicted, "It could be right in that period of time where it, I say, wash—it washes through. Other people don't like that term. But where it washes through."

Despite this, the president struck a completely different tune on March 17, when he told reporters, "This is a pandemic.… I felt it was a pandemic long before it was called a pandemic."

Another example of the administration's mixed messages: test distribution versus test completion.

On March 9, Vice President Mike Pence said, "We literally are going to see a dramatic increase in the available—availability of testing." This was in response to a question about the lack of testing. "Over a million tests have been distributed.… Before the end of this week, another 4 million tests will be distributed."

On April 27, President Trump said that 200,000 people were tested the previous Saturday and that more than 5.4 million tests had been conducted across the United States. ABC's Jon Karl—noting that Vice President Pence had mentioned weeks earlier that the country would be at the four-million-test mark by mid-March—asked why it took longer than expected to test that many people.

"I appreciate the question," Pence said, "but it represents a misunderstanding on your part and frankly the—a lot of people in the public's part—about the difference between *having* a test versus the ability to actually *process* the test."

Karl then asked, "So when you said 4 million tests, seven weeks ago, you were just talking about tests being sent out, not actually being—being completed?" Pence said that was "precisely correct."

The vice president added that had those four million tests gone out, people would "still be waiting on those tests to be done in many cases, because they were tests that were designed to be run in the old laboratory model." Why they were only seven weeks earlier touted by the vice president is unknown.

For months, health officials have emphasized that asymptomatic transmission plays a significant role in the spread of the virus—which is why testing was so desperately needed.

"Asymptomatic and mildly symptomatic transmission are a major factor in transmission for COVID-19," said Dr. William Schaffner, a professor at Vanderbilt University School of Medicine and longtime adviser to the CDC. "They're going to be the drivers of spread in the community."

Don't Drink the Disinfectants

During a press briefing on April 23, William Bryan, leader of the science and technology directorate of the Department of Homeland Security (DHS), told the media that recent DHS research showed that the "virus dies the quickest in the presence of direct sunlight" and also mentioned the testing of disinfectants that would quickly kill the virus on surfaces.

Trump then spoke about the powers of sunlight and disinfectant, turning at times to address Dr. Deborah Birx, the White House coronavirus response coordinator and a physician who specializes in vaccine research. Said Trump:

> A question that probably some of you are thinking of if you're totally into that world, which I find to be very interesting. So, supposing we hit the body with a tremendous, whether it's ultraviolet

or just very powerful light, and I think you said that hasn't been checked, but you're going to test it. And then I said supposing you brought the light inside the body, which you can do either through the skin or in some other way. And I think you said you're going to test that too. Sounds interesting, right? And then I see the disinfectant, where it knocks it out in a minute, one minute. And is there a way we can do something like that by injection inside or almost a cleaning, because you see it gets in the lungs and it does a tremendous number on the lungs. So it'd be interesting to check that. So that you're going to have to use medical doctors with, but it sounds interesting to me. So, we'll see, but the whole concept of the light, the way it kills it in one minute. That's pretty powerful.

After being thoroughly mocked for this statement, the next day, the president said that he was being "sarcastic." Nevertheless, the company that makes cleaners like Lysol® felt

A doctor gives a patient a vaccination to stave off illness. Vaccines work by introducing a dead or weakened virus, or part of a virus, into the body that won't make you sick but will stimulate your immune system to produce antibodies.

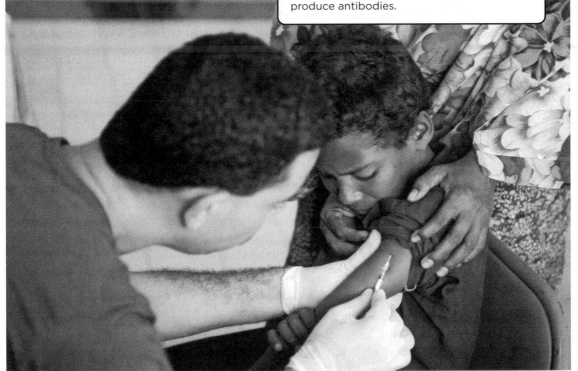

the need to warn that injecting or ingesting disinfectants is dangerous and potentially fatal. A Kansas man drank cleaning products, according to a Kansas health official, days after President Trump floated the disinfectant idea. The man survived.

The Kansas Poison Control Center saw a more than 40-percent increase in cases about cleaning products, the secretary of the Kansas Department of Health and Environment, Lee Norman, said. The New York City Poison Control Center reported 30 inquiries in an 18-hour period "specifically about exposure to Lysol, 10 cases specifically about bleach and 11 cases about exposures to other household cleaners," city health department spokesperson Pedro F. Frisneda told NPR.

Maryland governor Larry Hogan said that his state's health officials had received "hundreds" of inquiries about the safety of consuming or injecting cleaning products.

This isn't happening only in America, unfortunately. Iranian media reported that nearly 300 people have died and more than 1,000 sickened by drinking methanol in a country where drinking alcohol is banned and those who do drink rely on bootleggers. (Methanol is typically used in nondrinkable fluids like antifreeze.) Iranian doctor Hossein Hassanian told the Associated Press that the problem was even greater, giving a death toll of around 480 and 2,850 people sickened.

Quack remedies spread across social media in Iran, where people are deeply suspicious of the government after it also downplayed COVID-19 before the disease overwhelmed the country.

"Other countries have only one problem, which is the new coronavirus pandemic. But we are fighting on two fronts here," said Dr. Hassanian, an adviser to Iran's Health Ministry who gave the higher figures to the AP. "We have to both cure the people with alcohol poisoning and also fight the coronavirus."

Iranian social media accounts falsely suggested that a British schoolteacher and others cured themselves of the coronavirus with whiskey and honey, based on a tabloid story from early February. This, combined with stories about drinking alcohol-based hand sanitizers, led some to wrongly believe that drinking high-proof alcohol would kill the virus in their bodies.

That fear of the virus, poor education, and internet rumors left dozens sickened by drinking bootleg alcohol. Some bootleggers in Iran added a splash of bleach before selling it as drinkable.

In India, misconceptions about COVID-19 swept through the country primarily through Whatsapp but also with the help of the national government. In January, the Indian government, through the Ministry of AYUSH, which promotes alternative forms of medicine, published questionable advisories about homeopathy and Unani (a type of herbal practice). Homeopathy has been widely dismissed by public-health experts as not being effective for any health condition.

The Indian fact-checking website *Alt News* determined that "the homeopathic drug 'Arsenicum album 30' cannot prevent a COVID-19 infection as claimed by the Ministry of AYUSH," said Sumaiya Shaikh, a neuroscientist working in Sweden and science fact-checker for *Alt News*. Shaikh told *Time* magazine that she found an "immense number of faults" in these studies, including "data fudging" and "bad statistics." Homeopathy, which involves treatments that are heavily diluted, "will always be popular where there is distrust in the regular medical health system," Shaikh says. These remedies also tend to be cheap, she notes, which could explain homeopathy's popularity in India.

Elected officials from Prime Minister Narendra Modi's Bharatiya Janata Party (BHJP) have promoted unproven therapies, too. Suman Haripriya, a BJP lawmaker in Assam, suggested that cow urine and dung could be used to cure the coronavirus. The chief minister of Uttar Pradesh, Yogi Adityanath, suggested that COVID-19 and other diseases could be overcome with the help of yoga.

Alt News debunked a tweet from the spokesperson of Indian People's Party in Maharashtra, which linked to an article alleging that China was seeking a court's approval to kill more than 20,000 COVID-19 patients in order to contain the virus.

This Is the Deal

Of all the states in the United States, New York was the first to be hit hard by COVID-19. In March 2020, Governor Andrew Cuomo ordered residents to stay at home and all nonessential businesses to close. Similar orders have divided the American public. In the more rural states—Arkansas, Iowa, Nebraska, North Dakota, and South Dakota—governors held off on imposing stay-at-home orders as long as they could. Others, such as Alabama, Florida, Georgia, Mississippi, Missouri, Oklahoma, Pennsylvania, South Carolina, Texas, Utah, and Wyoming, have issued partial stay-at-home orders. (In addition, residents of Washington, D.C., and Puerto Rico have been urged to stay at home.)

Because the enemy is not visible, many people are not afraid of it, especially when their livelihood is at stake. Others see COVID-19 as an excuse for big, bad government to tighten its hold on Americans. Still others have called the lockdowns a threat to America's democracy. Christian pastor Jonathan Shuttlesworth of Pennsylvania referred to social distancers as "sissies" and "pansies"

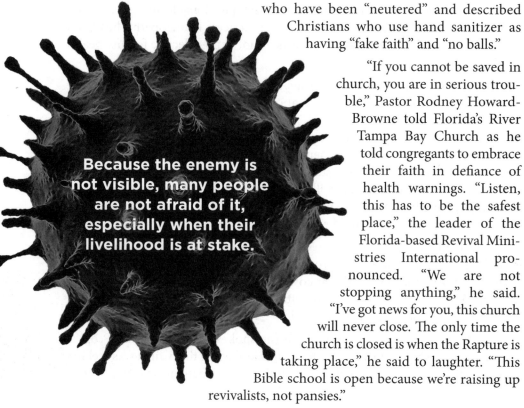

who have been "neutered" and described Christians who use hand sanitizer as having "fake faith" and "no balls."

Because the enemy is not visible, many people are not afraid of it, especially when their livelihood is at stake.

"If you cannot be saved in church, you are in serious trouble," Pastor Rodney Howard-Browne told Florida's River Tampa Bay Church as he told congregants to embrace their faith in defiance of health warnings. "Listen, this has to be the safest place," the leader of the Florida-based Revival Ministries International pronounced. "We are not stopping anything," he said. "I've got news for you, this church will never close. The only time the church is closed is when the Rapture is taking place," he said to laughter. "This Bible school is open because we're raising up revivalists, not pansies."

Some politicians, including Dan Patrick, lieutenant governor of Texas, and pundits like Glenn Beck and Brit Hume have suggested that older Americans should be willing to risk death to preserve the economy. In a sense: "Take it like a man."

Security was the promise of President Franklin D. Roosevelt's first inaugural address in 1933. The goal of his New Deal in 1935 was "the security of the men, women, and children of the nation against certain hazards and vicissitudes of life." After the New Deal took hold, many conservatives railed against it. In 1949, Strom Thurmond, the governor of South Carolina and presidential candidate the previous year, said, "Nothing could be more un-American and more devastating to a strong and virile nation than to encourage its citizens to expect government to provide security from cradle to grave."

"We must preserve the American tradition of freedom to take a chance—to lose your shirt, if you want to," Eric Johnston of the U.S. Chamber of Commerce said in 1943. "Freedom is not for weaklings," H. W. Prentis of the National Association of Manufacturers said in 1942. Only "ultra-liberal and socialistic

PLAGUES, PANDEMICS AND VIRUSES

critics" misguidedly and dangerously "put security first," thereby threatening American liberty.

For most Americans, and for most people around the world, COVID-19's lockdown exemplifies the loss of basic rights: to go where you want, see whom you want, and earn your keep.

Demonstration after demonstration against the shutdown measures were plastered on everything from Instagram to the nightly news, with scores of people—some masked, most not—carrying "Don't Tread on Me" flags as well as Confederate flags. Although many of these residents do not live in what had been Confederate states, the flag symbolizes a rebellious spirit—it's what separated us from England, but it's also what divided us during the Civil War.

Protesters march at the state capital of Olympia, Washington, to complain about orders to stay at home to avoid the spread of the COVID-19 virus. Protests like this in Kentucky resulted in spikes in virus cases.

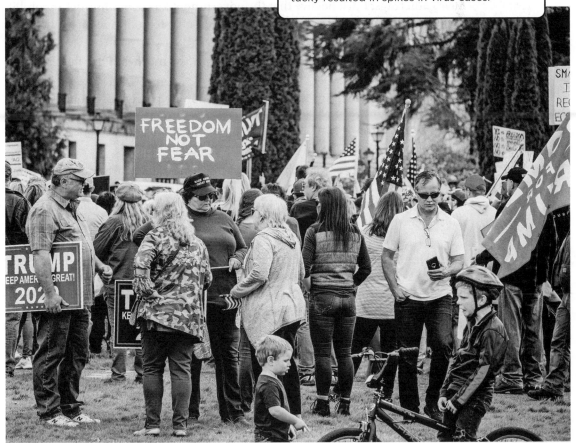

"We believe that the state governor has gone beyond his constitutional authority in shutting down businesses and ordering people to stay at home," Washington State protest organizer Tyler Miller told the BBC. In mid-March, Washington governor Jay Inslee announced an emergency proclamation that included closing restaurants and bars and banning large gatherings.

Washington protesters said that that was unconstitutional. "The state constitution says that the right of the people to peaceably assemble shall never be abridged. We believe that the … proclamations that the governor here ordered violate that."

Miller said that he was not protesting against the recommendations from the public-health bodies and respected the need to flatten the curve. ("Flattening the curve" means slowing the spread of the virus so that hospitals are not overwhelmed with too many patients at the same time.) "I even self-quarantined for 14 days.… The fact I am protesting does not mean I think it is a good idea to have gatherings, I just believe that the government has no authority to prohibit them." Throughout the crisis, Miller has been able to continue his work as an engineering technician with the U.S. Navy.

So, how does COVID-19 compare with the more familiar flu virus and the 1918 pandemic?

Seasonal flu strains kill on average about 0.1 percent of people who become infected. The 1918 flu was far more contagious and had a much higher fatality rate, around 2 percent, which sounds small but equaled tens of millions of people.

Early estimates from China about the death rate were around 2 percent, just like the 1918 outbreak, but a new report on 1,099 cases from various parts of China, published on February 28, 2020, in *The New England Journal of Medicine*, records it at 1.4 percent.

The potential financial costs and death tolls from a modern-day pandemic in the United States suggest an initial cost of several hundred billion dollars and the deaths of hundreds of thousands to several million people. Cities are likely to have greater mortality rates than rural areas. Compared to 1918, however, urban and rural areas are more connected today—this may decrease the difference in mortality rates between cities and rural areas. Similarly, a greater percentage of the U.S. population is now considered urban (about 80 percent) compared to the U.S. population at the time of the previous pandemic (51 percent in 1920).

Blaming the Asians

Meanwhile, just as the Jewish community was blamed for the Black Death, Asians as a whole are being blamed for COVID-19. In London, England,

DRACONIAN MEASURES

"Others question the cost of China's containment, and are asking if it's worth turning to draconian measures...."—*Time*, March 13, 2020

"China's coronavirus gamble: What should we learn from Beijing's draconian response to COVID-19?"—*New York Daily News*, March 15, 2020

"Chinese City Adopts Draconian Measures after a Student from New York 'Imported' Coronavirus Infecting 70 People"—*Science Times*, April 24, 2020

"Queensland's top health official lauds cooperation amid 'draconian' measures"—*News7 Australia*, April 30, 2020

The word "draconian" comes from "Draco." Draco was the first Athenian legislator in ancient Greece and was responsible for implementing a written legal code in c. 621 B.C.E. Prior to Draco, the system was one of oral law. This was an early—and brutal—manifestation of Athenian democracy.

Although the full Draconian constitution no longer exists, severe punishments were reportedly meted out to those convicted of offenses as minor as stealing an apple. It's possible that only one penalty, execution, existed for all convicted violators of the Draconian constitution, and the laws were said to be written in blood instead of ink. These legends have become part of the English language, with the adjective "draconian" referring to unusually harsh punishment. In the case of COVID-19, it usually refers to how government has responded to the pandemic by taking away people's civil liberties and is frequently quoted along with the norm in communist China and what Americans fear will become the norm in the United States.

Jonathan Mok, a 23-year-old student from Singapore, was left with multiple fractures to his face after a racist assault in London by a man shouting, "I don't want your coronavirus in my country!" Also, in Great Britain, a 24-year-old tax consultant from Thailand was attacked and robbed by a gang yelling, "Coronavirus!"

In France, Twitter users of Asian descent began the hashtag #jenesuispasunvirus—"I am not a virus." In Italy, Chinese Italian activists blamed misinformation from anti-immigration politicians on a rise of assaults on Asian people and boycotts of Chinese businesses. In the United States, Asian Americans have reported physical attacks and racial slurs.

One person, who said in a Facebook group that they suffer from asthma, said that they were followed by a group of teenage males yelling "diseased Asian" and "corona Asian." Another person said that a man pushed him off a bicycle, telling him, "You're Chinese, all Chinese people have the coronavirus."

A Korean woman, who lives in the Netherlands, said she woke up in the morning and discovered a swastika scratched in the hallway outside her home. Only her Korean family and another family, who are white and Dutch, live in the building.

In Italy, Chinese Italian activists blamed misinformation from anti-immigration politicians on a rise of assaults on Asian people and boycotts of Chinese businesses.

Fox News commentator Jesse Watters upped the ante with his demand for an apology from the Chinese: "I would like to just ask the Chinese for a formal apology," Watters said. "This coronavirus originated in China, and I have not heard one word from the Chinese. A simple 'I am sorry' would do."

As the rest of his colleagues appeared somewhat embarrassed and tried to laugh off his rant, Watters then insisted that the virus originated from the Chinese eating diseased uncooked animals.

"Let me tell you why it happened in China," he declared. "They have these markets where they were eating raw bats and snakes."

"No, Jesse," cohost Dana Perino pleaded.

"They are very hungry people," Watters continued, causing more laughter. "The Chinese communist government cannot feed the people. And they are desperate, this food is uncooked, it is unsafe. And that is why scientists believe that's where it originated from.

"And according to *The New York Times*, Dana, the Chinese government has been very deceitful and deceptive in communicating the extent of the infections to the world," Watters concluded. "So, as I said, tomorrow I will expect an apology."

Watters, meanwhile, has a history of making culturally insensitive remarks and innuendo, particularly about Asians. In a 2016 segment, Watters took to the streets of New York City's Chinatown to ask Asians—some of whom didn't speak English—if they do karate, where he can buy some homeopathic herbs for "performance," or whether he's "supposed to bow to say hello," all the while playing Carl Douglas' song "Kung Fu Fighting" in the background.

Asians around the world are suffering economically, too. Chinese-owned businesses and restaurants in particular have been hit hard by coronavirus panic. As Jenny G. Zhang wrote on *Eater.com*, the panic has had a "decidedly dehumanizing effect, reigniting old strains of racism and xenophobia that frame Chinese people as uncivilized, barbaric 'others' who bring with them dangerous, contagious diseases."

Looking for someone to blame, some misguided people have actually attacked Asian Americans, wrongfully blaming all Chinese people for the virus outbreak. Asians who are not Chinese have also been attacked.

Jiye Seong-Yu, a 29-year-old Korean interpreter who lives in the Hague, was almost punched by a white man while biking home and wrote about the incident on her Facebook page: "So yes, this kind of shit is happening. Yes people are actually physically attacking Asians. So please don't question us when we say it does," she wrote. "We're really tired of this shit."

Blaming the LGBTQ Community

Some evangelical leaders think that the LGBTQ community is somehow linked to COVID-19.

Right-wing pastor, E. W. Jackson said on his radio show that the "homovirus" is devastating the American family and society. "The last thing in the world the black community needs is more destruction of the family, more attacks on the family, and that's all this whole homosexual movement amounts to," Jackson said. "It is a virulent, violent attack. You know what? I'm going to get in trouble for this one, but this is right off the presses: It is the homovirus for the family.

"Of course, I am speaking from a spiritual and a psychological perspective," he clarified. "I hope that no one misunderstands my little putting together of two things, because you know we're talking about this coronavirus. I'm not talking about physical illness. I'm not talking about pronouncing any physical curses on people," Jackson added.

Reverend Steven Andrew said in a press release that "God's love shows it is urgent to repent, because the Bible teaches homosexuals lose their souls and God destroys LGBT societies." As pastor of USA Christian Church, Andrew is "focused on pastoring the nation to reaffirm covenant that the USA serves the Lord, with pastors nationwide," according to his website.

"Our safety is at stake, since national disobedience of God's laws brings danger and diseases, such as coronavirus, but obeying God brings covenant protection (Exodus 15:26)," Andrew said. "God protects the USA from danger as the country repents of LGBT, false gods, abortion and other sins."

Israeli Rabbi Meir Mazuz said that a recent gay pride parade was "a parade against nature, and when someone goes against nature, the one who created nature takes revenge on him." He then claimed that countries all over the world are being called to account because of their gay pride events "except for the Arab countries that don't have this evil inclination." That was why, he said—falsely suggesting that only one case of infection has occurred in the Arab world—they have not seen a spread of coronavirus.

Wash Your Hands

To fend off COVID-19, your first defense is protecting yourself against pathogens—your skin. Soap is made of molecules that have receptors at the top that are hydrophilic (meaning they like water) and bind to water in the same way that virus receptors bind to cells. The soap molecules also have hydrocarbon chains at the other end that look like a tail, which are hydrophobic (meaning they don't like water). This tail binds to oils and fats—essentially, the components of dirt. When soap, combined with water, comes into contact with dirt, the soap molecules arrange into ball-shaped formations called micelles, with heads out and tails in, almost like soldiers going into battle. Micelles then pick up the dirt and take it away.

Similarly, when you wash your hands, pathogens on your skin become surrounded by micelles. The molecule tails, because they don't like water, cram themselves into the fatty covering of certain viruses, ripping them apart.

This covering, called a lipid membrane, is what holds the virus proteins in place, allowing them to infect cells. Not all viruses have them, but COVID-19 does in addition to HIV, the Ebola virus, the Zika virus, and bacteria that attack the lungs and intestines.

It's important to thoroughly wash your hands to make sure that no traces of viruses or bacteria remain on your skin.

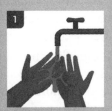

1 WET HANDS

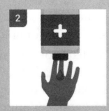

2 APPLY SOAP

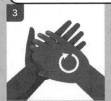

3 RUB HANDS PALM TO PALM

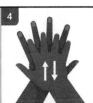

4 LATHER THE BACKS OF YOUR HANDS

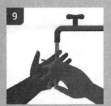

5 SCRUB BETWEEN YOUR FINGERS

6 RUB THE BACKS OF FINGERS ON THE OPPOSING PALMS

7 CLEAN THUMBS

8 WASH FINGERNAILS AND FINGERTIPS

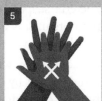

9 RINSE HANDS

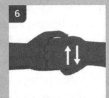

10 DRY WITH A SINGLE USE TOWEL

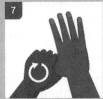

11 USE THE TOWEL TO TURN OFF THE FAUCET

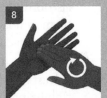

12 YOUR HANDS ARE CLEAN

APPLICATION OF HAND SANITIZER

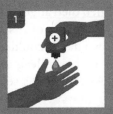

1 APPLY THE PRODUCT ON THE PALM OF ONE HAND

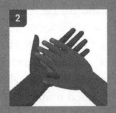

2 RUB HANDS TOGETHER

3 COVER ALL SURFACES UNTIL HANDS FEEL DRY (20 SEC)

PLAGUES, PANDEMICS AND VIRUSES

According to the CDC, this is the most effective way to wash your hands during the pandemic: "Wet your hands with clean, running water (warm or cold), turn off the tap, and apply soap. Lather your hands by rubbing them together with the soap. Be sure to lather the backs of your hands, between your fingers, and under your nails. Scrub your hands for at least 20 seconds."

The molecular tails of the soap "act like crowbars and destabilize the whole system," said Professor Pall Thordarson, acting head of chemistry at the University of New South Wales. Essential proteins spill from the ruptured membranes into the surrounding water, killing the bacteria and rendering the viruses useless.

In tandem, some soap molecules disrupt the chemical bonds that allow bacteria, viruses, and grime to stick to surfaces, lifting them off the skin. Micelles can also form around particles of dirt and fragments of viruses and bacteria, suspending them in floating cages. When you rinse your hands, all the microorganisms that have been damaged, trapped, and killed by soap molecules are washed away.

On the whole, hand sanitizers are not as reliable as soap. Sanitizers with at least 60 percent ethanol do act similarly, defeating bacteria and viruses by destabilizing their lipid membranes. (For the love of God, though, don't drink them.) However, they cannot easily remove microorganisms from the skin. Some viruses do not depend on lipid membranes to infect cells, nor do some types of bacteria that protect their delicate membranes with sturdy shields of protein and sugar. Examples include bacteria that can cause meningitis, pneumonia, diarrhea, and skin infections as well as the hepatitis A virus, poliovirus, rhinoviruses, and adenoviruses (frequent causes of the common cold).

These more resilient microbes are generally less susceptible to the chemical onslaught of ethanol and soap, but vigorous scrubbing with soap and water can still expunge these microbes from the skin, which is partly why hand washing is more effective than sanitizer. Alcohol-based sanitizer is a good backup, though, when soap and water are not accessible.

Hand washing has only been a worldwide practice relatively recently. In the 1840s, Dr. Ignaz Semmelweis, a Hungarian physician, discovered that if doctors washed their hands, far fewer women died after childbirth. At the time, microbes were not widely recognized as vectors of disease, and many doctors scoffed at the idea that washing their own hands could be responsible for avoiding their patients' deaths. Ostracized by his colleagues, Dr. Semmelweis was eventually committed to an asylum, where he was severely beaten by guards and died from infected wounds.

Florence Nightingale, an English nurse and statistician, also promoted hand washing in the mid-1800s, but it was not until the 1980s that the CDC issued the world's first nationally endorsed hand hygiene guidelines.

Washing with soap and water is one of the key public-health practices that can significantly slow the rate of a pandemic and limit the number of infections, preventing a disastrous overburdening of hospitals and clinics, but the technique works only if everyone washes their hands frequently and thoroughly: Work up a good lather, scrub your palms and the backs of your hands, interlace your fingers, rub your fingertips against your palms, and twist a soapy fist around your thumbs.

Canadian health officer Bonnie Henry said it best: "Wash your hands like you've been chopping jalapeños and you need to change your contacts."

Social Distancing

Saying it is easier than doing it. The difficulties lie in timing and compliance. Analysis of when cities in 1918 closed schools, saloons, and theaters; banned public events; and urged social distancing and the like demonstrated that intervening early, before a virus spreads throughout the community, did flatten the curve. That's why states across the country closed down to one degree or another until the numbers of fatalities decrease for fourteen consecutive days.

However, this raises another issue: compliance. The need for early intervention was well known in 1918. The Army surgeon general demanded that "influenza be kept out" of the basic-training camps, where new soldiers were being prepared to fight in World War I. "Epidemics of the disease can often be prevented," he said, "but once established they cannot well be stopped." He barred civilians from the camps and ordered that soldiers entering them be quarantined, soldiers showing symptoms be isolated, and whole units be quarantined if several soldiers were ill.

COVID-19's average incubation period is more than double that of influenza's, so compliance may have to be sustained for months....

However, an Army study found no difference in morbidity and mortality between camps that did and did not follow orders because, over time, most became sloppy. Further investigation found that only a tiny number of camps rigidly enforced measures.

In 1918, many cities imposed restrictions, lifted them too soon, then reimposed them. COVID-19's average incubation period is more than double that of influenza's, so compliance may have to be sustained for months, and openings and closings may also have to be repeated. For the public to comply over time, they will have to be led, inspired, or compelled. That brings us back to the most important lesson of 1918: tell the truth.

Remember that in 1918, under pressure to maintain morale during World War I, neither national nor local government officials told the truth. The disease was called the "Spanish flu"—a kind of exotic otherness that made it sound like it would stay in the Iberian Peninsula, plus the statement from Health Commissioner Dr. Royal S. Copeland, who said that "there was no cause for alarm over the presence of the disease."

One of the precautions for reducing the spread of COVID-19 is to try to keep a distance of six feet (two meters) between yourself and other people. This has been tough on many people. Human beings are, after all, social creatures.

COVID-19, like all pandemics, doesn't announce when it's about to strike, so most people—aside from the ones who study it for a living—are caught by surprise when it does, and massive pandemics are usually spread far enough apart that those who can remember one are usually gone by the time the next one hits. Combine that with the idea of a pandemic being something from medieval times, with carts full of dead bodies, or the plot to films like *I Am Legend*: leadership that wavers between telling people it's the same as the flu, then proceeding with state lockdowns; leadership that agrees it's a pandemic but incites citizens to protest the lockdowns; and the fact that the sun is shining, birds are chirping, and warm weather is coming—it can't be a pandemic if we don't see anyone dying in the streets, right?

Also, social distancing—which is standing at least 6 feet apart—has meant businesses closing, except for the ones deemed essential. This has also meant that people have lost their livelihood, and when that happens, fear begins—and we've seen in the past what fear leads to.

COVID-19 Strikes the Poor

Nonwhite groups in the United States have a greater chance of dying because roughly 90 percent of all nonwhites live in urban areas (compared to about 77 percent of whites). This correlates with lower-income individuals being more likely to die—nonwhite (excluding Asians) households have a lower median income ($30,858 in 2005) compared to white households ($50,784 in 2005). Similarly, only 10 percent of whites were below the poverty level in 2005 compared to more than 20 percent for various minority groups (except Asian).

This also means that people of color are likely to have, on average, less access to quality health care. Nearly 19 percent of city populations have zero health coverage. The question remains as to the affordability of health care and whether

---

BURYING THE DEAD

Health care only matters if systems are in place to ensure that a pandemic will not knock it out and prevent the rapid disposal of the dead in the cities. Such an event happened in Philadelphia, where deaths occurring after a parade held during the 1918 pandemic were exacerbated by medical services sent overseas during World War I. More than 12,000 people died.

---

free-service health-care providers, clinics, and emergency rooms (the most likely choices for the uninsured) are able to handle victims of the pandemic.

In an op-ed for *The New York Times*, writer Charles Blow—himself a man of color—offered the following:

> People like to say that the coronavirus is no respecter of race, class or country, that the disease COVID-19 is mindless and will infect anybody it can.
>
> In theory, that is true. But, in practice, in the real world, this virus behaves like others, screeching like a heat-seeking missile toward the most vulnerable in society. And this happens not because it prefers them, but because they are more exposed, more fragile and more ill.
>
> What the vulnerable portion of society looks like varies from country to country, but in America, that vulnerability is highly intersected with race and poverty. Early evidence from cities and states already shows that black people are disproportionately affected by the virus in devastating ways. As ProPublica reported, in Milwaukee County, Wis., as of Friday morning, 81 percent of the deaths were black people. Black people make up only 26 percent of that county.
>
> As for Chicago, WBEZ reported Sunday that "70 percent of COVID-19 deaths are black," and pointed out about surrounding Cook County, "While black residents make up only 23 percent of the population in the county, they account for 58 percent of the COVID-19 deaths."
>
> *The Detroit News* reported last week, "At least 40 percent of those killed by the novel coronavirus in Michigan so far are black, a percentage that far exceeds the proportion of African-Americans in the Detroit region and state."
>
> If this pattern holds true across other states and cities, this virus could have a catastrophic impact on black people in this country.
>
> And yet, we are still not seeing an abundance of news coverage or national governmental response that center on these racial disparities. Many states haven't even released race-specific data on cases and deaths. The federal government hasn't either.
>
> Partly for this reason, we are left with deceptive and deadly misinformation. The perception that this is a jet-setters' disease, or a spring breakers' disease, or a "Chinese virus" as President Trump

likes to say, must be laid to rest. The idea that this virus is an equal-opportunity killer must itself be killed.

And, we must dispense with the callous message that the best defense we have against the disease is something that each of us can control: We can all just stay home and keep social distance.

As a report last month by the Economic Policy Institute pointed out, "less than one in five black workers and roughly one in six Hispanic workers are able to work from home."

As the report pointed out, "Only 9.2 percent of workers in the lowest quartile of the wage distribution can telework, compared with 61.5 percent of workers in the highest quartile."

Until April 10, 2020, the death toll in St. Louis, Missouri, had only been black residents—then, on that day, a Latina woman in her fifties, a white man in his nineties, and a woman in her eighties whose race wasn't identified were reported to have died of the virus.

Statistics show that the disproportionate impacts of coronavirus on the black population continue to be felt across the country. St. Louis is not unique. Lori Lightfoot, the mayor of Chicago—where 72 percent of the deaths have been black residents—told CBS's *Face the Nation* that COVID-19 was devastating African American communities. These communities comprise 30 percent of Chicago's population. An inequity in access to health care and economic opportunity due to the history of systemic racism in the United States has made many African Americans far more vulnerable to the virus. Black adults are more likely to be uninsured and also suffer from higher rates of obesity, diabetes, and asthma—conditions that make them more susceptible to COVID-19."

They also often report that medical professionals take their ailments less seriously when they seek treatment. "The answer that we believe is right is because of the underlying conditions that people of color and particularly black folks suffer from, whether it's diabetes, heart disease, upper respiratory illnesses, the kind of things that we've been talking about for a long time that plague black Chicago, that lead to life expectancy gaps," Lightfoot said.

One particularly vulnerable community is the poor community, especially because private health care is expensive and inaccessible to many, while public hospitals lag behind in quality. According to the U.S. Census, in 2018 Native Americans had the highest poverty rate among minorities: 25.4 percent (over 700,000 people) lived below the poverty line. Immigrants living in the United States without legal permission are particularly vulnerable in the COVID-19 pandemic crisis: federal-relief efforts are not reaching this population.

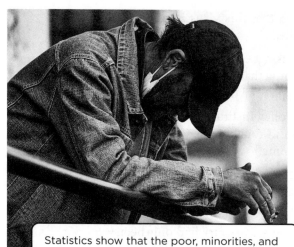

Statistics show that the poor, minorities, and immigrants in America are disproportionately affected by COVID-19.

Meanwhile, stimulus checks sent by the federal government to help ease the financial burden of tax-paying Americans were able to bypass easing the financial burden of tax-paying immigrants by insisting that checks only go to people with Social Security numbers. Instead of an SSN, many immigrants have an ITIN: individual tax identification number.

"At the federal level what we are pushing is that the ITIN, or the individual taxpayer identification number, and the individuals who pay taxes be included in the stimulus," said Angelica Salas, executive director of the Coalition for Humane Immigrant Rights.

However, California started taking applications for a onetime cash benefit of $500 per undocumented adult, capped at $1,000 per household. California has an estimated two million undocumented immigrants.

An estimated eleven million immigrants in the United States are undocumented, many of whom are now working the essential jobs. The Migration Policy Institute estimates that six million immigrant workers (a figure that does not take into account legal status) are in jobs on the frontlines of COVID-19 response, while another six million are in industries hardest hit by the pandemic. In normal times, undocumented labor is a pillar of the U.S. economy. In these extraordinary times, immigrant advocates say that lawmakers must recognize the contributions that essential undocumented workers are making.

Meanwhile, according to the ACLU and National Immigration Law Center, the Families First Act excluded tens of millions of people (among them Deferred Action for Childhood Arrivals [DACA] recipients and Temporary Protected Status holders) from testing and treatment by making it unavailable under emergency Medicaid. The stimulus package included funding for testing at community health centers, which undocumented immigrants can go to for services regardless of their status. The catch is the fear that their undocumented status—especially if they test positive—will get them deported, so the virus keeps spreading.

COVID-19 Strikes the Rich

"Wealth is the vector" is what sociologist Tressie McMillan Cottom tweeted on March 24, 2020, in reference to the spread of COVID-19. By this,

McMillan Cottom meant that while money doesn't cause outbreaks, it does spark them in isolated areas. It happened during the Black Death, it happened during the Great Plague of London, and it happened from Sun Valley, Idaho, to the north shore of Lake Superior.

In contrast to the poor getting sick because they're living in poor conditions with poor health, the rich have caused "super-spreading events," like in the wealthy town of Westport, Connecticut. About 50 guests gathered on March 5 at a lavish home for a fortieth birthday party with a guest list that included a friend visiting from South Africa. They shared food and viruses. Then, the party ended.

Now known as Party Zero, it showed how the "haves" can spread COVID-19 to the four corners of the globe—or just in one town. Westport, population 28,000, did not have a single known case of COVID-19 on the day of the party. It had 85 cases eleven days later.

All over the United States, people were escaping cities for the country. Some of them owned second homes there; others are renting at exorbitant prices. They could do this because, as per Charles Blow's op-ed, "61.5 percent of workers in the highest quartile" can work remotely.

Since no federal guidelines had been put into place about domestic travel, locals became citizens on patrol. In Oregon's Skamania County, signs spray-painted with "STAY OUT—LOCALS ONLY" were posted around town. (The local hardware store also offered free toilet paper with the purchase of a firearm.)

In the outer banks of North Carolina, police set up a checkpoint to turn back anyone, even a homeowner who is not a full-time resident. The island of North Haven, Maine, banned all visitors, including people who own property.

Locals in Vinalhaven, Maine, tried to forcibly quarantine three men whose car had New

> In contrast to the poor getting sick because they're living in poor conditions with poor health, the rich have caused "super-spreading events"....

Jersey plates by downing a tree across their street, but officials on Vinalhaven—an island only accessible by ferry—said that the incident wasn't representative of the tight-knit community of about one thousand year-round residents, who have come together during the global COVID-19 pandemic.

"To have those stories out there at a time like this only incites fear. We're trying to comfort people to some extent and come together as a community," Vinalhaven town manager Andrew Dorr told the *Bangor Daily News*.

After the cable went out at the house where the New Jersey plates were spotted, one of the three men staying there went to check out what was wrong, only to find that a tree had been cut down and dragged across the roadway leading to the house, according to the Knox County Sheriff's Office.

"While investigating the downed tree, a neighbor started yelling at him and a group of people showed up and began to gather around. Believing the group may be there to harm him, [he] fled to his residence and told his roommates what he had found," a statement from the Knox County Sheriff's Office read. "The trio decided to stay put in the residence, utilized a VHF radio to hail the Coast Guard for assistance, they had no other means of communication, and utilized their drone to keep an eye on the group until law enforcement could arrive to help them."

Police were unable to identify or locate the group of people who cut down the tree and allegedly yelled at the out-of-state resident. They learned that some island residents believed that the individuals needed to be quarantined because they came from out of state and could have COVID-19.

Deputies learned that the trio had been residing on Vinalhaven for about a month, meaning that they had been on the island prior to the state issuing any guidance surrounding travel restrictions. None have any symptoms consistent with COVID-19, according to the sheriff's office.

Most outsiders aren't thinking about how fear had affected these communities. They also didn't know the size of the hospitals and the limitations of the supply chain for food.

COVID-19 will spread through retirement homes, as it has in Lander, Wyoming, and decimate the disproportionately elderly populations that fill these rural states. It will spread through Native American reservations, where many extended families live together in one home. It will strike the rural South, where people are often uninsured and living in poverty. It will come to the dozens of counties whose hospitals have closed as their governors continue to refuse Medicaid expansion.

ANDREW CUOMO RISES TO THE CHALLENGE

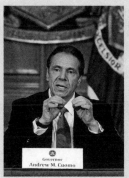

New York's Governor Andrew Cuomo.

New York governor Andrew Cuomo, with his furrowed brow and brusque manner, was never America's sweetheart. He didn't want to be. He sparred with opponents, a favorite being New York City mayor Bill de Blasio, and pulled no punches, but then, COVID-19 hit—something that even he was powerless against. It was not a position that Cuomo—the son of former New York governor Mario Cuomo—was used to being in, and yet, as they say, he leaned into it.

As with President Trump, Cuomo's press conferences were held daily. Both men were clearly the stars, but each struck a different tone. Cuomo admitted he didn't have all the answers. He again pulled no punches when it came to the federal government. The hashtag #cuomocrush started trending, and it wasn't solely in reference to his conventionally good-looking brother, CNN anchor Chris Cuomo. Andrew and Chris became to the media what the Property Brothers were to home flippers.

According to genomic analysis of New York infections, it's likely the virus was present in New York in mid-February, weeks prior to the first confirmed cases. "We get numbers in from every hospital at night, which tells you about the death rate and the infection rate. So that is what every day looks like ... *Groundhog Day*," Cuomo said, referring to the Bill Murray film where he lives the same day over and over again.

As COVID-19 works its way through the United States, millions of Americans face stay-at-home orders, but whether you have to stay in or can go outside depends largely on which state you live in.

An Interview with Dr. Anthony Fauci

President Trump's daily press briefings caused their own kind of spillover event. Dr. Anthony Fauci has been the head of the NIH's National Institute of

Allergy and Infectious Diseases since 1984 and had worked under six presidential administrations beginning with Ronald Reagan during the AIDS epidemic, when his became a household name. On the left, he's "America's Doctor." On the right, he's working with Bill Gates to undermine the president and profit on the development of a vaccine. Here is Dr. Fauci in his own words for *Plagues, Pandemics, and Viruses*:

On His Background

I was a Classics major in high school, and I was a Classics major in college. And I also had a degree of scientific interest and aptitude that I didn't realize I had. And my interest in Classics means that I'm very much a "people person"—interested in the human species and how that interacts with history, and how that interacts in many ways. So what I did when I was trying to figure out what I was going to do with my life, and I thought one of the ways to combine a deep interest in humans with a career that might have me interacting with people as opposed to products, as opposed to money, as opposed to gimmicks, would be to be very closely involved with people at the same time as pursuing a scientific career. To me the most obvious profession that fulfilled both those criteria was to be a physician. And that's the reason why I transitioned from being a Classics major interested in philosophy, history, languages, Greek, Latin, to somebody who not only became a physician, but a physician-scientist. So, it seemed to be a natural evolution in my career. The fact that I became a researcher was just something that happened, later on, after my pure medical training—because when I graduated from medical school I did the usual multi-years of internship and residency, and then I did a fellowship at the NIH, and it was that fellowship that put me in contact with fundamental, basic, and clinical science, and I found out that I was not only good at it, I liked it! So that's when my career veered more toward doing clinical research.

And then what happened was I was involved in both infectious diseases and immunology. I was, I guess you could say, over-trained because I was trained and board certified in both infectious diseases and in immunology—namely the interface between the body's immune system that protects you against infection and a variety of infections that are out there. And I did that for a few years until my life and the direction of my career was dramatically changed when they reported the first cases of what turned out to be HIV/AIDS in the summer of 1981. And that was my firsthand experience. I love history and I would read history of outbreaks like the pandemic flu of 1918 and the plagues of the thirteenth and fourteenth centuries and the measles outbreak among the Aztecs.... That always fascinated me, but I didn't think that's what I would be doing with my life until HIV/AIDS came along, which was an outbreak that was insidious in its recognition and in its onset, which over the last 39 years has turned out to be one of the most impactful outbreaks of infectious disease in history, if you look at the total number of people have been infected, and the total number of them who died and the total number that are currently infected.

So then as I went from being a researcher—fundamentally patients, fundamentally basic research—to 1984, when I became the director of the Institute. And it was then because I was anchored in HIV/AIDS I became not only

The director of the National Institutes of Allergy and Infectious Diseases since 1984, Dr. Anthony Fauci is an immunologist who was called on to lead President Trump's Coronavirus Task Force in January 2020.

acutely aware of but fascinated with the concept that outbreaks have always occurred in our history. Profound, impactful outbreaks occur at intervals far enough between each other that generationally most people don't remember them. There aren't very many people around today who were there when the 1918 pandemic came, and there are a number of people, but not a lot of people, who were there when the polio scare was around, when we were children and everybody was afraid of being paralyzed from polio.

On Outbreaks

Outbreaks have occurred forever. They occur now and they will continue to occur. If you look at what I've been through you know

I've been through the outbreak of AIDS in the beginning. Then there was the threat of pre-pandemic flus that fortunately never happened. There was Zika, there was Ebola, there was the resurgence of measles, so it's something that's there with us all the time. People used to ask me, "What is your biggest nightmare?" If you go back and look at my quotes from 25, 20, 15, 10, 5 years ago, it was the outbreak of a brand-new virus that's respiratory-borne, easily transmissible, and has a high degree of morbidity and mortality that could be influenza or that could be a virus that's not influenza but that's still a respiratory-borne virus. And here we are in 2020 in the middle of what's going to turn out to be an historic pandemic.

On Vaccines

Well, history tells us that there are some vaccines that if you induce a less than optimal response you can actually have the paradoxical effect of when someone gets infected after they're vaccinated. Namely, the vaccine wasn't effective enough to prevent infection but it did induce a suboptimal response, and paradoxically that antibody response, that suboptimal, could actually bind to the virus and enhance its ability to make you very sick. We have evidence of that with Dengue. We have evidence of that with respiratory syncytial virus. This has occurred and can occur, so the one thing you don't want to do is you don't want to give a vaccine to tens if not hundreds of millions of people, and you don't know if in fact it's safe and you don't know if it's effective.

Where He Was When He Heard about the Virus

I was sitting right where I'm sitting right now, in my office. I think it came out there was an announcement, I can't even remember whether it was from WHO or it was just from news reports, that there was a strange new virus that was seen in China. And then a few days later they identified it as a coronavirus. I mean, I thought it was a coronavirus as soon as I heard the way it was acting, because we'd had experience with coronaviruses before. Mainly SARS in 2002 which was a coronavirus just like this novel coronavirus now. It infected eight thousand people and killed almost eight hundred with a fatality rate of about 10 percent. It was not nearly as efficiently transmitted as this virus is. This virus is highly efficiently transmitted in addition to having a serious degree of morbidity and mortality. We also had experience with MERS, the Middle East respiratory syndrome,which came in 2012. That didn't infect as many people. That had about a 30 percent fatality. Neither of those were as efficiently transmitted as this one. Very soon as we got into January and February. It became clear from China and then from Europe and now from the United States, that this is a very very transmissible virus, unfortunately for us.

On Viruses

Viruses mutate and figure out ways to survive. So, if you want to make it a metaphor, you could say they're very clever and the tool they have is their ability to rapidly replicate. And when you're rapidly replicating and you have the capability of mutating, you can change. You know, you can change your clothes, you can change your appearance; you can do a lot of things. So, you know you always have people saying viruses are really smart. Well, they're not. They don't have a brain. But what they do have is the capability of rapidly replicating and mutating.

On Whether Working on SARS Has Helped Here

Of course, we're using similar platforms, and the more experience you have with a given vaccine platform—we used the DNA platform for SARS, but we're using a message RNA platform here—the better. And some companies are using a DNA platform. So yes, any experience you have with a related virus, particularly a virus that's of the same class or family, it always puts you in good stead for the next time you experience it, always.

On What Future Generations Should Know

Well, first of all, I think future generations, even the current generation, should know what I've been saying for all of my professional career: that pandemics have always occurred. You know in history we tend to forget about them. Pandemics occur now and pandemics will occur in the future. They're unpredictable. We don't know when, they have no rhythm to them, but they do occur. Seventy-five percent of all new infections evolved from jumping from an animal species, very similar to what we've seen here with the COVID-19. And one needs to be prepared. The only trouble is when you're in-between pandemics, to the get the momentum to prepare for a pandemic is often not optimal because people have other priorities of dealing with things that are currently going on. So preparing for something that has not happened yet is often very difficult. We've tried to do that with our pandemic preparedness plan, but often that falls short. And then you have to play catch-up when it really happens.

Dr. Fauci also said that we're moving at "warp speed" from a virology perspective to develop a vaccine. More on that in the next section.

Vaccines

In the winter of 1976, a novel influenza caused hundreds of respiratory infections at Fort Dix, a New Jersey Army post. This virus appeared to be closely related to the 1918 flu pandemic that killed over one hundred million people globally and struck Army bases filled to the brim because of World War I. These coincidences caused health officials to start planning for what could conceivably become large and deadly outbreaks, if not an actual pandemic, as the cold weather progressed.

The WHO took a "wait and see" attitude to track the number of emerging infections before crying, "Pandemic!" However, then president Gerald Ford's administration took a different tack—a zealous campaign to vaccinate every American STAT. In late March, President Ford announced the government's plan to vaccinate "every man, woman, and child in the United States." Emergency legislation for the "National Swine Flu Immunization Program" was signed shortly thereafter on April 15, 1976, and six months after the virus first appeared, high-profile photos of celebrities and even President Ford were photographed getting vaccinated. This was the dawn of a new day in modern medicine.

Except that it wasn't. Within ten months, nearly 25 percent of Americans, or 45 million people, were vaccinated, but due to the pressure of creating immunizations for a brand-new virus, the government used a weakened "live" virus for the vaccine instead of an inactivated or "killed" virus. With President Ford's reelection campaign looming, the vaccination campaign began to be seen as politically motivated rather than in the public's best interest. It turned out that the flu wasn't even related to the 1918 virus, and, indeed, those who were infected with the flu only suffered from a mild illness, while more than 450 people who were vaccinated developed Guillain-Barré syndrome. (GBS is the paralyzing disorder researchers now believe was the cause of FDR's paralysis.)

At a media event on March 2, 2020, President Trump pressured the heads of various pharmaceutical companies into giving a definite timeline for a COVID-19 vaccine. Producing a vaccine means conducting trial after trial before it can be sent out into the world, so they had no definite answer. The president also asked whether the flu vaccine could be used to combat coronavirus.

The answer to that is no—most assuredly because during a briefing on March 2, WHO officials said that they didn't know how COVID-19 behaves; it's not like influenza, and they didn't know how it was transmitted and what treatments would work to keep it from spreading. This was in stark contrast to the assurances that it only spreads through close contact.

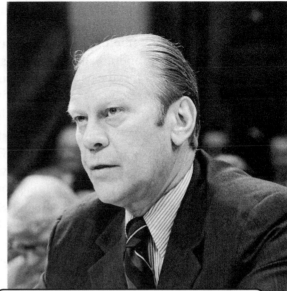

President Gerald Ford ordered an aggressive vaccination program to stop the spread of a 1976 outbreak of a virus that started in Fort Dix, New Jersey. He might have jumped the gun, however, when it turned out that the flu variant was not that severe.

They also raised the topic of the virus's mortality rate. "Globally, about 3.4% of reported COVID-19 cases have died," WHO director-general Tedros Adhanom Ghebreyesus said from WHO's headquarters in Geneva, Switzerland. In comparison, a seasonal flu generally kills far fewer than 1 percent of those infected, he said.

It was a dangerous way to prove the point that vaccines take time. According to Dr. Fauci:

> Vaccines are given to healthy people to prevent them from getting sick. So paramount then in all vaccines is safety and whether it works. So, in order to prove that, most of the time that takes several years to do. If you look at the history of how you develop vaccines when you're in an emergency situation like this, I think we are going faster than we have ever gone in the history of vaccinology.

> It was only 62 days from the time that the sequence of the [SARS-CoV-2] virus was identified to the time we went into Phase I Trial.

But since safety is as important in many respects as efficacy because you don't want to hurt anybody, that process takes several months. So the fastest that we can go is about a year to a year-and-a-half. That's warp speed compared to historically. And that's just the nature of needing to identify, prove safety, proof efficacy and make enough vaccine to distribute. That's just the reality of what we have available to us.

A government-funded study found that patients who took remdesivir—the drug that prevents SARS-CoV-2 from replicating—recovered faster than patients who did not. It improved recovery time for coronavirus patients from 15 to 11 days. That's similar to the effect that Tamiflu has on the flu. Tamiflu also doesn't cure patients quickly but can reduce how long they are sick. "The data shows that remdesivir has a clear-cut, significant, positive effect in diminishing the time to recovery," said Dr. Fauci.

About 1,090 people participated in the trial internationally, Fauci said, calling it "the first truly high-powered randomized placebo-controlled trial." The U.S. Food and Drug Administration made plans to announce an emergency-use authorization for remdesivir, according to *The New York Times*.

A government-funded study found that patients who took remdesivir—the drug that prevents SARS-CoV-2 from replicating—recovered faster than patients who did not.

Though promising, CNN senior medical correspondent Elizabeth Cohen said that it was important to clarify that remdesivir is not a cure. People taking this drug still died. "There is a legitimate fear that people will hear about this drug and will think, 'Oh my goodness, there is a cure. We don't need to worry about it. We don't need to social distance,'" she said. "That's not the case. It cut the duration of the illness basically by four days. That's important and it shows that the drug works and it allows scientists to do further research in this area. But we haven't seen remdesivir save lives yet. People are still taking this drug and dying. That's still happening. So we need to keep that in mind as we talk more about this drug."

The WHO

In an abrupt about-face concerning his feelings toward the way China handled COVID-19 (one tweet had said that China "has everything under control"), President Trump announced on April 14 that he was halting funding to the WHO.

At more than $400 million per year, the United States contributes more to the international organization than any other country. While the medical community—and scores of leaders around the world—said that the move would undercut global efforts to combat a pandemic reaching its peak, Trump said that denying funding would hold the WHO accountable.

> The World Health Organization (WHO) is a United Nations agency with headquarters in Geneva, Switzerland. In 2020, President Trump, critical of the WHO response to COVID-19, stopped U.S. payments to the organization.

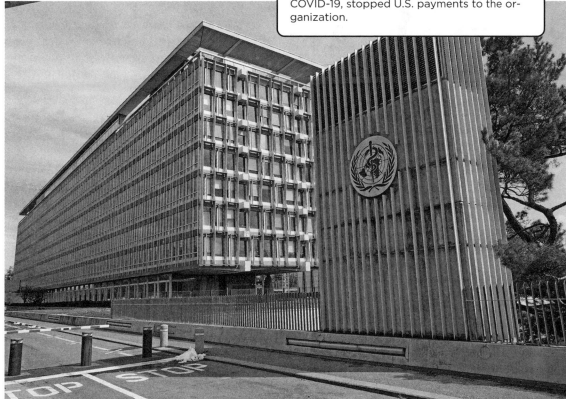

Trump accused the WHO of "severely mismanaging and covering up the spread of the coronavirus" and called its opposition to U.S. travel restrictions on China in the outbreak's early months "disastrous."

"The WHO was willfully working with the [Chinese Communist Party] to mislead the rest of the world as to what was going on," said Jason Miller, a 2016 Trump campaign senior communications adviser. Miller went on to say that conservatives have always held a degree of suspicion toward international organizations that receive U.S. money, such as the United Nations.

"Fighting a global pandemic requires international cooperation and reliance on science and data," said Patrice Harris, president of the American Medical Association, who urged the administration to reconsider.

Ironically, earlier that day, one of Trump's top health officials praised Chinese officials for swiftly alerting the United States to the virus in early January. "Now, some of the assessments that the Chinese made at that time, were obviously not accurate," said Robert Redfield, director of the CDC, on SiriusXM's "Doctor Radio" show. "But you know, it's a testament to them that within a short period of time, as you know, they identified a new coronavirus, which they basically almost immediately shared online, and allowed us to develop the diagnostic test … that gave us eyes on this outbreak."

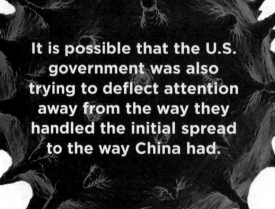

It is possible that the U.S. government was also trying to deflect attention away from the way they handled the initial spread to the way China had.

Many Trump supporters agreed that the WHO should not get any more money from the United States until the organization's director, Dr. Tedros Adhanom Ghebreyesus, steps down.

This is in tandem with conspiracy theories about COVID-19. The office of the director of national intelligence said that it had ruled out the possibility of the virus being man-made but was still investigating the precise source of the global pandemic.

PLAGUES, PANDEMICS AND VIRUSES

Scientific evidence pointed to the different conclusion that the coronavirus was transmitted from animals to humans. That is the way it's been spread for a millennia and the way it will probably continue to be spread for millennia. The lab theory, while possible, is unlikely and difficult to prove, but the "escape from a lab" conspiracy pits the coronavirus in a moral struggle against communism rather than as a matter of public health. When it comes to battling COVID-19, it seems, you're either with the communists or against them.

Trump, however, claimed to have seen evidence to support the theory that the origin was an infectious disease lab in Wuhan and said that the United States now "is finding how it came out."

"It's a terrible thing that happened," the president said. "Whether they made a mistake or whether it started off as a mistake and then they made another one, or did somebody do something on purpose?"

The intel statement said that the federal agencies concur "with the wide scientific consensus that the COVID-19 virus was not manmade or genetically modified. The IC will continue to rigorously examine emerging information and intelligence to determine whether the outbreak began through contact with infected animals or if it was the result of an accident at a laboratory in Wuhan."

It is possible that the U.S. government was also trying to deflect attention away from the way it handled the initial spread to the way China had responded. In addition to the lab theories, Trump had also threatened to sue China, joined on April 28 by the state of Missouri, holding China and a series of state and nonstate health agencies "responsible for the enormous death, suffering, and economic losses they inflicted on the world, including Missourians."

How to Stay Healthy

Epidemiologist Anita Ghatak has this advice:

In the absence of a vaccine or proven effective treatment, the key basic strategy to staying healthy would be to limit (or ideally, prevent) exposure. The recommendations are:

- Stay at home.
- Limit travel to include only essential activities (such as getting food and medicine).
- Social distancing: Do not allow anyone normally not residing in your home to enter your home or to have any contact with your immediate family members. This includes your grandparents, aunts, uncles, cousins, friends, your child's girlfriend/boyfriend, or neighbors, to name a

few. This also includes personal physical contact—no hugs, kisses, handshakes, fist bumps, or high fives. This is a critical and essential component of social distancing, as any exposure (intentional or unintentional) that these individuals may have had in the last 14 days with others can affect the health and wellness of you and your family. Because it is impractical to conduct the contact tracing of all those you may encounter, it is better to have a no-contact approach.

- Keep a minimum of a six-foot distance between you and nonfamily members at all times; this includes during outdoor activities that have been deemed safe and allowable by the local or state authorities (such as walks, bike rides, or jogging).

- After exposure, wash your hands with soap and water for a minimum of 20 seconds. Any soap will effectively kill the virus, provided the duration and technique of handwashing is sufficient. Antibacterial soap is not necessary. In the absence of soap and water, hand sanitizer with a greater than 60 percent alcohol content is a good temporary measure, but at the first possible opportunity, hands should be washed with soap and water.

- Limit contact with items from the outside environment, such as mail, deliveries, takeout food, and the like. When these items come into your home, good preventive measures would call for quarantining of items for the appropriate amount of time for the virus to die off the given surface and/or disinfecting the surfaces. If the items cannot be disposed of, consider disinfecting them. If, for any reason, a person who does not reside in your home comes into your home (such as a service worker or health-care worker), disinfect surfaces that he/she may have touched or come into contact with (like doorknobs and handles, remote controls, phones, tabletops, and faucets).

- Wear a mask in situations where you may be in the presence of others where social distancing may be difficult to maintain. Certainly, the most effective are N95 masks or surgical masks, should you already own one. However, given the current shortage of masks for health-care providers, the public is asked not to purchase these masks but instead to create homemade masks. Certain fabrics are more effective than others. The most effective materials are tightly woven and are not transparent or sheer. An additional barrier, such as a coffee filter or a paper towel, may be inserted between the layers of fabric. Those wearing masks need to realize that these homemade masks are not intended as a measure of protection from infection. Rather, these masks are to *slow* the transmission from you to others in the event that you are infected and asymptomatic and are unaware of your illness. A mask is not an excuse to resume normal activities and should not be cause for relaxing social distancing restrictions.

- Cover your mouth and nose when sneezing or coughing with the crook of your elbow, not with your hands or into the air. Good practice would be to immediately wash your hands and throw away tissues if used.

- Gloves may add a level of protection if used correctly, but without truly understanding the potential for cross-contamination, they may cause a greater potential for spread, not containment.

- After any and all exposure, prior to entering your home, remember not to touch anything (but if you do, simply disinfect it) and remove all contaminated clothing items, placing them directly in the washing machine to wash in hot water and detergent. This may require you to remove clothing while in view of other family members, depending upon the location of your washing machine. You may wish to ask family to give you a few moments of privacy and/or cover your body with a robe or towel while walking to the bathroom for your shower/bath. Keep in mind that the robe and towel used as a cover will then also be contaminated and will need to be washed as well. Shoes should be kept in a remote location, perhaps outside, in the garage, or in the mudroom, to avoid spreading the virus to the interior surfaces of your home.

Essential workers: follow steps outlined above and any or all of the following:

- Be vigilant about wearing PPE at all times when at work and follow all guidelines appropriate to your workplace.

- Diligently wash hands throughout the day at work and at home. Wash hands prior to leaving work and then upon returning home.

- Social distancing within the home: stay/sleep in separate quarters and limit physical contact for added security measures if warranted by the nature of your work.

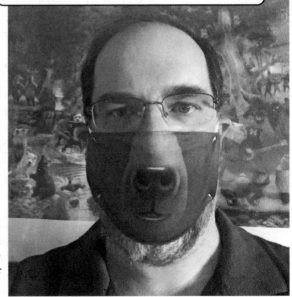

Hey, if you have to wear a mask, you might as well have fun with it! Many people are buying custom masks to wear in public places.

- If a safer home environment for a loved one is available (i.e., one with lower or no exposure), consider sending family members to those locations. This may include sending children or parents to live temporarily at some distance, but this is safer for all involved.

- Use good judgment and always opt for safe, conservative measures over potentially reckless ones.

A Nurse's Story

Jeanette Mallett, RN, talked about working at Hartford, Connecticut's Medical Oncology & Hematology Infusion Suite during the pandemic:

> I went from not being worried about it in the sense that I'm 45, it'll suck but it'll be OK—I was more worried about my parents. Now they're doing OK because they're finally listening to me. They're finally ordering groceries. I saw them almost two weeks ago. I stayed downstairs. In the car I took two masks from work—one for myself and one for my father, who has cancer.
>
> But more and more young people are getting it and ending up in the hospital and dying. I don't know if they have other things going on, if they're smokers.
>
> Our entire surgical unit is completely shut down unless it's emergency surgery. Our surgical nurses were told, "You are now taking care of COVID-19 patients."
>
> My friend, Rachel, bought me ten packs of masks. And I'm OK with rationing, but you should have a new mask every day. N95s are essentially almost airtight. They suck to wear. They're uncomfortable, they're very tight to your face, it's not as easy to breathe normally. Every year we're required to do fit testing. So the hospital spends money on N95s, but when we're in a situation where we need them, training for how to put them on and take them off, we're being asked to reuse them.
>
> I also get really angry at the leadership at my hospital. The CEOs are doing a job that I would not want to do, but at the same time they spend money on the dumbest shit. We're under the Hartford Health Care Umbrella. They took artwork down that was donated by a patient's family and they put up ugly custom Hartford Health Care wallpaper. They spend money on that, but they don't think

of the janitors that are cleaning the rooms that might contract COVID-19.

[Hartford Health Care] also created a COVID-19 command center to call if you think you've been exposed. I feel like the command center is being inconsistent in what they're telling everyone. One of our doctors had two friends over for dinner, and one of the friends ended up at Yale [New Haven Hospital]. They told the doctor to stay home till he got the test. It came back positive, but he had no symptoms, so they told him he could come back to work.

I take care of immune-compromised people. One of our patients with lung cancer is now in the hospital with COVID. The nurse who was taking care of her was sent home for two weeks. That doctor should've been sent home. Why are some sent home but others aren't? Don't we have a moral responsibility?

I got a lot of pushback about wearing PPE (personal protective equipment). It lessens the odds that you and the patient are going to get sick, especially if you're taking care of a COVID patient. I got a lot of pushback about it. And now we're all wearing masks. We were given one to use until it gets soiled. One of the girls, her mother made us reusable ones, so we have those. Anytime you're going in a room where you're putting on PPE, the mask should be changed.

When I leave work, I take a plastic bag and I fill it with a few CaviWipes. And I scrub my shoes before I get into my car. And I'm doing this with gloves on. When I get home, I put on a new pair of gloves, wipe down everything in my car, take my sneakers off, put on a new pair of gloves and clean the doorknobs. I take a shower as soon as I get home, too.

I feel badly for those who work in the grocery who also don't have this stuff. All those cashiers, everyone should be wearing masks. Everything should be wiped down. I want to see them cleaning those grocery carts. It's not like me where I have a sink by me all the time. Hand washing is the best thing that you can do. A cashier does not have that access. I'm a pretty vigorous hand scrubber.

Cancer during COVID-19

Disease doesn't stop and let a pandemic take center stage. Some people, including New Jersey governor Phil Murphy, were battling illnesses like cancer and going through treatment while much of the country was on lockdown. Kristen Ficarra Huetz talked about her young niece's cancer treatments—a heartbreak at any time and seemingly impossible during a pandemic:

> My niece, Sophie, is almost nine, and when she was diagnosed in November [2019] it was very shocking, though she'd been complaining about stomach pains. She'd been to different kinds of doctors, gastroenterologists, and was starting to develop little kid PTSD.
>
> After they'd treated her for constipation, my sister—who had just been laid off and was on her way to a job interview—got the phone call.... It was Stage 4 neuroblastoma that had metastasized to a bone on my niece's hip.
>
> When Sophie was first diagnosed, we were crushed. But the town came together for this child and there was fundraiser after fundraiser. Absolutely touching and beautiful, and they started meal chains and at Christmas organized a caterer who did the whole meal, and women decorated and bought tons of presents for the kids, and everything was just gorgeous.
>
> Sophie has just completed her fifth round of chemo, which caused hearing loss which is likely permanent. She is now getting hearing aids. Next comes the toughest round of chemo, and then two rounds of stem cell transplant. This is a new kind that results in mouth sores and skin rashes. Then she comes home, and they do it again. Six months of immunotherapy. Before the pandemic we got to go in and decorate her room. Now her family is wearing masks and being as cautious as they can be. Sophie's parents are incredibly graceful through all this—I wish I could film every minute of the way they are with her when she gets scared. She has to get shots and transfusions and catheters and cries and gets nervous. But the way they are so calm and gentle, they are incredible human beings.

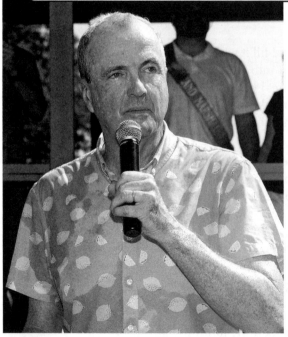

Governor Phil Murphy of New Jersey contracted COVID-19 while also battling kidney cancer. People who have other illnesses such as cancer, diabetes, or diseases that impair the immune system are particularly vulnerable.

My sister doesn't sleep much at all. Sophie is a wonderful, sweet, beautiful child, but it's a challenge. Sophie had gotten through two nights without vomiting, then she barfed all over herself and wouldn't move. My sister held her and sat in the vomit and urine. She said to me, "You know I don't complain about this because it's not about me, but this really tested me to sit in vomit and chemo urine." After 90 minutes she finally agreed to allow herself to be changed—but that's the level of devotion that's beyond what most people could do.

It's really hard not being able to see them; the sense of helplessness was there anyway because I can't even distract Sophie and give her a break. Sophie loves to play poker! And do crafts and we'd just do stuff together. And the hospital the doctors and nurses are incredible. It's upsetting when you look at the way things happen … and adding a pandemic to the mix was not what anybody in the world expected. I feel like one family should not have that many terrible things happening. They would always let me into her room to decorate because they recognized that that was just as important but that's all gone.

COVID-19 Coparenting

If you think coparenting is difficult enough as it is, try navigating it during a pandemic. Some parents who share custody with their ex-spouses or partners find that it can throw a huge wrench into the idea of sheltering in place.

"My ex asked if I wanted him to take the boys while they were [home from school]," said one mom of three. "Here in New Hampshire, that's at least April 3rd. But if the world is falling apart and people are dying, there is NO WAY I'm going to be apart from them. So … we're still splitting time.

"If it were just my boys going back and forth between me and their dad, it would be one thing. But my step-kids go to their mom's too. And my ex-husband has a serious girlfriend with a son who spends time with *his* dad … so really our social distancing and isolation is this long chain of family pods, and we can only hope that all of the other parents are being as vigilant as we are and not letting them hang with friends or go play laser tag."

For Haley and John (names have been changed), "it ended up being the opposite experience than we thought," said Haley.

"We both have a biological child. I have a son who's ten and John has a daughter, Beth, who has special needs—both have an autism spectrum diagnosis, but she's less functioning verbally and struggles with communicating.

"Maybe once a week I've been on Facebook and co-parents are very 50/50—half are keeping schedules as they are and the other half doing it as we are. John reached out to the pediatrician office and I reached out to Kids First Center [a nonprofit organization that has 'classes & groups for parents to learn how to put the needs of their children first while dealing with the legal & financial pressures of divorce & separation'].

"I asked, 'What are the recommendations?' and there really aren't a whole lot. The guidance is kind of, 'Well, do your best to follow your co-parent agreement.' It puts people in tense co-parenting situations without any evidence to back it up, though states with stay-in-place orders have that decision made for people.

"I've been dealing with my ex for eight years, since kindergarten," said John. "The only way it's gotten better is through the courts. I kept getting more responsibility and now have all the parental rights. [My ex] is not mentally healthy. Beth could benefit from medication and [my ex] refused and refused and refused, and it took the court switching that to at least try it. I try and make decisions based on what's best for Beth and not for me."

Continued Haley, "I laid out for [my ex] all the facts—not saying what I thought *should* happen but that the CDC is recommending social distancing, and the recommendation is that people stay in [for several more weeks]. I do think it's valuable and healthy for Paul to spend time with his dad, and … he did then take a step back and kind of say he understands it's stressful for everybody and offered a switch to stay with him at Easter. I responded with, 'That's fine as long as going in everyone understands that then Paul then can't come back to me until school starts again or until June.' My ex said, 'Well that seems like a long time to be away from you.' His wife works from home and he says they're following social distancing, but he does often send Paul to his grandmother.

"The vibe I get from him about this is that he understands it's serious but thinks it's going to go away soon—it's very difficult to convince someone who sees it that way. As much as I dislike my ex-husband, he is my son's father, and my son loves him very much and he should have time with him. It's difficult."

The guidelines by the American Academy of Matrimonial Lawyers said that parenting plans should be observed during the pandemic. Like many aspects of high-conflict divorce, guidelines are not the law, but even if they were mandated—like one that's signed off on by the judge—they can't do a lot to enforce a parenting plan.

The Division of Family Services has also had to change tactics in addressing children whose home life needs to be monitored. Caseworkers are essential employees but in addition to dealing with parents who have addiction and other mental health problems, they now had to worry about getting COVID-19 and bringing it home to their own children.

One caseworker in Delaware said, "We have masks and gloves. We can do virtual contact as much as possible through Google Duo and FaceTime, but there are some occasions where we need to see a kid in the house. Also, our supervisors just told us there are now 67 unmanned cases sitting on desks because people are quitting, and investigation workers are not getting out and doing cases. Our clients have day care that's shutting down. Vulnerable populations are sitting together in these little houses.

"The good news is our unit is really on top of it so we just have to take up the slack. For my families in crisis I've already established a relationship going back years, but for new ones we're not going in as a helper. It's a different whole set of interviewing and assessing the kids to see if the kids are safe. The supervisors say, 'Tell them to meet you outside,' but how am I supposed to assess new houses if I can't go in? But I know they're not going to be happy to see a new person; they might spit on me."

Where Is God?

Three clergy members—a pastor, an imam, and a rabbi—talk about what they tell their congregation when a question like this comes up in times like these or, indeed, in any trying times.

Methodist Pastor Stephen C. Butler (ret.):

I believe that God is not a creator of evil things, God has created the world and He has given us free will—He cannot control how we move around in life, so because of this, any evil that happens is because of what the hands of men have put forth. And that ultimately a lot of times we see within this a lot of negativity and blame God. But pain doesn't equal punishment—perhaps God is relieving us on the other side. Pain is transient. We're travelers in this word and everything we do in this life is for tomorrow—we go to school to become educated. Within that education is the ability to take care of my family, a responsibility that I am blessed with.

The bigger objective is the hereafter and the afterlife. According to Prophet Job, who suffered for 18 months or 18 years—he only had his wife by his side. He lost everything, but he didn't lose faith in God. God healed him.

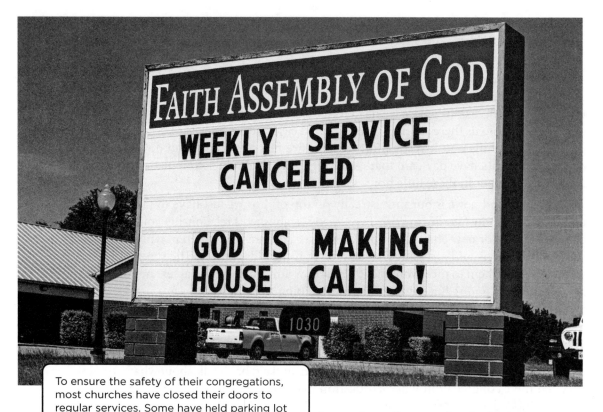

To ensure the safety of their congregations, most churches have closed their doors to regular services. Some have held parking lot services or presented sermons over the internet.

I complain of my grief to God because He's the only one who can understand what I'm going through. As though, when you need me call upon me and I'm here to take care of you. He wants to be there for us. If you think, "I've been doing that and God doesn't answer," there are different ways to look at this. It doesn't mean He's not listening, but He knows best when to answer in a time that's going to be better. God hasn't turned away from us and there's always something better to look forward to.

I look at where they are at that moment—what's their level of faith and commitment to God? Sometimes people come up with answers to their own issues. Some may need more guidance than others, but there are others where just asking that question in the right manner leads to an answer. I'm very careful—I like to listen more than I give advice in the beginning. There are times I'll contact a psychologist or therapist and ask, "What do you advise?" and synergize the religious and psychotherapy side of it.

Imam Wesley Lebron:

I believe that we don't want to place false trust in God—that's reckless—don't be reckless. Faith is about protecting lives and being respectful.

But that is the unsolvable problem of every religion. If God is good, then why is there evil? Theologians divide it between natural evil and moral evil—what people do along with perceived evil. The whole Book of Job is written to study the problem of why is there evil. God says to Job, "You'll never understand." Job yells at God, "Where were you?" Finally, Job is just stunned into silence. "I'm doing things that you cannot comprehend." The Book of Romans 8:28: "In all things, God works for good." God does not send evil to make something good. That makes no sense. God does not control everything. He's a force for good in everything. The virus was always there, sooner or later it's going to coming out. The more you can tolerate ambiguity you can see more possibilities. The community is our patient.

Rabbi Ariann Weitzman:

My movement is Deconstructionism: God doesn't control nature or making minute decisions in people's lives. God is the holy presence that brings comfort and rhythm and love into our lives to hold us during those moments. You see that in all religious communities—I think one of the best gifts of being part of this community is coming together and being there for each other in a physical way and emotional and spiritual way. The day after we decided we weren't holding services from the next day [because of the lockdown] we set up a call list and who's going to go shopping … that's where our minds go first, and at the same time offering prayer, physical and spiritual sustenance is part of the whole.

When I lost my father I was allowed as a clergy person to really fall apart, and that permission to be totally vulnerable and totally taken take of—sometimes we bifurcate spiritual and physical stress and we've all experienced spiritual stress.

I don't believe in a personal God, a God who acts as a person, who chooses, "I like this guy but not that guy." That's not the God I preach about. God is accessible no matter what. You don't develope a strong spiritual connection from these off moments—and when we're thrown off rhythm—that religious life is grounding and helpful. If you align yourself with the order of fixed prayer, you'll be ready and you'll have the words for when you need to pray. I'm primed and ready to see things and express things and experience awe and gratitude.

About this moment—this is unique. On the one hand you can't learn all the profound lessons from experience but you have to learn from every experience. I hope I am able to give more attention to my immediate family. Be less outward facing. We all have obligations that are outside of our family that we balance or don't balance, and on one hand it's terrible because there's only so much family that you can take! For those of us who have safe and loving families it's an opportunity to provide more emotional and spiritual needs.

Conclusion

Poverty and starvation play a role as much as quarantines and lockdowns. Over 820 million people are hungry, some of them poor and desperate for any kind of food. These factors are unprecedented on planet Earth: we know from the fossil record that no large-bodied animal has ever been nearly as abundant as humans are now, and consequences of this population spike are ecological disturbances and increasing viral exchanges—first from animal to animal, then animal to human, then human to human, sometimes on a pandemic scale.

We invade the wild, which harbors so many species of animals and plants—and also so many unknown species of viruses and bacteria. We cut down trees, burn jungles, destroy ecosystems, encage animals, and let these viruses loose. When that happens, viruses need a new host. Often, it's us.

This goes hand in hand with governments that deal in denial and concealment. The distance from Wuhan or the Amazon to Paris, Toronto, or Washington is short for some viruses, measured in hours, given how well they can ride within airplane passengers.

Long term: When the coronavirus is over, it must not be classified as a novel event or a misfortune that befell us; it's simply part of a pattern of choices that we continue to make. Insanity is doing the same thing over and over again and expecting different results. With the coronavirus, we can stop being stark raving mad.

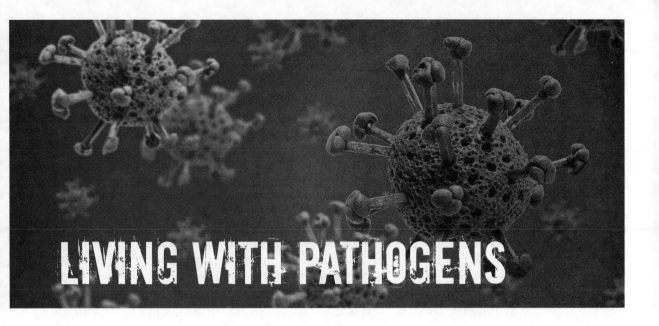

LIVING WITH PATHOGENS

In Season 3 of *The Simpsons*, Bart Simpson's fourth-grade class is forced to watch a film called *A World without Zinc*. In it, a young man named Jimmy wishes for a zinc-less world but discovers a world without zinc is no world for him—no battery to start his car, no rotary phone to call his girlfriend, and no firing pin in his gun when he tries to kill himself. Happily, in the end we see it was just a nightmare, and Jimmy rejoices in the fact that he lives among car batteries, telephones, handguns … and other things made of zinc.

Who cares about zinc? And yet we actually do need it! Without zinc our wounds wouldn't heal and our blood wouldn't clot. Sometimes it's these seemingly inconsequential things that mean more than we realize.

Now let's look at something bigger (that's small). Who wants to live in a world without viruses? Would it be a cleaner world, a happier world, a safer world?

About 90% of living creatures in the ocean are microscopic. Every day, viruses kill about 20% of them and about 50% of all oceanic bacteria. This clears the way for plankton to get enough food—and therefore energy—to undertake high rates of photosynthesis, thereby producing oxygen and ultimately ensuring much of life on Earth continues—and for plankton to also become food for whales.

LIKE IT OR NOT, WE NEED VIRUSES

"If all viruses suddenly disappeared, the world would be a wonderful place for about a day and a half, and then we'd all die—that's the bottom line," Tony Goldberg, an epidemiologist at the University of Wisconsin—Madison, told the BBC. "All the essential things they do in the world far outweigh the bad things."

The fact that life is so dependent on death, and yet we do our best to forestall it, is one of our great paradoxes. The study of viruses is biased toward the ones that harm us. Why spend time and money researching pathogens that leave us alone? And while thousands of viruses have been classified, there may be millions more we don't know about. Perhaps we don't want to.

So does this mean there are "good" viruses and "bad" viruses? Viruses, for being so biologically simple, are quite complex when it comes to philosophical questions. "Good" or "bad" depends on one's perspective, not on the virus itself. Even though it's in our nature to anthropomorphize what we study—and also fight—it's still crucial to remember that it's nothing personal. Remember, all a virus wants to do is replicate. It doesn't particularly want to help us, either, but oncology researchers are developing therapies that use viruses instead of chemotherapy and radiation to kill cancer cells. A virus targets particular cells; chemotherapy and radiation kill cancerous and noncancerous cells alike, which causes terrible side effects. Over the past two decades, viruses from many different families have been tapped to be used as anticancer agents:

- *Adenoviridae* causes everything from pink eye to respiratory infections
- *Herpesviridae* causes herpes and chicken pox
- *Rhabdoviridae* causes rabies
- *Parvoviridae* causes rashes and arthritis in humans, and can be fatal in dogs
- *Picornaviridae* causes polio, meningitis, and hepatitis
- *Poxviridae* causes smallpox

But due to their ability to attack tumors and kill cancer cells without harming noncancerous cells, these viruses (which have been genetically modified, or coded, to be "good") are referred to as oncolytic viruses—from the Greek *ónkos*, meaning "mass," and *lytikos*, meaning "to loosen." They literally tear apart cancer cells, releasing cancer antigens and causing immune responses that seek and destroy any remaining tumor cells nearby and anywhere else in the body.

GOOD BACTERIA

Now let's widen the net and include a world without bacteria. Illnesses ranging from food poisoning to plague wouldn't exist if there were no bacteria. We would have freedom from moldy bread and bad breath. But now imagine what would happen to all the world's dead—after all, microbes don't kill everything. All that lives still has to die. Bacteria, for example, recycle the nutrients of dead plants and animals back into the ground so the next generation of plants can grow. Without them, dead people, dead plants, dead giraffes, dead sharks, and dead azaleas, would keep piling atop each other. Since their nutrients aren't going anywhere, plants don't grow, we all starve, we die, and the pile gets bigger and bigger and bigger.

In soil and in the ocean, bacteria are also major players in decomposing organic matter and recycling it into critical chemical elements like carbon and nitrogen. In your body, bacteria help you break down plant-based foods like fruits and vegetables that you have a tough time doing on your own, also helping you get more nutrition. Outside your body, those stories of bacteria crawling all over your skin are creepy but true. There are roughly 200 different species of bacteria living on your body, standing guard to keep harmful bacteria from being able to take hold, while also eating your dead skin cells.

And, inside or out, exposure to all types of bacteria, both "good" and "bad," is important in developing a healthy immune system. It gets the immune system ready from the moment you're born to respond to pathogens every second throughout your life. As counterculture writer Stewart Brand once said, "If you don't like bacteria, you are on the wrong planet."

So, pathogens—can't live with 'em, can't live without 'em. The best we can do is eradicate the ones that harm us and turn others into microscopic agents of infectious change. As mentioned, genetic modifications to certain viruses may convert them into our best defense against cancer. In 2015, the U.S. Food and Drug Administration approved the use of Imlygic® as the first—and as of now, the only—available oncolytic viral therapy. It's for patients with melanoma. Imlygic® is a genetically modified version of the herpes simplex virus type 1— the kind that causes cold sores—that treats melanoma lesions in the skin and lymph nodes that can't be removed surgically. Imlygic® is programmed to replicate within tumors and cause cell lysis, or death, which ruptures tumors, releasing the antigens that cause an anti-tumor immune response. This is especially crucial because melanoma continues to be one of the most difficult-to-treat cancers, as it often does not respond to chemotherapy, can be highly aggressive, and can require several different types of treatment, depending on the stage and location of the disease and health of the patient.

Meanwhile, since bacteria were able to be seen years before viruses, doctors and researchers have been studying them as a means of cancer therapy since the nineteenth century. Dr. William B. Coley, who worked at the New York Hospital (which later became the Memorial Sloan Kettering Cancer Center) in the late 1800s, noticed that tumors began to shrink in cancer patients who also had streptococcal infections. One patient who had a cancerous tumor nearly died from a post-op bacterial skin infection yet was able to both eradicate the infection and the tumor with his own immune response. His tumor disappeared, and he was still alive years later when Coley tracked him down at his home on the Lower East Side of Manhattan.

Coley decided to test if infecting patients with the bacteria from this infection could also cause their tumors to shrink. He performed the first inoculation in 1891 on a man named Zola, who was given only weeks to live due to a tumor "the size of a small hen's egg" in his right tonsil. The experiment worked: Zola's tumor shrank, and he lived another eight years.

By 1892, Coley had generated a variety of "anti-tumor vaccines" to bring about the symptoms of an infection—like fever and inflammation—that hindered tumor development but without risking an actual infection. These vaccines became known as "Coley's toxins" and were given to patients with sarcomas, carcinomas, lymphomas, and melanomas.

Bacterial cancer therapies date back to at least 2600 B.C.E., when Egyptian physician Imhotep treated tumors by applying a poultice, then an incision, to let an infection get in the desired location and cause tumors to shrink. So why have we not been using "bad" bacteria for good?

A couple reasons. One is that Coley's toxins are not easy to make. It's not a one-size-fits-all form of immunotherapy, just like there isn't a single type of cancer. So different "toxins" created by different laboratories had differing levels of efficacy and needed to be tailored to each individual patient in order to induce and sustain a fever but not an infection.

Second, Coley's work came at the dawn of radiotherapy, which the medical community—and Coley's superior, pathologist James Ewing—saw as the answer to fighting cancer. By comparison, Coley's toxins were deemed too dangerous, inconsistent, and bordering on folkloric. Just because certain practices were carried out in ancient Egypt didn't mean they worked. The point was to look ahead for treatment, so Coley was forced to cease production of his toxins due to claims of inconsistent data in favor of radiotherapy, which became the cancer therapy of choice even today, along with chemotherapy. It also helped that wealthy mining engineer James Douglas, who was a radium advocate, bestowed a healthy endowment to the hospital.

Sixteen different types of Coley's toxins have been used since 1892, but his work gradually fell out of favor, and by 1962 the FDA refused to approve any of Coley's toxins, except for one: Bacillus Calmette-Guerin (BCG). BCG is the only bacterial agent approved by the FDA. It's been used to treat early stage bladder cancer since the late 1970s. BCG is a weakened strain of *Mycobacterium bovis*, which causes tuberculosis in cattle and is related to *Mycobacterium tuberculosis*, which causes tuberculosis in humans. Patients typically receive repeated doses of live bacteria directly into the bladder as treatment.

THE LAST WORD

When it comes to pathogens, the one thing we can be certain of, to use an old chestnut, is that we cannot be certain of anything. Their sheer number, diversity, and biology is too vast for us to fully grasp. That's why this chapter about the future of pathogens delves so much into the past. If we are to deal with future pandemics—whether keeping them at bay or preventing them from erupting in the first place—along with whatever else nature has in mind, it's critical to know pathogens' beneficial and harmful qualities. And, if they are intrinsically "bad," if there's any way to make them "good." Pathogens are always going to be with us, side by side, invisible, yet powerful. Once we realize that it's often the pathogens that call the shots and not the government or the media, then we may begin healing.

FURTHER READING

"184 Cases Influenza in New York." *The Philadelphia Inquirer,* September 17, 1918.

Adedeji, W.A. "The Treasure Called Antibiotics." *National Center for Biotechnology Information.* https://www .ncbi.nlm.nih.gov/pmc/articles/PMC5354621/. Accessed July 10, 2019.

Amirian, E. Susan. "Potential Fecal Transmission of SARS-CoV-2: Current Evidence and Implications for Public Health." 2020. *International Journal of Infectious Diseases.* https://www.ijidonline.com/article/S1201- 9712(20)30273-3/pdf. Accessed April 30, 2020.

Anonymous. *Alcoholics Anonymous: The Big Book, Fourth Edition.* New York, NY: Alcoholics Anonymous World Services, Inc., 2004.

Armstrong, Dorsey. "The Black Death." *History.com.* https://www.history.com/topics/ancient-americas/aztecs. Accessed March 3, 2020.

Baird, Woody. "Spirit Thrives After 41 Years in Iron Lung." *Los Angeles Times,* October 13, 1991.

Barry, John M. *The Great Influenza: The Story of the Deadliest Pandemic in History.* New York, NY: Penguin Books, 2005.

Bartlett, Kenneth. *The Civilization of the Italian Renaissance: A Sourcebook, Second Edition.* Toronto, ON: University of Toronto Press, 2011.

Bauer, Ralph, translator. *An Inca Account of the Conquest of Peru.* Boulder, CO: University Press of Colorado, 2005.

Belluz, Julia. "Plague Is Spreading at an Alarming Rate in Madagascar. Yes, Plague." *Vox.* https://www.vox.com/ science-and-health/2017/10/6/16435536/plague-madagascar-epidemic-2017. Accessed August 14, 2019.

Biello, David. "Ancient Athenian Plague Proves to Be Typhoid." *Scientific American.* https://www.scientific- american.com/article/ancient-athenian-plague-p/. Accessed March 3, 2020.

Blow, Charles M. "Social Distancing Is a Privilege." *New York Times,* April 5, 2020.

Bostock, John. *Pliny the Elder: The Natural History.* London, UK: Taylor & Francis, 1855.

Boundy, Donna. "Program for Cocaine-Abuse Under Way." *New York Times,* November 17, 1985.

Brammer, John Paul. "Three Decades Later, Men Who Survived the 'Gay Plague' Speak Out." *NBC News.* https://www.nbcnews.com/feature/nbc-out/three-decades-later-men-who-survived-gay-plague-speak-out- n825621. Accessed March 18, 2019.

Bray, R.S. *Armies of Pestilence: The Impact of Disease on History*. New York, NY: Barnes & Noble, 2003.

Brinton, Daniel B., translator. *The Annals of the Cakchiquels*. Seattle, WA: Amazon Services, LLC, 2010.

Brockell, Gillian. "Sir Isaac News Did His Best Work While Working from Home." *Washington Post*, March 12, 2020.

Browne, David. "Music's Fentanyl Crisis: Inside the Drug That Killed Prince and Tom Petty." *Rolling Stone*. https://www.rollingstone.com/music/music-features/musics-fentanyl-crisis-inside-the-drug-that-killed-prince-and-tom-petty-666019/. Accessed May 15, 2019.

Brüssow, Harald. "On Viruses, Bats and Men: A Natural History of Food-Borne Viral Infections." *National Center for Biotechnology Information*. https://www.ncbi.nlm.nih.gov/pmc/articles/PMC7121238/. Accessed April 2, 2020.

Buckley, Chris and Steven Lee Myers. "As New Coronavirus Spread, China's Old Habits Delayed Fight." *New York Times*, February 1, 2020.

Buczek, Monica. "Where Did Zika Go (And Will It Come Back)?" *American Study for Microbiology*. https://www.asm.org/Articles/2018/September/Where-Did-Zika-Go-And-Will-It-Come-Back. Accessed January 20, 2020.

Bump, Phillip. "The Circumstances Are Wildly Different. Trump's Response Is the Same." *Washington Post*, April 5, 2020.

Butler, S. Interview with Heather Quinlan with Heather Quinlan. March 31, 2020.

Byrne, Katherine. *Tuberculosis and the Victorian Literary Imagination*. Cambridge, UK: Cambridge University Press, 2013.

Caradonia, Jackie. "How These Medical Centers Beat the 'Revolving Door' of Healthcare with a Wellness-Oriented Approach." *Yahoo! Finance*. https://finance.yahoo.com/news/medical-centers-beat-revolving-door-200048308.html. Accessed May 23, 2019.

Caraman, Philip. *Henry Morse: Plague Priest of London*. London: Longmans, Green, 1957.

Carey, John. *Eyewitness to Science*. Cambridge, MA: Harvard University Press, 1995.

Castell-Rodrìguez, Andres, and others. "Dendritic Cells: Location, Function, and Clinical Implications." *Biology of Myelomonocytic Cells*. https://www.intechopen.com/books/biology-of-myelomonocytic-cells/dendritic-cells-location-function-and-clinical-implications. Accessed July 13, 2019.

"Carlo Urbani: A 21st Century Hero and Martyr." *Molecular Biology and Pathogens*. https://norkinvirology.wordpress.com/2014/02/11/carlo-urbani-a-21st-century-hero-and-martyr-2/. Accessed April 2, 2020.

"Carolina Researchers Playing a Key Role in the Development of New COVID-19 Treatment." *The University of North Carolina at Chapel Hill*, May 6, 2020. https://www.unc.edu/posts/2020/04/06/carolina-researchers-key-role-in-the-development-of-new-covid-19-treatment/.

Cartwright, Mark. "Cuzco." *Ancient History Encyclopedia*. https://www.ancient.eu/Cuzco/. Accessed August 20, 2019.

———. "Templo Mayor." 2017. *Ancient History Encyclopedia*. https://www.ancient.eu/Templo_Mayor/. Accessed August 20, 2019.

Centers for Disease Control and Prevention. "Antibiotic Use: Questions and Answers." https://www.cdc.gov/antibiotic-use/community/about/should-know.html. Accessed February 5, 2020.

———. "Biggest Threats and Data." https://www.cdc.gov/drugresistance/biggest-threats.html .Accessed February 1, 2020.

———. "History of Smallpox." https://www.cdc.gov/smallpox/history/history.html. Accessed August 12, 2019.

———. "Methicillin-resistant *Staphylococcus aureus* (MRSA)." https://www.cdc.gov/mrsa/index.html. Accessed February 1, 2020.

Char, Sherie. "Hawaii's Father Damien: From Priesthood to Sainthood." 2009. *Hawai'i Magazine*, October 10, 2020.

Chew, Suok Kai. "SARS: How a Global Epidemic Was Stopped." 2007. *World Health Organization*. https://www.ncbi.nlm.nih.gov/pmc/articles/PMC2636331/. Accessed March 2, 2020.

Choi, David. "'They Are a Very Hungry People': Fox News Host Fuels Racist Tropes about Chinese over Coronavirus Outbreak." *Business Insider*. https://www.businessinsider.com/fox-news-jesse-watters-chinese-demands-apology-racism-2020-3. Accessed March 8, 2020.

Coe, Michael D. *Breaking the Maya Code*. London, UK: Thames & Hudson, 1992.

Cohen, Elizabeth. "Infected People without Symptoms Might Be Driving the Spread of Coronavirus More Than We Realized." *CNN*. https://www.cnn.com/2020/03/14/health/coronavirus-asymptomatic-spread/index.html. Accessed March 19, 2020.

"Crack Epidemic Still Going Strong." *Rehabs America*. https://www.rehabsamerica.org/blog/crack-epidemic-still-going-strong-19. Accessed February 13, 2020.

Darville, Toni, and Ingrid J. G. Rours. "Chlamydia trachomatis." *ScienceDirect*. https://www.sciencedirect.com/topics/medicine-and-dentistry/chlamydiae. Accessed May 4, 2020.

Darwin, Charles. *On the Origin of Species by Means of Natural Selection; or, The Preservation of Favoured Races in the Struggle for Life*. London, UK: John Murray Publishers. 1859.

Daunt, Tina. "Written in Pain." *Los Angeles Times,* March 16, 2005.

Davis, Gerald J., translator. *Gilgamesh: The New Translation*. Sacramento, CA: Insignia Press. 2014.

Davis, Simon. "Solving the Mystery of an Ancient Epidemic." *The Atlantic*, September, 2015. https://www.theatlantic.com/health/archive/2015/09/disease-plague-of-athens-ebola/403561/

Dean, Heather. "Paediatrics Child Health." *Journal of Developmental Origins of Health and Disease*. https://www.ncbi.nlm.nih.gov/pmc/articles/PMC2735379/. Accessed June 15, 2019.

DeCroes Jacobs, Charlotte. *Jonas Salk: A Life*. Oxford, UK: Oxford University Press, 2017.

Delahoyde, Michael. "The Pardoner's Tale." https://public.wsu.edu/~delahoyd/chaucer/ParT.html. Accessed April 3, 2020.

Dewing, H. B., translator. *History of the Wars Vol. I.* By Procopius. Cambridge, MA: Harvard University Press, 1914.

DeWitte, S. Interview with Heather Quinlan, April 7, 2020.

Diamond, Jared. *Guns, Germs, and Steel: The Fates of Human Societies*. New York, NY: W. W. Norton & Company. 2005.

DiMarco, Vincent. *It Has Helped to Admiration: Eighteenth-Century Medical Cures from the Kitchen Book of Bridget Lane, 1737*. iUniverse, 2010.

Ditunno, John F. Jr., and others. "Franklin Delano Roosevelt: The Diagnosis of Poliomyelitis Revisited." National Center for Biotechnology Information. https://pubmed.ncbi.nlm.nih.gov/27178375/. Accessed February 19, 2019.

Doucleff, Micaheleen. "Last Person to Get Smallpox Dedicated His Life to Ending Polio." *NPR.* https://www.npr.org/sections/health-shots/2013/07/31/206947581/last-person-to-get-smallpox-dedicated-his-life-to-ending-polio. Accessed May 2, 2020.

"Dr. Fauci Discusses Ending the HIV Epidemic from the 2019 IAS Conference on HIV Science." HIV.gov. https://www.hiv.gov/blog/dr-fauci-discusses-ending-hiv-epidemic-2019-ias-conference-hiv-science. Accessed July 5, 2020.

"Dr. Jonas Edward Salk." *One Dream Foundation.* http://onedreamfoundation.com/read-more/. Accessed September 11, 2019.

Dronke, Ursula, translator. *The Poetic Edda*, Volume II. Oxford, UK: Clarendon Press, 1997.

"Drug Resistant Tuberculosis." *World Health Organization.* https://www.who.int/tb/areas-of-work/drug-resistant-tb/en/. Accessed February 24, 2020.

Earnest, Mark. "On Becoming a Plague Doctor." *New England Journal of Medicine.* https://www.nejm.org/doi/full/10.1056/NEJMp2011418. Accessed May 20, 2020.

Endrst, James. "New Rock Hudson Biography Reveals the Secrets the Closeted Star Tried to Hide." *USA Today*, December 4, 2018.

Fauci, A. Interview with Heather Quinlan, April 22, 2020.

"Fauci Voices Optimism about Remdesivir as Treatment For COVID-19 Infection." *CBS News.* https://www.cbsnews.com/news/fauci-remdesivir-coronavirus-treatment/. Accessed May 1, 2020.

Fawcett, Kirstin. "Doctors Didn't Actually Wear Beaked Masks during the Black Plague." *Mental Floss.* https://www.mentalfloss.com/article/505090/doctors-didnt-actually-wear-beaked-masks-during-black-plague. Accessed November 30, 2019.

Ficarra Huetz, K. (2020, April 4). Interview with Heather Quinlan.

Fisher Coughlin, B. (2020, April 4). Interview with Heather Quinlan.

Ford, Talitha. "Disease, Death and Darwin: Dr. Sharon DeWitte on Her Upcoming Talks." *Little Village: Iowa City/Cedar Rapids News, Culture & Events.* https://littlevillagemag.com/disease-death-and-darwin-dr-sharon-dewitte-on-her-upcoming-talks/. Accessed April 6, 2020.

Fowler, Dave. "Flagellants and the Black Death." *The Black Death.* https://blackdeathfacts.com/flagellants/. Accessed April 14, 2020.

Frerichs, Ralph R. "Competing Theories of Cholera." *UCLA Department of Epidemiology: John Snow.* https://www.ph.ucla.edu/epi/snow/choleratheories.html. Accessed May 2, 2020.

Froggatt, Peter. "John Snow, Thomas Wakely, and *The Lancet.*" *Anaesthesia.* http://www.ph.ucla.edu/epi/snow/anaesthesia57_667_75_2002.pdf. Accessed May 1, 2020.

Galvin, G. Interview with Heather Quinlan, March 28, 2020.

Garrett, Laurie. *The Coming Plague: Newly Emerging Diseases in a World Out of Balance.* New York, NY: Penguin Books ,1995.

Gasquet, Frances. *The Black Death.* Seattle, WA: Jovian Press/Amazon Services, 2016.

Geggus, David. *Yellow Fever in the 1790s: The British Army in Occupied Saint Domingue*. Cambridge, UK: Cambridge University Press, 1979.

Ghatak, A. Interview with Heather Quinlan, April 13, 2020.

Ghosh, Bobby. "China's Internet Got a Strange And Lasting Boost from the SARS Epidemic." *Quartz*. https://qz.com/662110/chinas-internet-got-a-strange-and-lasting-boost-from-the-sars-epidemic/. Accessed May 21, 2020.

Gibbons, Ann. "Ancient DNA Traces the Black Death to Russia's Volga Region." *Science*. https://www.science-mag.org/news/2019/10/ancient-dna-traces-black-death-russia-s-volga-region. Accessed January 14, 2020.

Gill, Richardson B. *The Great Maya Droughts*. Albuquerque, NM: University of New Mexico Press, 2001.

Glickman, Lawrence. "The Conservative Campaign against Safety." *Atlantic*. https://www.theatlantic.com/ideas/archive/2020/03/conservative-campaign-security/608986/. Accessed March 30, 2020.

Godeke, Gert-Jan et al. "Middle East Respiratory Syndrome Coronavirus Neutralising Serum Antibodies in Dromedary Camels: A Comparative Serological Study." *The Lancet*. https://www.thelancet.com/journals/laninf/article/PIIS1473-3099(13)70164-6/fulltext. Accessed April 4, 2020.

Golden, Timothy. "Though Evidence Is Thin, Tale of C.I.A. and Drugs Has a Life of Its Own." *New York Times*, October 21, 1996, p. A14.

Goliber, Thomas. "The Status of the HIV/AIDS Epidemic in Sub-Saharan Africa." *Population Reference Bureau*. https://www.prb.org/thestatusofthehivaidsepidemicinsubsaharanafrica/. Accessed July 13, 2019.

"Gonorrhea—CDC Fact Sheet." *Centers for Disease Control and Prevention*. https://www.cdc.gov/std/gonorrhea/stdfact-gonorrhea-detailed.htm. Accessed May 4, 2020.

Gorman, James. "How Do Bats Live with So Many Viruses?" *New York Times*, January 28, 2020.

Grady, Denise. "An Ebola Doctor's Return from the Edge of Death." *New York Times*, December 7, 2014.

———. "The Mystery Behind an Eye That Changed Color." *New York Times*, May 7, 2015.

Green, David B. "This Day in Jewish History 1348: Jews Aren't Behind the Black Death, Pope Clarifies." *Haaretz*. https://www.haaretz.com/jewish/.premium-1348-jews-aren-t-behind-the-black-death-pope-clarifies-1.5405782. Accessed November 12, 2019.

Green, Hank. "Your Immune System: Natural Born Killer." *Crash Course Biology #32*. https://www.youtube.com/watch?v=CeVtPDjJBPU. Accessed July 10, 2019.

Green, John. "Disease!" *Crash Course World History 203*. https://www.youtube.com/watch?v=1PLBmUVYYeg. Accessed July 10, 2019.

———. "The Silk Road and Ancient Trade." *Crash Course World History #9*. https://www.youtube.com/watch?v=vfe-eNq-Qyg. Accessed November 11, 2019.

Greenhalgh, Hugo. "Religious Figures Blame LGBT+ People for Coronavirus." *Reuters*, March 9, 2020.

Greshko, Michael. "Colossal Volcano Behind 'Mystery' Global Cooling Finally Found." 2019. *National Geographic*, August, 2019.

Gross, Terry. "'All That Heaven Allows' Examines Rock Hudson's Life as a Closeted Leading Man." *NPR's Fresh Air*. https://www.npr.org/2018/12/05/673696589/all-that-heaven-allows-examines-rock-hudsons-life-as-a-closeted-leading-man. Accessed July 9, 2019.

Gunderman, Richard. "How Smallpox Devastated the Aztecs—And Helped Spain Conquer an American Civilization 500 Years Ago." *The Conversation*. https://theconversation.com/how-smallpox-devastated-the-aztecs-and-helped-spain-conquer-an-american-civilization-500-years-ago-111579. Accessed July 12, 2019.

Guthke, Karl S. *The Gender of Death: A Cultural History in Art and Literature*. Cambridge, UK: Cambridge University Press, 1999.

Hadhazy, Adam. "How Has Magic Johnson Survived 20 Years with HIV?" *Live Science*. https://www.livescience.com/16909-magic-johnson-hiv-aids-anniversary.html. Accessed March 20, 2020.

Hannaford, Alex. "The CIA, the Drug Dealers, and the Tragedy of Gary Webb." *The Telegraph*, March 21, 2015.

Harris, Patrice A. "AMA Statement on Halting World Health Organization Funding." *American Medical Association*. https://www.ama-assn.org/press-center/ama-statements/ama-statement-halting-world-health-organization-funding. Accessed April 20, 2020.

Harvey, Gideon. *A Discourse of the Plague Containing the Nature, Causes, Signs, and Presages of the Pestilence in General, Together with the State of the Present … Medicines Both for Rich and Poor (1665)*. Cincinnati, OH: EEBO Editions, ProQuest, 2010.

"He Warned of Coronavirus. Here's What He Told Us Before He Died." *New York Times*, February 7, 2020.

Heaney, Seamus, and Ted Hughes. *The Rattle Bag*. London, UK: Faber & Faber, 2005.

Heitman, Kristin. "Of Counts and Causes: The Emergence of the London Bills of Mortality." *Folger Shakespeare Company*. https://collation.folger.edu/2018/03/counts-causes-london-bills-mortality/. Accessed February 21, 2020.

Hempel, Sandra. *The Strange Case of the Broad Street Pump: John Snow and the Mystery of Cholera*. Berkeley, CA: University of California Press, 2007.

Henig, Robin Marantz. "AIDS: A New Disease's Deadly Odyssey." *New York Times,* February 6, 1983, Section 6, p. 28.

Hernandez, Bernat. "Guns, Germs, and Horses Brought Cortes Victory Over the Mighty Aztec Empire." *National Geographic*. https://www.nationalgeographic.com/history/magazine/2016/05-06/cortes-tenochtitlan/. Accessed August 4, 2019.

Herring, Francis. *Preservatives Against the Plague, or, Direction; Advertisements for This Time of Pestilential Contagion with Instructions for the Poorer People When They Shall Be Visited (1665)*. Ann Arbor, MI: EEBO Editions, ProQuest, 2010.

"HIV and AIDS in East and Southern Africa Regional Overview, 2018." *Avert*. https://www.avert.org/professionals/hiv-around-world/sub-saharan-africa/overview. Accessed June 12, 2019.

Hobbes, Thomas, translator. *The Peloponnesian War by Thucydides*. Chicago, IL: University of Chicago Press, 1989.

Holbein, Hans. *The Dance of Death*. London, UK: Random House UK, 2016.

"Hollywood's Rock Hudson Admits AIDS Diagnosis on This Day in 1985." *VOA*. https://www.voanews.com/arts-culture/hollywoods-rock-hudson-admits-aids-diagnosis-day-1985. Accessed October 12, 2019.

"Homologous Recombination within the Spike Glycoprotein of the Newly Identified Coronavirus May Boost Cross-Species Transmission from Snake to Human." *Physicians Weekly*. https://www.physiciansweekly.com/homologous-recombination-within-the-spike-glycoprotein-of-the-newly-identified-coronavirus-may-boost-cross-species-transmission-from-snake-to-human/. Accessed January 22, 2020.

Horrox, Rosemary. *The Black Death*. Manchester, UK: Manchester University Press, 1994.

Hu Wei-Shau and Stephen H. Hughes. "HIV-1 Reverse Transcription." *National Center for Biotechnology Information*. https://www.ncbi.nlm.nih.gov/pmc/articles/PMC3475395/. Accessed July 24, 2019.

Hudson, Myles. "Battle of Tenochtitlán." 2019. *Britannica*. https://www.britannica.com/event/Battle-of-Tenochtitlan

Hussain, Aneela Naureen. 2019. "Smallpox." Accessed May 2, 2020. Accessed September 30, 2019. https://emedicine.medscape.com/article/237229-overview

Hurston, Zora Neale. *Their Eyes Were Watching God*. New York, NY: Amistad Books, 2006.

"'Immunity Passports' in the Context of COVID-19." World Health Organization. https://www.who.int/news-room/commentaries/detail/immunity-passports-in-the-context-of-covid-19. Accessed April 30, 2020.

"Increased Drug Availability Is Associated with Increased Use and Overdose." *National Institution on Drug Abuse*. https://www.drugabuse.gov/publications/research-reports/prescription-opioids-heroin/increased-drug-availability-associated-increased-use-overdose. Accessed November 2, 2019.

Jabr, Ferris. "Why Soap Works." *New York Times*, March 13, 2020.

James, C.L.R. *The Black Jacobins: Toussaint L'Ouverture and the San Domingo Revolution*. New York, NY: Vintage, 1989.

Johnson, Brian D. "How a Typo Created a Scapegoat for the AIDS Epidemic." *Maclean's*. https://www.macleans.ca/culture/movies/how-a-typo-created-a-scapegoat-for-the-aids-epidemic/. Accessed March 18, 2020.

Johnson, Dirk. "Ryan White Dies of AIDS at 18; His Struggle Helped Pierce Myths." *New York Times*, April 9, 1990, p. D10.

Karimi, Nasser, and Jon Gambrell. "Industrial Alcohol Coronavirus 'Cure' Kills Hundreds of Iranians." *New York Daily News*, March 28, 2020.

Kharsany, Ayesha B. M., and Quarraisha A. Karim. "HIV Infection and AIDS in Sub-Saharan Africa: Current Status, Challenges and Opportunities." *National Center for Biotechnology Information*. https://www.ncbi.nlm.nih.gov/pmc/articles/PMC4893541/. Accessed July 20, 2019.

Kiger, Patrick J. "Did Colonists Give Infected Blankets to Native Americans as Biological Warfare?" *History*. https://www.history.com/news/colonists-native-americans-smallpox-blankets. Accessed September 12, 2019.

Knegt, Peter. "Killing Patient Zero: How a Quebec Flight Attendant Was Falsely Accused of Bringing AIDS to America." CBC. https://www.cbc.ca/arts/killing-patient-zero-how-a-quebec-flight-attendant-was-falsely-accused-of-bringing-aids-to-america-1.5224906. Accessed March 18, 2020.

Knopf, Sigard Adolphus. *Pulmonary Tuberculosis: Its Modern Prophylaxis and the Treatment in Special Institutions and at Home*. Mishawaka, IN: Palala Press, 2016.

Kolata, Gina. *Flu: The Story of the Great Influenza Pandemic of 1918 and the Search for the Virus That Caused It*. New York, NY: Farrar, Straus & Giroux, 2011.

Kormann, Carolyn. "From Bats to Human Lungs, the Evolution of a Coronavirus." *New Yorker*, March 27, 2020.

Kourtis, Athena P., and others. "Ebola Virus Disease." 2015. *National Center for Biotechnology Information*. https://www.ncbi.nlm.nih.gov/pmc/articles/PMC4666536/. Accessed April 22, 2020.

Kreston, Rebecca. "The Public Health Legacy of the 1976 Swine Flu Outbreak." *Discover*. https://www.discovermagazine.com/health/the-public-health-legacy-of-the-1976-swine-flu-outbreak. Accessed March 30, 2020.

Krishnan, Arjun Sai. "Codex Aubin: History in Reprint." *McGraw Commons*. http://commons.princeton.edu/wp-content/uploads/sites/35/2019/11/Codex-Aubin-Final.pdf. Accessed August 28, 2019.

Kroll, David. "Heartbreaker: Tom Petty Died from an Accidental Overdose of Opioids and Benzodiazepines." *Forbes*, January 19, 2018.

Kupferschmidt, Kai. "Bats Really Do Harbor More Dangerous Viruses Than Other Species." *Science*. https://www.sciencemag.org/news/2017/06/bats-really-do-harbor-more-dangerous-viruses-other-species. Accessed February 1, 2020.

Lady Mary Wortley Montagu, "Lady Mary Wortley Montagu on Small Pox in Turkey [Letter]." *Children and Youth in History, Item #157*. http://chnm.gmu.edu/cyh/items/show/157. Accessed August 12, 2019.

Lahman, Maria K. E. *Ethics in Social Science Research: Becoming Culturally Responsive*. New York, NY: SAGE Publications, 2017.

Langreth, Robert. "Coronavirus Outbreak Likely Began with Bats, an Omen for Next Epidemic." *Bloomberg*. February 3, 2020.

Lebron, W. Interview with Heather Quinlan, March 31, 2020.

Lembke, Anna. *Drug Dealer, MD: How Doctors Were Duped, Patients Got Hooked, and Why It's So Hard to Stop*. Baltimore, MD: Johns Hopkins University Press, 2016.

Lewis, Jon E. *London: The Autobiography*. London, UK: Robinson Publishing, 2012.

Lima, Maurizio. "A Trail of Zika-Borne Anguish." *New York Times*, March 9, 2016.

Lopez, German. "America's Huge Problem with Opioid Prescribing, in One Quote." 2017. *Vox*. https://www.vox.com/science-and-health/2017/9/18/16326816/opioid-epidemic-keith-humphreys. Accessed May 15, 2019.

Lovgren, Stefan. "Jared Diamond: Lessons from Hunter-Gatherers." *National Geographic*. https://www.nationalgeographic.com/science/2005/07/news-guns-germs-steel-jared-diamond-interview/. Accessed August 4, 2019.

MacDonald, Fiona. *The Plague and Medicine in the Middle Ages*. New York, NY: Gareth Stevens Publishing, 2005.

Maestri, Nicoletta. "Huitzilopochtli." *Thought Co*. https://www.thoughtco.com/huitzilopochtli-aztec-god-of-the-sun-171229. Accessed August 20, 2019.

Mallett, J. Interview with Heather Quinlan, April 22, 2020.

Mansoor, Sanya. "India Is the World's Second-Most Populous Country. Can It Handle the Coronavirus Outbreak?" *Time*. https://time.com/5801507/coronavirus-india/. Accessed March 31, 2020.

Maqbool, Aleem. "Coronavirus: The US Resistance to a Continued Lockdown." 2020. *BBC News*. https://www.bbc.com/news/world-us-canada-52417610. Accessed May 31, 2020.

Marcus, Jacob Rader. *The Jew in the Medieval World: A Source Book: 315-1791*. Rev. ed. Cincinnati, OH: Hebrew Union College Press, 1999.

Marineli, Filio, and others. "Mary Mallon (1869–1938) and the History of Typhoid Fever." 2013. *National Center for Biotechnology Information*. https://www.ncbi.nlm.nih.gov/pmc/articles/PMC3959940/. Accessed September 12, 2019.

Markel, Howard. "Remembering Ryan White, the Teen Who Fought Against the Stigma of AIDS." 2016. https://www.pbs.org/newshour/health/remembering-ryan-white-the-teen-who-fought-against-the-stigma-of-aids. Accessed July 9, 2019.

Marshall, Joseph M. III. *The Journey of Crazy Horse: A Lakota History*. New York, NY: Penguin Books, 2005.

Mayo Clinic. "HIV/AIDS." https://www.mayoclinic.org/diseases-conditions/hiv-aids/symptoms-causes/syc-20373524. Accessed June 28, 2019.

———. "Smallpox." https://www.mayoclinic.org/diseases-conditions/smallpox/symptoms-causes/syc-20353027. Accessed June 28, 2019.

"Mayor Lori Lightfoot Discusses Coronavirus on *Face the Nation*." *CBS Face the Nation*. April 12, 2020.

Mazumdar, Tulip. "Why Plague Caught Madagascar Unaware." *BBC News*. https://www.vox.com/science-and-health/2017/10/6/16435536/plague-madagascar-epidemic-2017. Accessed August 14, 2019.

McEwan, Gordon. *The Incas: New Perspectives*. New York, NY: W.W. Norton & Co., 2016.

McGovern, George. *Terry: My Daughter's Life and Death Struggle with Alcoholism*. New York, NY: Villard, 1997.

McKenna, Stacey. "What Immunity to COVID-19 Really Means." Scientific American. https://www.scientificamerican.com/article/what-immunity-to-covid-19-really-means/. Accessed April 14, 2020.

McNeil, Donald G. Jr. "H.I.V. Arrived in the U.S. Long Before 'Patient Zero.'" *New York Times*, October 26, 2016.

McWilliam, G. H., translator. *The Decameron*. By Giovanni Bocaccio. New York, NY: Penguin Classics, 2004.

Medians, Linda E. *The Secret Malady: Venereal Disease in Eighteenth-Century Britain and France*. Lexington, KY: The University Press of Kentucky, 1996.

Meier, Allison. "A Lost 15th-Century Mural That Depicted Death's Indiscriminate Dance." *Hyperallergic*. https://hyperallergic.com/331875/lubeck-danse-macabre-chapel/. Accessed April 14, 2020.

———. "How Tuberculosis Symptoms Became Ideals of Beauty in the 19th Century." *Hyperallergic*. https://hyperallergic.com/415421/consumptive-chic-a-history-of-beaty-fashion-disease/. Accessed February 14, 2019.

Miller, Kathleen. *The Literary Culture of Plague in Early Modern England*. London, UK: Palgrave Macmillan, 2017.

Milne, Gustav. *The Great Fire of London*. Whitstable, UK: Historical Publications, Ltd UK, 1986.

Minster, Christopher. "Treasure of the Ancient Aztecs." 2019. *Thought Co*. https://www.thoughtco.com/the-treasure-of-the-aztecs-2136532. Accessed July 12, 2019.

Molho, Anthony. *Marriage Alliance in Late Medieval Florence*. Cambridge, MA: Harvard University Press, 1994.

Monster, Christopher. "The Capture of Inca Atalhuapa." *Thought Co*. https://www.thoughtco.com/capture-of-inca-atahualpa-2136546. Accessed August 20, 2019.

Morrison, Theodore, translator. *The Portable Chaucer*. By Geoffrey Chaucer. New York, NY: Viking Press, 1949.

Moughty, Sarah. "20 Years After HIV Announcement, Magic Johnson Emphasizes: 'I Am Not Cured.'" 2011. *PBS*. https://www.pbs.org/wgbh/frontline/article/20-years-after-hiv-announcement-magic-johnson-emphasizes-i-am-not-cured/. Accessed March 30, 2020.

Mozes, Allen. "Reports Warn of Growing Opioid Crisis Among Seniors." *Penn State Hershey*. http://penn statehershey.adam.com/content.aspx?productId=35&gid=3220. Accessed May 20, 2020.

Munkhoff, Richelle. Interview with Heather Quinlan, April 21, 2020.

———. "Searchers of the Dead: Authority, Marginality, and the Interpretation of Plague in England, 1574–1665." *Gender and History*, April, 1999, pp. 1–29.

"Naming the Coronavirus Disease (COVID-19) and the Virus That Causes It." *World Health Organization*. https://www.who.int/emergencies/diseases/novel-coronavirus-2019/technical-guidance/naming-the-coronavirus-disease-(covid-2019)-and-the-virus-that-causes-it. Accessed March 12, 2020.

Narayan, Adi. "Side Effects of 1918 Flu Seen Decades Later." *Time*. http://content.time.com/time/health/article/0,8599,1929814,00.html. Accessed April 1, 2020.

National Institute of Allergy and Infectious Diseases. "The Evidence That HIV Causes AIDS." https://aidsinfo.nih.gov/news/528/the-evidence-that-hiv-causes-aids. Accessed June 20, 2019.

Nealon, Tom. *Food Fights and Culture Wars: A Secret History of Taste*. South Oxfordshire, UK: The British Library Publishing Division, 2016.

———. "John Snow Redux." MedPage Today. https://www.medpagetoday.com/blogs/inotherwords/38472. Accessed May 1, 2020.

Nix, Elizabeth. "This Is Why the Maya Abandoned Their Cities." *History*. https://www.history.com/news/why-did-the-maya-abandon-their-cities. Accessed August 17, 2019.

Normile, Dennis. "Coronavirus Infections Keep Mounting After Cruise Ship Fiasco in Japan." *Science*. https://www.sciencemag.org/news/2020/02/coronavirus-infections-keep-mounting-after-cruise-ship-fiasco-japan. Accessed February 26, 2020.

Ntreh, Nii. "Haiti Paid Over $20 Billion In Present-Day Money to Free Itself from France. Here's Why." https://face2faceafrica.com/article/haiti-paid-over-20-billion-in-present-day-money-to-free-itself-from-france-heres-why. Accessed February 22, 2020.

Nuwer, Rachel. "To Prevent Next Coronavirus, Stop the Wildlife Trade, Conservationists Say." *New York Times*, February 19, 2020.

Ó Mongáin, Colm. "Why Has Coronavirus Infected So Many People in Italy?" 2020. *RTÉ News*. https://www.rte.ie/news/2020/0305/1120469-why-has-coronavirus-infect-so-many-people-in-italy/. Accessed March 10, 2020.

Okie, Susan. "Crack Babies: The Epidemic That Wasn't." *New York Times*, January 26, 2009.

Ollstein, Alice Miranda. "Trump Halts Funding to World Health Organization." 2020. *Politico*. https://www.politico.com/news/2020/04/14/trump-world-health-organization-funding-186786. Accessed April 14, 2020.

Opal, J. M., and Steven M. Opal. "How the Spanish Flu Could Have Changed 1919's Paris Peace Talks." The World. https://www.pri.org/stories/2019-01-02/how-spanish-flu-could-have-changed-1919s-paris-peace-talks. Accessed January 11, 2020.

Opdycke, Sandra. *The Flu Epidemic of 1918: America's Experience in the Global Health Crisis*. Oxford: Abingdon Press, 2014.

"Opioid Addiction 2016 Facts and Figures." *American Society of Addiction Medicine*. https://www.asam.org/docs/default-source/advocacy/opioid-addiction-disease-facts-figures.pdf. Accessed May 28, 2019.

PLAGUES, PANDEMICS AND VIRUSES

Ordoñez, Franco. "Pence Says His Earlier Comments about Testing Were Misunderstood." *NPR*. April 28, 2020.

Orme, Nicholas. *Medieval Children*. New Haven, CT: Yale University Press, 2001.

Ortiz, Aimee. "'Group of Local Vigilantes' Try to Forcibly Quarantine Out-of-Towners, Officials Say." *New York Times*, March 29, 2020.

Oshinsky, David M. *Polio: An American Story*. Oxford: Oxford University Press, 2006.

Osler, William. *Principles and Practice of Medicine*. Seattle, WA: Amazon Services, 2006.

"A Pandemic Looks Likely." *Global Health Now*. https://www.globalhealthnow.org/2020-02/pandemic-looks-likely. Accessed February 11, 2020.

Park, Alice. "The Story Behind the First AIDS Drug." *Time*. https://time.com/4705809/first-aids-drug-azt/. Accessed July 14, 2019.

Pattani, Aneri. "A Dangerous, 'Silent Reservoir' for Gonorrhea: The Throat." *New York Times*, July 31, 2017.

Payne, Linda. "London's Bill of Mortality (December 1664–December 1665) [Official Document]." *Children & Youth in History*. http://chnm.gmu.edu/cyh/primary-sources/159. Accessed February 1, 2020.

Perry, Wayne. "Germ from Human Feces Makes Deadly Leap to Coral." *Live Science*. https://www.livescience.com/15625-coral-disease-wastewater.html. Accessed January 18, 2020.

Piot, Peter. *No Time to Lose: A Life in Pursuit of Deadly Viruses*. New York, NY: W. W. Norton, 2016.

"Plan More Hospitals for Influenza Victims." Philadelphia Inquirer, October 4, 1918, p. 13.

"Polio Disease and Polio Virus." *Centers for Disease Control and Prevention*. https://www.cdc.gov/cpr/polioviruscontainment/diseaseandvirus.htm. Accessed October 3, 2019.

Poore, G.V. "Address on London, Ancient and Modern, from a Medical Point of View." *The Lancet*. https://books.google.com/books?id=CYxPAAAAYAAJ&pg=PA316&lpg=PA316&dq. Accessed April 18, 2020.

Porter, Roy. *Medicine: A History of Healing*. London: Ivy Press, 1997.

"Prevalence of IgG Antibody to SARS-Associated Coronavirus in Animal Traders—Guangdong Province, China, 2003." *Centers for Disease Control and Prevention*. https://www.cdc.gov/mmwr/preview/mmwrhtml/mm5241a2.htm. Accessed May 3, 2020.

Pringle, Heather. "How Europeans Brought Sickness to the New World." *Science*. https://www.sciencemag.org/news/2015/06/how-europeans-brought-sickness-new-world. Accessed August 22, 2019.

Quammen, David. *Spillover: Animal Infections and the Next Human Pandemic*. New York, NY: W.W. Norton & Co., 2012.

Raaflaub, Kurt A., and Richard J. A. Talbert. *Geography and Ethnography: Perceptions of the World in Pre-Modern Societies*. Hoboken, NJ: Wiley-Blackwell, 2012.

Rajagopalan, Megha. "Men Yelling 'Chinese' Tried to Punch Her Off Her Bike. She's the Latest Victim of Racist Attacks Linked to Coronavirus." *Buzzfeed News*. https://www.buzzfeednews.com/article/meghara/coronavirus-racism-europe-covid-19. Accessed March 10, 2020.

Ramsay, Michael A. E. "John Snow, MD: Anaesthetist to the Queen of England and Pioneer Epidemiologist." *National Center for Biotechnology Information*. https://www.ncbi.nlm.nih.gov/pmc/articles/PMC1325279/. Accessed May 1, 2020.

Randel, Michael. *The Harvard Dictionary of Music*. Cambridge, MA: Belknap Press. 2003.

Reagan, Ronald. "We Owe It to Ryan." *Washington Post*, April 11, 1990.

"Remarks by President Trump in Address to the Nation." *Whitehouse.gov.* https://www.whitehouse.gov/briefings-statements/remarks-president-trump-address-nation/. Accessed May 22, 2020.

"Remarks by President Trump and Members of the Coronavirus Task Force in Meeting with Pharmaceutical Companies." *Whitehouse.gov.* https://www.whitehouse.gov/briefings-statements/remarks-president-trump-members-coronavirus-task-force-meeting-pharmaceutical-companies/. Accessed March 30, 2020.

"Remarks by President Trump, Vice President Pence, and Members of the Coronavirus Task Force in Press Briefing." *Whitehouse.gov.* https://www.whitehouse.gov/briefings-statements/remarks-president-trump-vice-president-pence-members-coronavirus-task-force-press-briefing-31/. Accessed April 25, 2020.

"Remdesivir Drug Shows Promise—But It Is Far from a Coronavirus Cure." *CNN.* http://lite.cnn.com/en/article/h_4fdee35da8e7f2fd788aabf38b9ab76d. Accessed May 2, 2020.

Reid, Ann H., and others. "Origin and Evolution of the 1918 'Spanish' Influenza Virus Hemagglutinin Gene." *Proceedings of the National Academy of Science.* https://www.pnas.org/content/96/4/1651. Accessed January 15, 2020.

Reinberg, Steven. "'Herd Immunity' May Be Curbing U.S. Zika Numbers." Chicago Tribune, August 17, 2017.

Reisman, David. *The Story of Medicine in the Middle Ages.* New York, NY: Paul B. Hoeber, Inc., 1935.

Résendez, Andrés. *The Other Slavery: The Uncovered Story of Indian Enslavement in America.* Boston, MA: Mariner Books, 2016.

Rettner, Rachel. "Rats May Not Be to Blame for Spreading the 'Black Death.'" 2018. *Live Science.* https://www.livescience.com/61444-black-death-cause-found-transmission.html. Accessed January 15, 2020.

Richards, Matt, and Mark Langthorne. *83 Minutes: The Doctor, the Damage, and the Shocking Death of Michael Jackson.* New York, NY: Thomas Dunne Books, 2016.

Rodriguez, Jafet A. Ojeda, and Chadi I. Kahwaji. "Vibrio Cholerae." *National Center for Biotechnology Information.* https://www.ncbi.nlm.nih.gov/. Accessed May 3, 2020.

Rogers, Katie. "Trump Now Claims He Always Knew the Coronavirus Would Be a Pandemic." *New York Times,* March 17, 2020.

Rollo-Koster, Joëlle. *Death in Medieval Europe: Death Scripted and Death Choreographed.* Abingdon: Routledge Press, 2016.

Roos, Dave. "Why the Second Wave of the 1918 Spanish Flu Was So Deadly." *History.* https://www.history.com/news/spanish-flu-second-wave-resurgence. Accessed March 8, 2020.

Ross, John J. *Shakespeare's Tremor and Orwell's Cough: The Medical Lives of Famous Writers.* New York, NY: St. Martin's Press, 2012.

Sanders, Robert. "Coronavirus Outbreak Raises Question: Why Are Bat Viruses So Deadly?" *Berkeley News.* https://news.berkeley.edu/2020/02/10/coronavirus-outbreak-raises-question-why-are-bat-viruses-so-deadly/. Accessed February 11, 2020.

"SARS and Public Health in Ontario." *The SARS Commission First Interim Report.* http://www.archives.gov.on.ca/en/e_records/sars/report/v4-pdf/Volume4.pdf. Accessed November 30, 2019.

Sayej, Nadja. "'These Aren't Extinct Cultures'—Indigenous Art Gets A Stage at the Met." *The Guardian,* November 27, 2018.

"Secretary Azar Declares Public Health Emergency for United States for 2019 Novel Coronavirus." *Health and Human Services.* https://www.hhs.gov/about/news/2020/01/31/secretary-azar-declares-public-health-emergency-us-2019-novel-coronavirus.html. Accessed May 4, 2020.

Seladi-Schulman, Jill. "What Is a Retrovirus?" *Healthline.* https://www.healthline.com/health/what-is-a-retrovirus. Accessed July 20, 2019.

Sellman, J. Douglas, and others. "DSM-5 alcoholism: A 60-Year Perspective." Australian and New Zealand Journal of Psychiatry. https://journals.sagepub.com/doi/abs/10.1177/0004867414532849?journalCode=anpa. Accessed May 3, 2019.

Shilts, Randy. *And the Band Played On: Politics, People, and the AIDS Epidemic.* Rev. ed. New York, NY: St. Martin's Griffin, 2007.

"Shocking Termination of a Marriage in France." *Brooklyn Daily Eagle*, August 8, 1855.

Siena, Kevin. *Rotten Bodies: Class & Contagion in 18th-Century Britain.* New Haven, CT: Yale University Press, 2019.

Silva, Manuel T., and Margarida Correia-Neves. "Neutrophils and Macrophages: The Main Partners of Phagocyte Cell Systems." *Frontiers in Immunology.* https://www.frontiersin.org/articles/10.3389/fimmu.2012.00174/full. Accessed July 28, 2019.

Simon, Scott. "Rats Blamed for Bubonic Plague, But Gerbils May Be the Real Villains." *NPR's Weekend Edition.* https://www.npr.org/2015/02/28/389595442/rats-blamed-for-bubonic-plague-but-gerbils-may-be-the-real-villains. Accessed January 15, 2020.

Sinclair, John D., translator. *Dante's Inferno.* By Dante Alighieri. New York, NY: Oxford University Press, 1978.

Smith, Robert C. *Encyclopedia of African-American Politics.* New York, NY: Facts on File, 2003.

Smith, Tara C. "The Animal Origins of Coronavirus and Flu." *Quanta Magazine.* https://www.quantamagazine.org/how-do-animal-viruses-like-coronavirus-jump-species-20200225/. Accessed April 14, 2020.

Snitzer, Zachary. "The Disease of Alcohol: A Bit of History." *Maryland Addiction Recovery Center.* https://www.marylandaddictionrecovery.com/the-disease-of-alcoholism-a-bit-of-history/. Accessed May 15, 2019.

Snow, John. *Mode of Communication of Cholera.* London: John Churchill, 1849.

Snowden, Frank. *Epidemics and Society: From the Black Death to the Present.* New Haven, CT: Yale University Press. 2019.

Sontag, Susan. *Illness as a Metaphor and AIDS and its Metaphors.* New York, NY: Farrar, Strauss & Giroux, 2013.

Spinney, Laura. *Pale Rider: The Spanish Flu of 1918 and How It Changed the World.* New York, NY: PublicAffairs Books, 2017.

Steele, Paul Richard, and Catherine Jean Allen. *Handbook of Inca Mythology.* Santa Barbara, CA: ABC-CLIO. 2004.

Steinberg, Gary David. "Bacillus Calmette-Guérin Immunotherapy for Bladder Cancer Overview of BCG Immunotherapy." *Medscape.* https://emedicine.medscape.com/article/1950803-overview. Accessed June 14, 2020.

"Stocks Sink as Markets Open in China." *New York Times*, February 2, 2020.

"The Story of Polio." Canadian Public Health Association. https://www.cpha.ca/story-polio. Accessed April 2, 2020.

Sullivan, Robert. *Rats: Observations on the History & Habitat of the City's Most Unwanted Inhabitants.* New York, NY: Bloomsbury, USA, 2005.

Suryadevara, Uma, and others. "Opioid Use in the Elderly." Psychiatric Times. https://www.psychiatrictimes.com/view/opioid-use-elderly. Accessed May 15, 2019.

Sutherland, I. "John Graunt." *McGill Faculty of Medicine.* http://www.medicine.mcgill.ca/epidemiology/hanley/c609/Material/GrauntEoB.pdf. Accessed February 1, 2020.

"Syphilis—CDC Fact Sheet." *Centers for Disease Control and Prevention.* https://www.cdc.gov/std/syphilis/stdfact-syphilis.htm. Accessed June 24, 2019.

Target Health. "The Plague of Athens Leading to the Fall of the Golden Age of Greece." https://www.target health.com/post/the-plague-of-athens-leading-to-the-fall-of-the-golden-age-of-greece. Accessed March 3, 2020.

Terry, Mark. "Compare: 2009 H1N1 Pandemic Versus the 2020 Coronavirus Pandemic." 2020. BioSpace. https://www.biospace.com/article/2009-h1n1-pandemic-versus-the-2020-coronavirus-pandemic/. Accessed April 14, 2020.

"Thomas Wolfe at Harvard: Damned Soul in Widener (1958)." *The Harvard Crimson.* https://www.thecrimson.com/article/1958/10/18/thomas-wolfe-at-harvard-damned-soul/. Accessed October 19, 2019.

Thombs, Dennis L., and Cynthia J. Osborn. *Introduction to Addictive Behaviors.* 5th ed. New York, NY: Guilford Press, 2019.

Tisonick, Jennifer R., and others. "Into the Eye of the Cytokine Storm." *National Center for Biotechnology Information.* https://www.ncbi.nlm.nih.gov/pmc/articles/PMC3294426/. Accessed July 10, 2019.

Tomič, Zlata Blažina, and Vesna Blažina. "Expelling the Plague: The Health Office and the Implementation of Quarantine in Dubrovnik, 1377–1533." *Bulletin of the History of Medicine.* https://www.researchgate.net/publication/304779654_Expelling_the_Plague_The_Health_Office_and_the_Implementation_of_Quarantine_in_Dubrovnik_1377-1533_by_Zlata_Blazina_Tomic_Vesna_Blazina. Accessed June 30, 2019.

Tsebo, Khanye. *From Africa to America to The World.* Morrisville, NC: Lulu Press, 2019.

Tumpey, Terrence M., and others. "Characterization of the Reconstructed 1918 Spanish Influenza Pandemic Virus." *Science.* https://science.sciencemag.org/content/310/5745/77. Accessed January 15, 2020.

Tuthill, Kathleen. "John Snow and the Broad Street Pump: On the Trail of an Epidemic." *Cricket Magazine.* https://www.ph.ucla.edu/epi/snow/snowcricketarticle.html. Accessed May 1, 2020.

Uhler, Andy. "With No Federal Aid, Undocumented Immigrants Look to States, Philanthropy for Support." *Marketplace.* May 1, 2020.

Wang, Jessica. *Mad Dogs and Other New Yorkers: Rabies, Medicine, and Society in an American Metropolis, 1840–1920.* Baltimore, MD: Johns Hopkins University Press, 2019.

Wark, Lori. *Enhanced Classics: The Decameron.* Chevy Chase, MD: Enhanced Classics, 2020.

Watts, Sheldon. *Epidemics and History: Disease, Power, and Imperialism.* New Haven, CT: Yale University Press, 1997.

Weitzman, A. Interview with Heather Quinlan, March 31, 2020.

Wheelis, Mark. "Biological Warfare at the 1346 Siege of Caffa." *Centers for Disease Control and Prevention.* https://wwwnc.cdc.gov/eid/article/8/9/01-0536_article. Accessed November 11, 2019.

Whitley, Richard J. "Herpesviruses." *National Center for Biotechnology Information.* https://www.ncbi.nlm.nih.gov/books/NBK8157/. Accessed May 5, 2020.

"WHO MERS-CoV Global Summary and Risk Assessment." *World Health Organization.* https://www.who.int/emergencies/mers-cov/mers-summary-2016.pdf?ua=1. Accessed April 4, 2020.

Williamson, Elizabeth, and Kristin Hussey. "Party Zero: How a Soirée in Connecticut Became a 'Super Spreader.'" *New York Times*, March 23, 2020.

Wolf, Colin. "Florida Pastor Says He'll Keep Church Open During Coronavirus Outbreak, Claims to Have Most Sterile Building in America." *Orlando Weekly*, March 27, 2020.

Wolfe, Nathan: *The Viral Storm: The Dawn of a New Pandemic Age*. New York, NY: Henry Holt, 2011.

Wolfe, Thomas. *Look Homeward, Angel*. New York, NY: Scribner Books, 2006.

World Health Organization. "Drug-Resistant Tuberculosis." https://www.who.int/tb/areas-of-work/drug-resistant-tb/en/. Accessed February 1, 2020.

———. "HIV/AIDS." https://www.who.int/gho/hiv/en/. Accessed March 28, 2020.

"WHO's First Global Report on Antibiotic Resistance Reveals Serious, Worldwide Threat to Public Health." https://www.who.int/mediacentre/news/releases/2014/amr-report/en/. Accessed February 1, 2020.

Younai, Fariba S. "Thirty Years of the Human Immunodeficiency Virus Epidemic and Beyond." *Nature*. https://www.nature.com/articles/ijos201376. Accessed July 20, 2019.

Yuko, Elizabeth. "How the Tuberculosis Epidemic Influenced Modernist Architecture." *Bloomberg City Lab*. https://www.bloomberg.com/news/articles/2018-10-30/what-architecture-learned-from-tb-hospitals. Accessed February 15, 2019.

Zeigler, Philip. *The Black Death*. New York, NY: Harper & Row, 1969.

Zentner, McLaurine H. *The Black Death and Its Impact on Church and Religion*. [Unpublished master's thesis.] University of Mississippi. Sally McDonnell Barksdale Honors College, 2015.

Zronik, John Paul. *Francisco Pizarro: Journeys through Peru and South America*. New York, NY: Crabtree Publishing Books, 2005.

INDEX

Note: (ill.) indicates photos and illustrations

PLAGUES, PANDEMICS AND VIRUSES

PLAGUES, PANDEMICS AND VIRUSES

PLAGUES, PANDEMICS AND VIRUSES